Adipose-Derived Stromal/Stem Cells

Adipose-Derived Stromal/Stem Cells

Editor

Patrick C. Baer

MDPI • Basel • Beijing • Wuhan • Barcelona • Belgrade • Manchester • Tokyo • Cluj • Tianjin

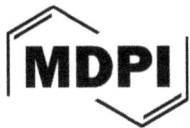

Editor
Patrick C. Baer
Goethe-Universitat Frankfurt am Main
Germany

Editorial Office
MDPI
St. Alban-Anlage 66
4052 Basel, Switzerland

This is a reprint of articles from the Special Issue published online in the open access journal *Cells* (ISSN 2073-4409) (available at: https://www.mdpi.com/journal/cells/special_issues/adipose_stem_cell).

For citation purposes, cite each article independently as indicated on the article page online and as indicated below:

LastName, A.A.; LastName, B.B.; LastName, C.C. Article Title. *Journal Name* **Year**, *Article Number*, Page Range.

ISBN 978-3-03943-282-0 (Pbk)
ISBN 978-3-03943-283-7 (PDF)

Cover image courtesy of Patrick Baer.

© 2020 by the authors. Articles in this book are Open Access and distributed under the Creative Commons Attribution (CC BY) license, which allows users to download, copy and build upon published articles, as long as the author and publisher are properly credited, which ensures maximum dissemination and a wider impact of our publications.

The book as a whole is distributed by MDPI under the terms and conditions of the Creative Commons license CC BY-NC-ND.

Contents

About the Editor vii

Patrick C. Baer
Adipose-Derived Stromal/Stem Cells
Reprinted from: *Cells* **2020**, *9*, 1997, doi:10.3390/cells9091997 1

Andreas Ritter, Alexandra Friemel, Susanne Roth, Nina-Naomi Kreis, Samira Catharina Hoock, Babek Khan Safdar, Kyra Fischer, Charlotte Möllmann, Christine Solbach, Frank Louwen and Juping Yuan
Subcutaneous and Visceral Adipose-Derived Mesenchymal Stem Cells: Commonality and Diversity
Reprinted from: *Cells* **2019**, *8*, 1288, doi:10.3390/cells8101288 5

Sanja Stojanović, Stevo Najman and Aleksandra Korać
Stem Cells Derived from Lipoma and Adipose Tissue—Similar Mesenchymal Phenotype but Different Differentiation Capacity Governed by Distinct Molecular Signature
Reprinted from: *Cells* **2018**, *7*, 260, doi:10.3390/cells7120260 29

Patrick C. Baer, Benjamin Koch, Elena Hickmann, Ralf Schubert, Jindrich Cinatl Jr., Ingeborg A. Hauser and Helmut Geiger
Isolation, Characterization, Differentiation and Immunomodulatory Capacity of Mesenchymal Stromal/Stem Cells from Human Perirenal Adipose Tissue
Reprinted from: *Cells* **2019**, *8*, 1346, doi:10.3390/cells8111346 51

Ting Ting Ng, Kylie Hin-Man Mak, Christian Popp and Ray Kit Ng
Murine Mesenchymal Stromal Cells Retain Biased Differentiation Plasticity Towards Their Tissue of Origin
Reprinted from: *Cells* **2020**, *9*, 756, doi:10.3390/cells9030756 69

Na-Eun Ryu, Soo-Hong Lee and Hansoo Park
Spheroid Culture System Methods and Applications for Mesenchymal Stem Cells
Reprinted from: *Cells* **2019**, *8*, 1620, doi:10.3390/cells8121620 83

Mathew Cowper, Trivia Frazier, Xiying Wu, J. Lowry Curley, Michelle H. Ma, Omair A. Mohiuddin, Marilyn Dietrich, Michelle McCarthy, Joanna Bukowska and Jeffrey M. Gimble
Human Platelet Lysate as a Functional Substitute for Fetal Bovine Serum in the Culture of Human Adipose Derived Stromal/Stem Cells
Reprinted from: *Cells* **2019**, *8*, 724, doi:10.3390/cells8070724 97

Natsuko Kakudo, Naoki Morimoto, Yuanyuan Ma and Kenji Kusumoto
Differences between the Proliferative Effects of Human Platelet Lysate and Fetal Bovine Serum on Human Adipose-Derived Stem Cells
Reprinted from: *Cells* **2019**, *8*, 1218, doi:10.3390/cells8101218 111

Agnieszka Smieszek, Katarzyna Kornicka, Jolanta Szłapka-Kosarzewska, Peter Androvic, Lukas Valihrach, Lucie Langerova, Eva Rohlova, Mikael Kubista and Krzysztof Marycz
Metformin Increases Proliferative Activity and Viability of Multipotent Stromal Stem Cells Isolated from Adipose Tissue Derived from Horses with Equine Metabolic Syndrome
Reprinted from: *Cells* **2019**, *8*, 80, doi:10.3390/cells8020080 123

Jerran Santos, Thibaut Hubert and Bruce K Milthorpe
Valproic Acid Promotes Early Neural Differentiation in Adult Mesenchymal Stem Cells Through Protein Signalling Pathways
Reprinted from: Cells 2020, 9, 619, doi:10.3390/cells9030619 143

Ewa Kuca-Warnawin, Urszula Skalska, Iwona Janicka, Urszula Musiałowicz, Krzysztof Bonek, Piotr Głuszko, Piotr Szczęsny, Marzena Olesińska and Ewa Kontny
The Phenotype and Secretory Activity of Adipose-Derived Mesenchymal Stem Cells (ASCs) of Patients with Rheumatic Diseases
Reprinted from: Cells 2019, 8, 1659, doi:10.3390/cells8121659 169

Margherita Di Somma, Wandert Schaafsma, Elisabetta Grillo, Maria Vliora, Eleni Dakou, Michela Corsini, Cosetta Ravelli, Roberto Ronca, Paraskevi Sakellariou, Jef Vanparijs, Begona Castro and Stefania Mitola
Natural Histogel-Based Bio-Scaffolds for Sustaining Angiogenesis in Beige Adipose Tissue
Reprinted from: Cells 2019, 8, 1457, doi:10.3390/cells8111457 185

Ann-Christin Klemenz, Juliane Meyer, Katharina Ekat, Julia Bartels, Selina Traxler, Jochen K. Schubert, Günter Kamp, Wolfram Miekisch and Kirsten Peters
Differences in the Emission of Volatile Organic Compounds (VOCs) between Non-Differentiating and Adipogenically Differentiating Mesenchymal Stromal/Stem Cells from Human Adipose Tissue
Reprinted from: Cells 2019, 8, 697, doi:10.3390/cells8070697 201

Nadja Zöller, Sarah Schreiner, Laura Petry, Stephanie Hoffmann, Katja Steinhorst, Johannes Kleemann, Manuel Jäger, Roland Kaufmann, Markus Meissner and Stefan Kippenberger
Collagen I Promotes Adipocytogenesis in Adipose-Derived Stem Cells In Vitro
Reprinted from: Cells 2019, 8, 302, doi:10.3390/cells8040302 215

Jana Plava, Marina Cihova, Monika Burikova, Martin Bohac, Marian Adamkov, Slavka Drahosova, Dominika Rusnakova, Daniel Pindak, Marian Karaba, Jan Simo, Michal Mego, Lubos Danisovic, Lucia Kucerova and Svetlana Miklikova
Permanent Pro-Tumorigenic Shift in Adipose Tissue-Derived Mesenchymal Stromal Cells Induced by Breast Malignancy
Reprinted from: Cells 2020, 9, 480, doi:10.3390/cells9020480 229

Teresa Raquel Tavares Serejo, Amandda Évelin Silva-Carvalho,
Luma Dayane de Carvalho Filiú Braga, Francisco de Assis Rocha Neves,
Rinaldo Wellerson Pereira, Juliana Lott de Carvalho and Felipe Saldanha-Araujo
Assessment of the Immunosuppressive Potential of INF-γ Licensed Adipose Mesenchymal Stem Cells, Their Secretome and Extracellular Vesicles
Reprinted from: Cells 2019, 8, 22, doi:10.3390/cells8010022 249

Patrick C. Baer, Julia Sann, Ruth Pia Duecker, Evelyn Ullrich, Helmut Geiger, Peter Bader, Stefan Zielen and Ralf Schubert
Tracking of Infused Mesenchymal Stem Cells in Injured Pulmonary Tissue in Atm-Deficient Mice
Reprinted from: Cells 2020, 9, 1444, doi:10.3390/cells9061444 265

About the Editor

Patrick C. Baer is a Cell Biologist and Associate Professor of Experimental Medicine at the Hospital of the Goethe University in Frankfurt/M. He completed his studies in Biochemistry at the Technical University of Darmstadt and received his doctorate and habilitation at the Goethe University of Frankfurt/M. P.C.B. has currently published 96 research articles, including three book chapters and three patents. The research areas of P.C.B. focus on the isolation, culture, and differentiation of adipose-derived mesenchymal stromal/stem cells (ASCs) and the transplantation of ASCs or their derivatives (conditioned medium, extracellular vesicles) to improve renal regeneration. For 25 years, P.C.B. has also been working with cell culture models of renal proximal and distal tubular epithelial cells to study regeneration processes in the renal epithelium and to investigate the effects of drugs.

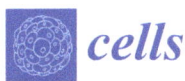

Editorial
Adipose-Derived Stromal/Stem Cells

Patrick C. Baer

Division of Nephrology, Department of Internal Medicine III, University Hospital, Goethe-University, 60596 Frankfurt am Main, Germany; patrick.baer@kgu.de or p.baer@em.uni-frankfurt.de; Tel.: +49-69-6301-5554; Fax: +49-69-6301-4749

Received: 21 August 2020; Accepted: 25 August 2020; Published: 30 August 2020

Adipose tissue is a rich, ubiquitous, and easily accessible source for multipotent mesenchymal stromal/stem cells (MSCs), so-called adipose-derived stromal/stem cells (ASCs). Primary isolated ASCs are a heterogeneous preparation consisting of several subpopulations of stromal/stem and precursor cells. Donor-specific differences in ASC isolations and the lack of culture standardization hinder the comparison of results from different studies. Nevertheless, ASCs are already used in different in vivo models and clinical trials to investigate their ability to improve tissue and organ regeneration. Many questions concerning their counterparts and biology in situ, their differentiation potential in vitro and in vivo, and also the mechanisms of regeneration (paracrine effects including regeneration promoting factors and extracellular vesicles, differentiation, immunomodulation) are not completely understood or remain unsolved. For this reason, this special edition aims to expand current knowledge about the extremely diverse potential of ASCs.

This Special Issue covers research articles investigating various adipose tissues as a source for ASC isolation [1–3], specific cultures methods to enhance proliferation or viability [4–7], and the differentiation capacity [8–12]. Furthermore, other studies highlight aspects of various diseases [13,14], the immunosuppressive potential of ASCs and their derivates [15] or the in vivo tracking of transplanted ASCs [16].

Ritter and co-workers analyzed the functional similarities and differences of ASCs isolated from different adipose depots [3]. The authors described that ASCs isolated from subcutaneous and visceral fat share multiple cellular features, but significantly differ in their functions. The functional diversity of ASCs depends on their origin, cellular context, and surrounding microenvironment within adipose tissues. Stojanović and co-workers characterized the molecular signature and the differentiation capacity of ASCs isolated from lipoma [2]. A study by our group from the nephrological research laboratory summarized the isolation and culture of ASCs from perirenal adipose tissue, characterized the cultured cells, and demonstrated their immunomodulatory potential and their high permissiveness for human cytomegalovirus [1].

Platelet lysate has been shown to be an effective replacement for serum in the culture, expansion, and differentiation of ASCs [4,7]. Metformin has been shown as a preconditioning agent that stimulates proliferative activity and viability of ASCs [6]. The addition of metformin improved metabolism and viability, correlated with higher mitochondrial membrane potential, and reduced apoptosis. As a possible alternative to standard cell culture, Ryu and co-workers reviewed spheroid culture systems that could provide a physicochemical environment similar to that in vivo by facilitating cell-cell and cell-matrix interaction, thereby overcoming the limitations of traditional monolayer cell culture [5].

The findings of Ng and co-workers suggest that the epigenetic state of MSCs is associated with the biased differentiation plasticity towards its tissue of origin, proposing a mechanism related to the retention of epigenetic memory [11]. This result could improve the selection of optimal tissue sources for MSCs for therapeutic applications. Others studied various effects of differentiation events induced by differentiation-inducing agents. Using valproic acid, the induced neural differentiation of ASCs was demonstrated by the upregulation of characteristic neuro-specific factors [8]. Zöller and co-workers showed that collagen I was able to modulate lipogenesis and adiponectin expression, and hypothesized that this could contribute to age-related metabolic disorders [10]. Klemenz and co-workers determined volatile organic compounds during adipogenic differentiation of ASCs in order to avoid cell destruction during monitoring of cell status [9]. Their data indicated that measuring these compounds could be a useful, non-invasive tool for the metabolic monitoring of cells in vitro. Di Somma and co-workers tested the ability of Histogel, a natural mixture of glycosaminoglycans, to sustain the differentiation of ASCs into brown-like cells and brown adipose tissue [12]. A study by Plava and co-workers identified that ASCs are permanently altered in the presence of tumor breast tissue and have the potential to increase tumor cell invasive ability through the activation of epithelial-to-mesenchymal transition in tumor cells [13]. Another study characterized ASCs isolated from patients with rheumatoid arthritis and described their altered phenotype and secretory activity compared to ASCs from healthy donors [14].

In recent years, several in vitro preconditioning (also called pretreatment or licensing) strategies have been investigated to enhance the regenerative and immunomodulatory potential of ASCs. Serejo and co-workers investigated how a preconditioning regime with interferon-γ affects the immunomodulatory functions of ASCs and examined their secretome and released extracellular vesicles [15]. Preconditioned ASCs showed a higher immunosuppressive potential compared to unlicensed ASCs. Another study by our group from the nephrological research laboratory shows in vivo tracking of luciferase-transgenic ASCs after transplantation in a model of inflammatory lung disease [16]. In vivo imaging demonstrated a significantly longer retention time of transplanted ASCs in the injured lung parenchyma compared to healthy wild type mice, which could indicate increased regeneration of the damaged tissue.

Funding: The author received no funding for this editorial.

Conflicts of Interest: The author declares no conflict of interest.

References

1. Baer, P.C.; Koch, B.; Hickmann, E.; Schubert, R.; Cinatl, J.; Hauser, I.A.; Geiger, H. Isolation, Characterization, Differentiation and Immunomodulatory Capacity of Mesenchymal Stromal/Stem Cells from Human Perirenal Adipose Tissue. *Cells* **2019**, *8*, 1346. [CrossRef] [PubMed]
2. Stojanović, S.; Najman, S.; Korać, A. Stem Cells Derived from Lipoma and Adipose Tissue-Similar Mesenchymal Phenotype but Different Differentiation Capacity Governed by Distinct Molecular Signature. *Cells* **2018**, *7*, 260. [CrossRef] [PubMed]
3. Ritter, A.; Friemel, A.; Roth, S.; Kreis, N.-N.; Hoock, S.C.; Safdar, B.K.; Fischer, K.; Möllmann, C.; Solbach, C.; Louwen, F.; et al. Subcutaneous and Visceral Adipose-Derived Mesenchymal Stem Cells: Commonality and Diversity. *Cells* **2019**, *8*, 1288. [CrossRef] [PubMed]
4. Cowper, M.; Frazier, T.; Wu, X.; Curley, L.; Ma, M.H.; Mohuiddin, O.A.; Dietrich, M.; McCarthy, M.; Bukowska, J.; Gimble, J.M. Human Platelet Lysate as a Functional Substitute for Fetal Bovine Serum in the Culture of Human Adipose Derived Stromal/Stem Cells. *Cells* **2019**, *8*, 724. [CrossRef] [PubMed]
5. Ryu, N.-E.; Lee, S.-H.; Park, H. Spheroid Culture System Methods and Applications for Mesenchymal Stem Cells. *Cells* **2019**, *8*, 1620. [CrossRef] [PubMed]
6. Smieszek, A.; Kornicka, K.; Szłapka-Kosarzewska, J.; Androvic, P.; Valihrach, L.; Langerova, L.; Rohlova, E.; Kubista, M.; Marycz, K. Metformin Increases Proliferative Activity and Viability of Multipotent Stromal Stem Cells Isolated from Adipose Tissue Derived from Horses with Equine Metabolic Syndrome. *Cells* **2019**, *8*, 80. [CrossRef] [PubMed]
7. Kakudo, N.; Morimoto, N.; Ma, Y.; Kusumoto, K. Differences between the Proliferative Effects of Human Platelet Lysate and Fetal Bovine Serum on Human Adipose-Derived Stem Cells. *Cells* **2019**, *8*, 1218. [CrossRef] [PubMed]
8. Santos, J.; Hubert, T.; Milthorpe, B.K. Valproic Acid Promotes Early Neural Differentiation in Adult Mesenchymal Stem Cells Through Protein Signalling Pathways. *Cells* **2020**, *9*, 619. [CrossRef] [PubMed]

9. Klemenz, A.-C.; Meyer, J.; Ekat, K.; Bartels, J.; Traxler, S.; Schubert, J.K.; Kamp, G.; Miekisch, W.; Peters, K. Differences in the Emission of Volatile Organic Compounds (VOCs) between Non-Differentiating and Adipogenically Differentiating Mesenchymal Stromal/Stem Cells from Human Adipose Tissue. *Cells* **2019**, *8*, 697. [CrossRef] [PubMed]
10. Zöller, N.; Schreiner, S.; Petry, L.; Hoffmann, S.; Steinhorst, K.; Kleemann, J.; Jäger, M.; Kaufmann, R.; Meissner, M.; Kippenberger, S. Collagen I Promotes Adipocytogenesis in Adipose-Derived Stem Cells In Vitro. *Cells* **2019**, *8*, 302. [CrossRef] [PubMed]
11. Ng, T.T.; Mak, K.H.-M.; Popp, C.; Ng, R.K. Murine Mesenchymal Stromal Cells Retain Biased Differentiation Plasticity Towards Their Tissue of Origin. *Cells* **2020**, *9*, 756. [CrossRef] [PubMed]
12. Di Somma, M.; Schaafsma, W.; Grillo, E.; Vliora, M.; Dakou, E.; Corsini, M.; Ravelli, C.; Ronca, R.; Sakellariou, P.; Vanparijs, J.; et al. Natural Histogel-Based Bio-Scaffolds for Sustaining Angiogenesis in Beige Adipose Tissue. *Cells* **2019**, *8*, 1457. [CrossRef] [PubMed]
13. Plava, J.; Cihova, M.; Burikova, M.; Bohac, M.; Adamkov, M.; Drahosova, S.; Rusnakova, D.; Pindak, D.; Karaba, M.; Simo, J.; et al. Permanent Pro-Tumorigenic Shift in Adipose Tissue-Derived Mesenchymal Stromal Cells Induced by Breast Malignancy. *Cells* **2020**, *9*, 480. [CrossRef] [PubMed]
14. Kuca-Warnawin, E.; Skalska, U.; Janicka, I.; Musiałowicz, U.; Bonek, K.; Głuszko, P.; Szczęsny, P.; Olesińska, M.; Kontny, E. The Phenotype and Secretory Activity of Adipose-Derived Mesenchymal Stem Cells (ASCs) of Patients with Rheumatic Diseases. *Cells* **2019**, *8*, 1659. [CrossRef] [PubMed]
15. Serejo, T.R.T.; Silva-Carvalho, A.É.; Braga, L.D.d.C.F.; Neves, F.d.A.R.; Pereira, R.W.; Carvalho, J.L.D.; Saldanha-Araujo, F. Assessment of the Immunosuppressive Potential of INF-γ Licensed Adipose Mesenchymal Stem Cells, Their Secretome and Extracellular Vesicles. *Cells* **2019**, *8*, 22. [CrossRef] [PubMed]
16. Baer, P.C.; Sann, J.; Duecker, R.P.; Ullrich, E.; Geiger, H.; Bader, P.; Zielen, S.; Schubert, R. Tracking of Infused Mesenchymal Stem Cells in Injured Pulmonary Tissue in Atm-Deficient Mice. *Cells* **2020**, *9*, 1444. [CrossRef]

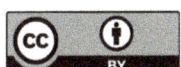

© 2020 by the author. Licensee MDPI, Basel, Switzerland. This article is an open access article distributed under the terms and conditions of the Creative Commons Attribution (CC BY) license (http://creativecommons.org/licenses/by/4.0/).

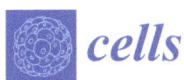

Article

Subcutaneous and Visceral Adipose-Derived Mesenchymal Stem Cells: Commonality and Diversity

Andreas Ritter *, Alexandra Friemel, Susanne Roth, Nina-Naomi Kreis, Samira Catharina Hoock, Babek Khan Safdar, Kyra Fischer, Charlotte Möllmann, Christine Solbach, Frank Louwen and Juping Yuan *

Division of Obstetrics and Prenatal Medicine, Department of Gynecology and Obstetrics, University Hospital, Goethe University, D-60590 Frankfurt, Germany; alexandra.friemel@kgu.de (A.F.); susanne.roth@kgu.de (S.R.); nina-naomi.kreis@kgu.de (N.-N.K.); samirahoock@gmx.de (S.C.H.); babek.safdar@hotmail.com (B.K.S.); kyra.fischer@kgu.de (K.F.); charlottejohanna.moellmann@kgu.de (C.M.); christine.solbach@kgu.de (C.S.); frank.louwen@kgu.de (F.L.)
* Correspondence: Andreas.Ritter@kgu.de (A.R.); Yuan@em.uni-frankfurt.de (J.Y.); Tel.: +49-069-6031-83297 (A.R.)

Received: 30 September 2019; Accepted: 17 October 2019; Published: 21 October 2019

Abstract: Adipose-derived mesenchymal stem cells (ASCs) are considered to be a useful tool for regenerative medicine, owing to their capabilities in differentiation, self-renewal, and immunomodulation. These cells have become a focus in the clinical setting due to their abundance and easy isolation. However, ASCs from different depots are not well characterized. Here, we analyzed the functional similarities and differences of subcutaneous and visceral ASCs. Subcutaneous ASCs have an extraordinarily directed mode of motility and a highly dynamic focal adhesion turnover, even though they share similar surface markers, whereas visceral ASCs move in an undirected random pattern with more stable focal adhesions. Visceral ASCs have a higher potential to differentiate into adipogenic and osteogenic cells when compared to subcutaneous ASCs. In line with these observations, visceral ASCs demonstrate a more active sonic hedgehog pathway that is linked to a high expression of cilia/differentiation related genes. Moreover, visceral ASCs secrete higher levels of inflammatory cytokines interleukin-6, interleukin-8, and tumor necrosis factor α relative to subcutaneous ASCs. These findings highlight, that both ASC subpopulations share multiple cellular features, but significantly differ in their functions. The functional diversity of ASCs depends on their origin, cellular context and surrounding microenvironment within adipose tissues. The data provide important insight into the biology of ASCs, which might be useful in choosing the adequate ASC subpopulation for regenerative therapies.

Keywords: adipose-derived mesenchymal stem cells; differentiation; migration; secretion; primary cilium; sonic hedgehog signaling

1. Introduction

For several decades, adipose tissue (AT) was thought to be a passive organ with functions in energy homeostasis, accumulation of lipids as energy-storage depot, and supplying energy-rich fat molecules for generating energy and membrane synthesis [1,2]. Nowadays, AT is known to be an important endocrine organ with diverse functions in multiple cellular processes. Cytokine and hormone signals convey immune functions and inflammatory responses that module the energy homeostasis by regulating the food intake, insulin sensitivity, and energy expenditure in tight association with other organs [3]. In line with these complex roles, the ATs of different depots display heterogeneity in their morphological, molecular, and metabolic profiles tightly adjusted to their biological context [4]. Visceral AT in the mesentery and omentum contains increased the numbers of inflammatory and immune cells, is more metabolically active, has an higher uptake of free fatty acids and glucoses, and is less sensitive to insulin [5]. By contrast, subcutaneous AT has a higher affinity for free fatty acids and triglycerides, and its primary function is the energy storage, protection against mechanical damage, and homeostatic heat control [6].

Adipocytes within AT originate from the differentiation process of multipotent progenitor cells, named adipose-derived mesenchymal stem cells (ASCs) [7]. These cells are key regulators of AT. They are involved in tissue homeostasis with their potent differentiation capacity in adipogenesis and angiogenesis. Additionally, ASCs coordinate and maintain the local and systemic environment by immunomodulation and damage repair through their paracrine signaling and direct cell-cell interaction [8,9]. These cells are considered to be useful for novel regenerative medicine applications due to their accessibility and their various functions concerning tissue remodeling and homeostasis and become the focus of many translational clinical studies [10].

Numerous studies have been conducted to analyze the key properties of ASCs isolated from different AT depots (visceral, subcutaneous, and preperitoneal) [11]. In particular, subcutaneous and visceral ASCs have received great attention. However, the results of these studies were inconsistent regarding their differentiation potential, proliferation, and paracrine signaling [11,12]. We have already investigated the interaction of ASCs with breast cancer cells [13], the effect of Polo-like kinase 1 (Plk1) inhibitors on ASCs [14], and the influence of obesity on ASCs [15,16]. During these studies, we have observed similarities and disparities between subcutaneous and visceral ASCs. In the present work, we focus on the features of both ASC subtypes and further analyze their main functions. Our results highlight similarities in their cell surface marker profile, cell viability, and cell cycle progression, and diversities in the motility, differentiation capacity, and the cilium related sonic hedgehog (Hh) signal pathway.

2. Materials and Methods

2.1. Human Visceral and Subcutaneous ASC Isolation and Cell Surface Marker Measurement

This work was approved by the Ethics Committee of the Johann Wolfgang Goethe University Hospital Frankfurt and informed written consent was obtained from all the participants. Visceral (omental) and subcutaneous (abdominal) adipose tissues were taken from women undergoing Caesarean section. Table 1 lists participant information. Their age ranged between 25 and 35 years. Body mass index (BMI) of both ASC subgroups was 24.1 ± 2.9. ASCs were isolated, as described previously [13,14]. After isolation, the cells were cultured and expanded for three passages. Cells were then stored at −80 °C until use. Early passages (P3 to P6) of ASCs were used for all analyses. All experiments, unless otherwise indicated, were independently performed with ASCs that were isolated from at least three different donors.

FACSCalibur™ (BD Biosciences, Heidelberg, Germany) was used for determining the surface markers of ASCs. The cells were harvested with 0.25% trypsin and fixed for 15 min. with ice-cold 2% paraformaldehyde (PFA) at 4°C. Cells were washed twice with flow cytometry buffer (FCB: PBS with 0.2% Tween-20, and 2% fetal calf serum (FCS)) and stained with the following antibodies from eBioscience/BD-Pharmingen (Frankfurt, Germany): FITC-conjugated anti-human cluster of differentiation 90 (CD90) (#11-0909-42), PE-conjugated anti-human CD73 (#550257), PE-conjugated anti-human CD 105 (#323206), PE-conjugated anti-human CD146 (#561013), PerCP-Cy5.5-conjugated anti-human CD14 (#555397), FITC-conjugated anti-human CD34 (#343504), APC-conjugated anti-human CD106 (#551147), and APC-conjugated anti-human CD31 (#17-0319-41). Anti-mouse Ig, κ/negative control compensation particles (eBioscience/BD-Pharmingen, #552843), flow cytometry setup beads (eBioscience/BD-Pharmingen, #340486 and #340487), and non-stained ASCs were used as negative controls for FACS gating.

2.2. Indirect Immunofluorescence Staining, Microscopy, Fluorescence Intensity Quantification, and Nocodazole Washout

Indirect immunofluorescence staining was performed, as reported [17]. Cells were seeded on Nunc™ Lab-Tek™ SlideFlask chambers from Thermo Fisher Scientific (Schwerte, Germany). Cells were fixed for 8–10 min. with methanol at −20 °C or with 4% PFA containing 0.2% Triton X-100 for 15 min. at room temperature, as described [16]. The following primary antibodies were used: mouse monoclonal antibody against acetylated α-tubulin (Sigma-Aldrich, Darmstadt, Germany, #T6793), mouse monoclonal antibody against CD90 (Abcam, Cambridge, UK, ab133350), rabbit monoclonal antibody against CD73 (GenTex, Eching, Germany, GTX101140), mouse monoclonal antibody against Smo (Santa Cruz Biotechnology, Heidelberg, Germany, #sc-166685), rabbit polyclonal antibody against phospho-histone H3 (pHH3, Ser10, Merck Millipore, Darmstadt, Germany, #06-570), mouse monoclonal antibody against phospho-focal adhesion kinase (p-FAK, Cell Signaling, Frankfurt, Germany, #3283), rabbit monoclonal antibody against FAK (Proteintech, Manchester, UK, 66258-1-Ig), mouse monoclonal antibody against paxillin (BD Transduction Laboratories™, Frankfurt, Germany, #610619), and rabbit polyclonal antibody against p-paxillin (Cell Signaling, Frankfurt, Germany, #2541). FITC-, Cy3-, and Cy5 conjugated secondary antibodies were obtained from Jackson ImmunoResearch (Cambridgeshire, UK). DNA was visualized by using DAPI (4′,6-diamidino-2-phenylindole-dihydrochloride, Roche, Mannheim, Germany). The filamentous actin (F-actin) cytoskeleton was stained while using phalloidin (Phalloidin-Atto 550; Sigma-Aldrich, Munich, Germany). The slides were examined while using an AxioObserver.Z1 microscope (Zeiss, Göttingen, Germany) and images were taken using an AxioCam MRm camera (Zeiss, Göttingen, Germany). The immunofluorescence stained slides were further examined by confocal laser scanning microscopy (CLSM) using Z-stack images with a HCXPl APO CS 63.0 x 1.4 oil objective (Leica CTR 6500, Heidelberg, Germany) in sequential excitation of fluorophores. A series of Z-stack images were captured at 0.5 μm intervals. All the images in each experiment were taken with the same laser intensity and exposure time. Representatives are generated by superimposing (overlay) individual images from confocal Z-sections.

Fluorescent intensity was measured while using line-scan-based analysis in ImageJ (National Institutes of Health), as described [15,18]. The average intensities over a three-pixel-wide line along the axoneme were measured and then normalized against cilium length by using the ImageJ plugin Plot Roi Profile. The intensity was measured from the axonemal base to its tip in 10% intervals. The mean values of thirty cilia from three different donors were obtained for each group within the intervals and were plotted to GraphPad Prism 7 (GraphPad software Inc., San Diego, USA).

We performed a nocodazole washout assay to analyze the dynamics (disassembly/reassembly) of focal adhesions (FAs). The cells were treated with nocodazole (10 μM; Sigma-Aldrich, Darmstadt, Germany) for 5 h to depolymerize microtubules (MTs) [19]. The drug was washed out with phosphate-buffered saline (PBS), and MTs were repolymerized in medium for different time periods (0, 30, 75 min.). Cells were fixed and stained for paxillin and p-FAK. The slides were examined while using an AxioObserver.Z1 microscope (Zeiss, Göttingen, Germany) and the images were taken using an AxioCam MRm camera (Zeiss, Göttingen, Germany).

2.3. Sonic Hedgehog Stimulation, Cytokine Array and ELISA

Cells were incubated with 200 nM smoothened agonist (SAG) (Bioscience, Wiesbaden, Germany) in the absence of FCS for 24 h for activating the Hedgehog (Hh) pathway. Immunofluorescence line-scan-based analysis and quantitative RT-PCR analysis were then performed [15].

For cytokine measurement, visceral and subcutaneous ASC in passage 3 were cultured for three days to a confluence of 90% and supernatants were taken. The levels of chemokines, cytokines, and growth factors in the supernatants were determined by applying a human cytokine antibody array according to the manufacturer's instructions (R&D, Wiesbaden, Germany). The chemiluminescent membranes were developed using the ChemiDoc™ MP System (Bio-Rad, Munich, Germany) and the signal intensity was assessed with ImageJ 1.49i software (National Institutes of Health, Bethesda, USA) by determining the pixel intensity of the detected spots. The signal value from the provided negative control was subtracted from every measured sample [13].

The 72 h supernatants of visceral or subcutaneous ASCs were also used for evaluating IL-6, IL-8, and TNFα via ELISA, as instructed by the manufacturers (PeproTech, Hamburg, Germany).

2.4. Cell Cycle Analysis and Cell Proliferation

The cell cycle distribution was analyzed using a FACSCalibur™ (BD Biosciences, Heidelberg, Germany), as reported [20]. Briefly, cells were harvested, washed with PBS, fixed in chilled 70% ethanol at 4 °C for 30 min., treated with 1 mg/mL of RNase A (Sigma-Aldrich, Munich, Germany) and stained with 100 µg/mL of propidium iodide (PI) for 30 min. at 37 °C. DNA content was determined.

Cell proliferation assays were carried out by using Cell Titer-Blue® Cell Viability Assay (BD Biosciences, Heidelberg, Germany) on treated cells in 96-well plates (Promega, Mannheim, Germany). 20 µL of CellTiter-Blue® reagent was added to each well and then incubated at 37 °C with 5% CO_2 for 4 h before fluorescence reading while using a Victor 1420 Multilabel Counter (Wallac, Finland), as reported [20].

2.5. ASC Differentiation And Western Blot Analysis

ASC differentiation was performed, as reported [13]. ASCs were cultured with StemMACS AdipoDiff media (Miltenyi Biotec, Gladbach, Germany) up to 14 days to induce adipogenic differentiation. Cells were then fixed and stained for adiponectin (Abcam, Cambridge, #ab22554) and analyzed for lipid droplets characteristic of adipocytes. For osteogenic differentiation, ASCs were incubated with StemMACS OsteoDiff media (Miltenyi Biotec, Gladbach, Germany) up to 14 days, fixed, and stained with 2% Alizarin Red S (pH 4.2) to visualize calcific deposition, a hallmark of osteogenic cells.

Western blot analysis was performed, as reported [21,22], with the following antibodies: mouse monoclonal antibodies against cyclin B1 (Santa Cruz Biotechnology, Heidelberg, Germany, GNS1), monoclonal mouse against p53 (Santa Cruz Biotechnology, Heidelberg, Germany, DO-8), and rabbit polyclonal antibodies against cyclin B1 (Santa Cruz Biotechnology, Heidelberg, Germany, H-433), mouse monoclonal antibodies against p21 (Cell Signaling, Frankfurt, Germany, DSC60), rabbit monoclonal antibodies against E-cadherin (Cell Signaling, Frankfurt, Germany, 24E10), mouse monoclonal antibodies against vimentin (Dako, Hamburg, Germany, M0725), rabbit monoclonal antibody against fibronectin (BD Biosciences, 1573-1), mouse monoclonal β-actin (A2228) (Sigma-Aldrich, Munich, Germany), and GAPDH (GTX627408) from GeneTex (Eching, Germany).

2.6. RNA Extraction And Real-Time PCR

Total RNAs of ASCs were extracted with RNeasy Mini kit (7Bioscience, Neuenburg, Germany). Reverse transcription was performed while using High-Capacity cDNA Reverse Transcription Kit (Promega, Mannheim, Germany), as instructed. All the probes for gene analysis were obtained from Applied Biosystems: ADIPOQ (#Hs00605917_m1), IL-6 (#Hs00985639_m1), IL-8 (#00175123_m1), IL-10 (#Hs00961622_m1), TNFα (Hs00174128_m1), PLK1 (#Hs00153444_m1), PLK4 (#Hs00179514_m1), KIF2A (#Hs00189636_m1), SMO (#Hs01090242_m1), GLI1 (#Hs00171790_m1), NANOG (#Hs04260366_g1), PTCH1 (#Hs00181117_m1), RUNX2 (#Hs01047973_m1), KLF4 (#Hs00358836_m1), c-MYC (#Hs00153408_m1), PPARγ (#Hs01115513_m1), LEPTIN (#Hs00174877_m1), SOX2 (#Hs01053049_s1), EpCAM (Hs0090188s_m1), VIM (#Hs00958111_m1), SNAIL1 (Hs00195591_m1), TWIST (Hs01675818_s1), ZEB1 (Hs01566408_m1), and GAPDH (#Hs02758991_g1). Real-time PCR was performed with a StepOnePlus Real-time PCR System (Applied Biosystems). The data were analyzed while using StepOne Software v.2.3 (Applied Biosystems), as described previously [23].

2.7. Cell Motility, Migration, Attraction, and Invasion

For motility assay, the cells were seeded into 24-well plates with a low confluency and they were imaged for 12 h at 5 min. time intervals. All time-lapse imaging was performed with an AxioObserver.Z1 microscope (Zeiss, Göttingen, Germany) and imaged with an AxioCam MRc camera (Zeiss, Göttingen, Germany) that was equipped with an environmental chamber to maintain proper environmental conditions (37 °C, 5% CO_2). The time-lapse movies were analyzed by using ImageJ 1.49i software (National Institutes of Health) with the manual tracking plugin, and Chemotaxis and Migration Tool (Ibidi GmBH, Munich, Germany). The tracks were derived from raw data points and they were plotted in GraphPad Prism 7 (GraphPad software Inc.). The accumulated distance was calculated by using the raw data points by the Chemotaxis and Migration Tool. Thirty random cells per experiment were analyzed and the experiments were independently repeated three times. The patterns of motility were evaluated, as described previously [15,16,24].

Cell migration assays were performed with culture-inserts from ibidi (Martinsried, Germany). Visceral or subcutaneous ASCs (6.5×10^4) cells were seeded in each well of the culture-inserts. Culture-inserts were gently removed after at least 8 h. The cells were acquired and imaged at indicated time points with bright-field images. Four pictures of each insert were taken (three inserts for each experimental condition) and the experiments were performed in triplicates. The open area was measured while using the AxioVision SE64 Re. 4.9 software (Zeiss, Göttingen, Germany).

For attraction assay, cells were placed in six-well plates and one well of each insert was filled with visceral or subcutaneous ASCs (5.5×10^4) or with the investigated cells (MCF-7 or MDA-MB-231). After 8 h, the culture-inserts were removed and the images were obtained at the indicated time points. Cellular movement toward other migration front was evaluated by measuring the distance between the cell nucleus and the outermost cellular protrusion using the AxioVision SE64 Re. 4.9 software (Zeiss, Göttingen, Germany). The experiments were independently performed three times.

Visceral or subcutaneous ASCs were seeded (7.5×10^4) in 24-well transwell matrigel chambers for invasion assay, according to the manufacturer's instructions (Cell Biolabs Inc, San Diego), as previously reported [13]. The cells were fixed with ethanol and stained with DAPI. The invaded cells were counted with a microscope. The experiments were independently performed three times.

2.8. Statistical Analysis

Student's t-test (two tailed and paired or homoscedastic) was used to evaluate the significance of difference between different groups for gene analysis, cell viability assay, cell cycle distribution, and ciliated cell population. An unpaired Mann–Whitney U test was used to perform the statistical evaluation of the single cell tracking assay, line-scan analysis, and the measurement of the cilium length (two tailed). Difference was considered to be statistically significant when $p < 0.05$.

3. Results

3.1. Subcutaneous and Visceral ASCs Have a Comparable Cell Surface Marker Profile and Proliferation Rate

For this study, subcutaneous and visceral ASCs were isolated from age and BMI matched donors undergoing Caesarean sections. Table 1 lists the clinical information.

Table 1. Clinical information of 16 participants.

	Age	Gestational Age (weeks)	Body Mass Index (BMI)	Birth Weight (g)
mean value	31.6 ± 4.6	37.7 ± 2.8	24.1 ± 2.9	2964 ± 581

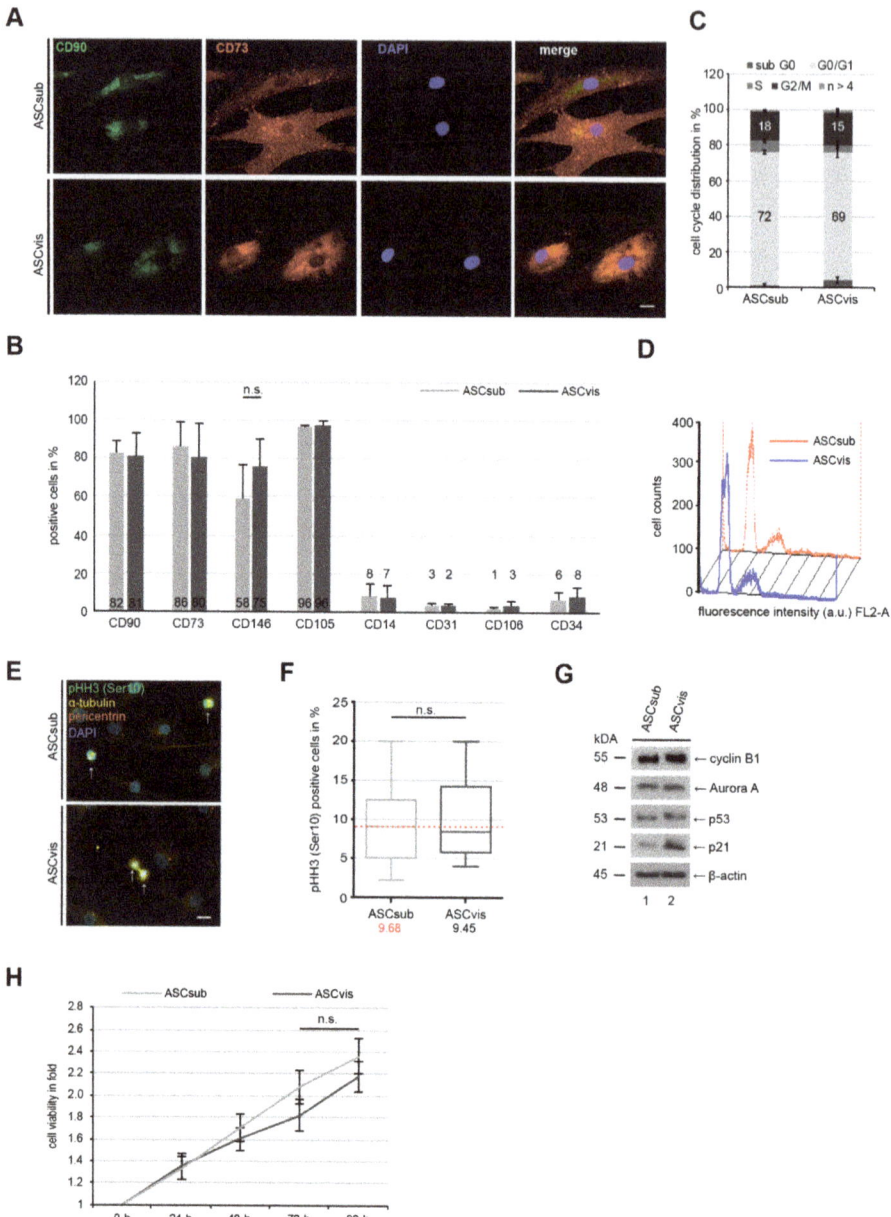

Figure 1. Subcutaneous and visceral adipose-derived mesenchymal stem cells (ASCs) display comparable cell surface marker profiles, cell cycle distribution and cell proliferation. (**A**) Immunofluorescence staining of mesenchymal stem cell surface markers CD90 (green) and CD73 (red), and DNA (DAPI, blue) in subcutaneous ASCs (ASCsub) and visceral ASCs (ASCvis). Scale: 20 μm. (**B**) Flow cytometric analyses of positive cell surface markers CD90, CD73, CD146, and CD105, and negative markers CD14, CD31, CD106, and CD34 for mesenchymal stem cells (MSCs). Values represent the percentages of ASCs expressing the indicated protein. The results from eight independent experiments (donors) are presented as mean ± standard error of the mean (SEM). (**C,D**) Cell cycle distribution was analyzed

using a FACSCalibur™. Profile examples were shown (**C**). Cell cycle phases of ASCs were presented in percentage and the results were derived from four independent experiments (**D**). (**E,F**) ASCs were stained for pHH3 (S10) (green), α-tubulin (yellow), pericentrin (red) and DNA (blue), and representatives are shown (**E**). Scale: 10 µm. pHH3 positive cells were quantified in ASCsub and ASCvis (**F**). The results are from three independent experiments with ASCs from three different donors and presented as median ± min/max whiskers in box plots. n.s. > 0.05. (**G**) Cellular extracts from ASCs were prepared for Western blot analyses with indicated antibodies. β-actin served as loading control. (**H**) ASCs were seeded in 96-well plates for 0, 24, 48, 72, and 96 h. Cell viability was measured via CellTiter-Blue® assay. The results are presented as mean ± SEM and statistically analyzed, showing no significant difference (n.s.).

The expression of cell surface markers was compared between subcutaneous ASCs (ASCsub) and visceral ASCs (ASCvis). The indirect immunofluorescence staining of CD90 and CD73, two important markers for mesenchymal stem cells (MSCs), including ASCs, showed positive signals to a comparable extent in both types of ASCs (Figure 1A). This was further underscored by flow cytometric analyses of CD90, CD73, CD146, and CD105 as positive markers and CD14, CD31, CD106, and CD34 as negative markers (Figure 1B), as described [25,26]. The percentages of cell surface markers were comparable between ASCsub and ASCvis (Figure 1B). Additionally, the cell cycle distribution of both ASC subtypes differed by only 3% in G0/G1-phase (ASCsub: 72%, ASCvis: 69%) and G2/M-phase (ASCsub: 18%, ASCvis: 15%) (Figure 1C,D). Furthermore, the cells were stained for phospho-histone H3 (pHH3 (Ser10)) (Figure 1E), a mitotic marker, for the evaluation of mitotic cells. No significant difference in the mitotic cell population was observed between two subtypes of ASCs (Figure 1F). ASCs were also harvested for Western blot analysis. The important mitotic proteins cyclin B1 and Aurora A showed no differences in their protein expression (Figure 1G, lane 1 and 2), whereas the cellular stress response proteins p53 and p21 were slightly elevated in visceral ASCs (Figure 1G, lane 4 and 5). Finally, the subcutaneous ASCs showed marginally increased cell viability upon 72 h and 96 h, which could not reach a significant level (Figure 1H, 72 h and 96 h). In summary, the results reveal no significant differences between matched ASCsub and ASCvis cells in the expression of their cell surface markers, cell cycle distribution, important mitotic regulators, and cell viability.

3.2. Both ASC Subtypes Display Comparable Migration and Invasion Rates but Different Modes of Motility

An important function of MSCs, to which ASCs belong, is their migration and homing ability to a target tissue or cell type [27]. Several assays were performed with ASCsub and ASCvis to investigate this issue in detail. At first, wound healing/migration assays were carried out, as previously described [13]. After 16 and 24 h, ASCsub cells showed a significantly increased migration capacity when compared to ASCvis (Figure 2A,B). Surprisingly, this pattern could not be observed in a single-cell tracking experiment, which analyzes the random movement of cells up to 12 h, as reported [14]. The results illustrated even a slightly increased accumulated distance in visceral ASCs with 523 µm as compared to 449 µm in subcutaneous ASCs (Figure 2C, left graph, and D). As calculated by time and distance, the velocity of these cells was also moderately elevated (ASCvis: 0.78 µm/min., ASCsub: 0.67 µm/min.) (Figure 2C, middle graph). In contrast, the intrinsic directionality of ASCvis was significantly reduced when compared to ASCsub (ASCvis: 0.23 d/D, ASCsub: 0.62 d/D) (Figure 2C, right graph), indicating that the ASCsub cells move in a directed fashion. To study the motility in a three-dimensional (3D) environment, invasion assays were carried out [13]. Interestingly, 39.6% of ASCsub and 40.3% of ASCvis were able to invade through the matrigel layer (Figure 2E,F) and no significant difference ($p = 0.49$) could be observed between both subpopulations.

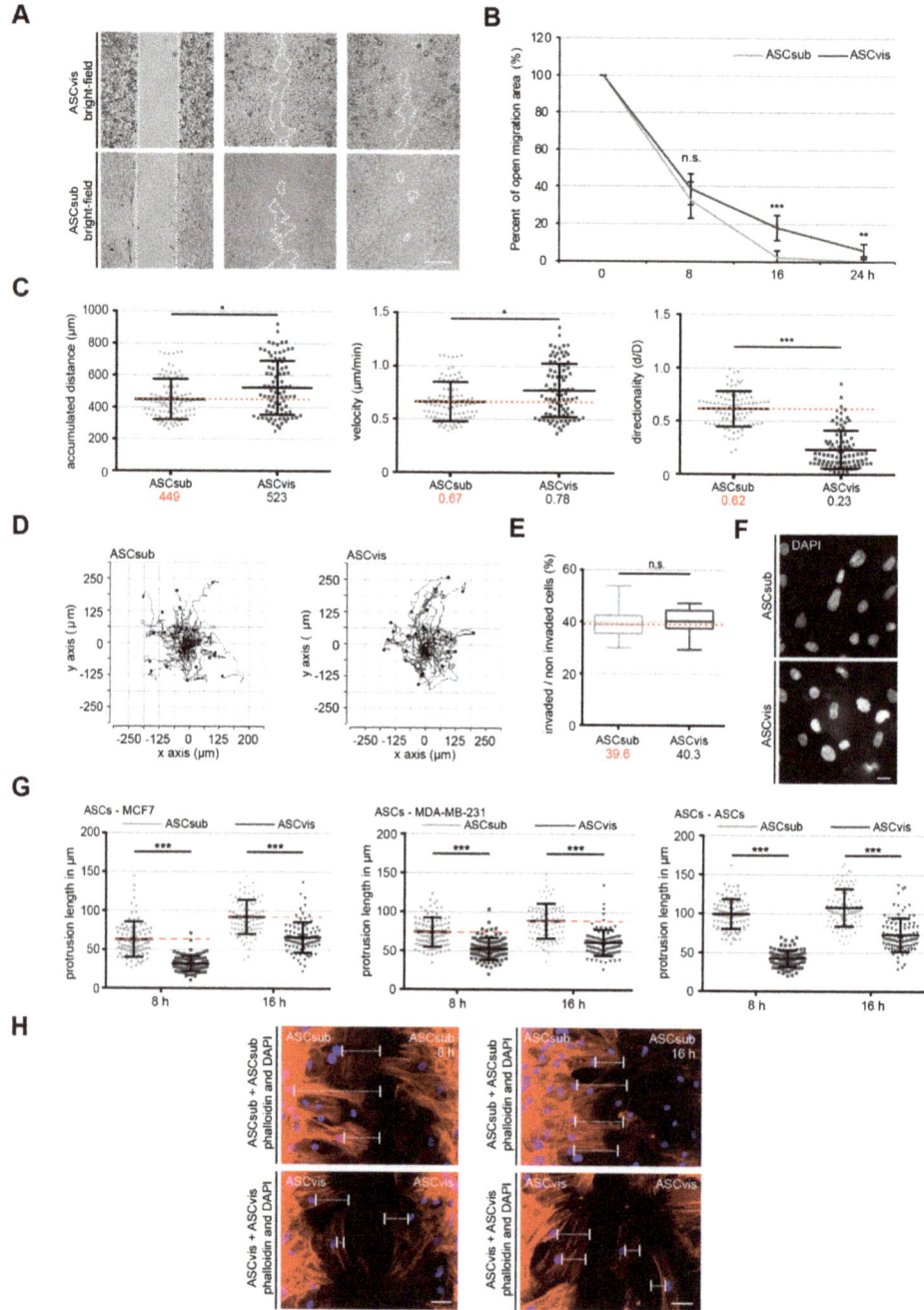

Figure 2. Both ASC subtypes display a comparable motility rate, but subcutaneous ASCs have a significantly higher directed migration capacity. (**A,B**) Wound healing/migration assays were performed with subcutaneous and visceral ASCs, and images were taken at indicated time points (0, 8, 16, 24 h) to document the migration front. (**A**) Representatives are shown. White dashed line depicts the migration front. Scale: 300 μm. (**B**) Quantification of the open area between both migration fronts at various time

points. The cell-free area at 0 h was assigned as 100%. The results from three independent experiments are presented as mean ± SEM. *** $p < 0.001$. (**C,D**) Time-lapse microscopy was performed with subcutaneous or visceral ASCs for up to 12 h. Random motility of these cells was analyzed. (**D**) Representative trajectories of individual cells ($n = 30$) are shown. (**C**) Evaluated accumulated distance (left), velocity (middle), and directionality (right) from three independent experiments are shown as box plots with variations. Unpaired Mann–Whitney *U*-test, * $p < 0.05$, *** $p < 0.001$. (**E,F**) Invasion assay. ASCs were seeded into transwells and starved for 12 h. The cells were released into fresh medium for 24 h and fixed for quantification. (**E**) Quantification of invaded cells per field in percent. The results from three independent experiments are presented as mean ± SEM. Student's t test was performed showing no significant difference (n.s. > 0.05). (**F**) Representatives of invaded ASCs are shown. Scale: 25 μm. (**G,H**) Homing assays. ASCs and breast cancer cells were seeded in separated chambers of a culture insert and cultured for 0, 8 and 15 h. (**G**) Evaluation of cell homing distance, the length between the nucleus and the outermost cell protrusion, in subcutaneous and visceral ASCs toward MCF-7 cells (left), MDA-MB-231 cells (middle), and ASC themselves (right). Each experiment was performed in triplicate, and the results are based on three independent experiments and presented as scatter plot showing mean ± SEM. (red dashed line indicates median value of ASCsub). ** $p < 0.01$, *** $p < 0.001$. (**H**) Representatives of ASCs on both migration fronts stained against phalloidin (red) and DAPI (blue) are depicted. White bars indicate cellular protrusion length. Scale: 50 μm.

Many studies have reported a tropism of ASCs toward cancer cells [28], which can be demonstrated via homing experiments [13]. Homing experiments were performed with ASCs and breast cancer cells seeded in separated chambers of a culture insert with a defined cell free gap to corroborate the observation that ASCsub cells move in a more directed fashion compared to ASCvis. We measured the cell homing distance, the length between the nucleus, and the outermost cell protrusion, including lamellipodia and filopodia, of ASCs toward distinct breast cancer cell lines MCF-7 and MDA-MB-231 demonstrating the tropism of ASCs at 8 h and 16 h. ASCsub showed a significantly increased homing ability after 8 h and 15 h toward MCF-7 and MDA-MB-231 cell lines as compared to ASCvis (Figure 2G, left and middle graphs). Interestingly, subcutaneous ASCs home even to their own cell type (Figure 2G,H, right graphs). In contrast, visceral ASCs were homing less efficiently toward other cell types (Figure 2G,H). Collectively, these results strongly suggest that subcutaneous ASCs have an extraordinarily directed mode of motility, whereas visceral ASCs seem to move in an undirected random fashion.

3.3. Subcutaneous ASCs Display Higher Gene Levels of Mesenchymal Transcription Factors and Have More Dynamic and Composition Altered FAs Compared to Visceral ASCs

Both subtypes of ASCs displayed distinct morphologies that are shown by staining with phalloidin, an actin cytoskeleton dye, and paxillin, a focal adhesion marker, especially in their early 3–4 passages. Subcutaneous ASCs were more "classical" mesenchymal-like, showing characteristics of a fibroblast-like morphology with a small and long cell body (Figure 3A, upper panel). Visceral ASCs were less mesenchymal-like with some likeness of apical-basal polarity and a large cell body (Figure 3A, lower panel). Western blot analyses corroborated this notion, by showing less protein levels of fibronectin and vimentin (Figure 3B, lane 1 and 3), mesenchymal cell markers, and higher levels of E-cadherin (Figure 3B, lane 2), an epithelial cell marker, in visceral ASCs as compared to subcutaneous ASCs (Figure 3B). In line with these data, the gene levels of zinc finger E-box-binding homeobox 1 (*ZEB1*), snail family transcriptional repressor 1 (*SNAIL1*), and twist family basic helix-loop-helix (bHLH) transcription factor 1 (*TWIST*), three important mesenchymal transcription factors, were enriched in ASCsub when compared to ASCvis (Figure 3C). Moreover, the epithelial cell adhesion molecule (*EpCAM*) gene was more demonstrative in ASCvis, while the expression of mesenchymal gene vimentin (*VIM*) encoding a type III intermediate filament was higher in ASCsub (Figure 3D, left) (Figure 3D, right). These results suggest that subcutaneous and visceral ASCs differ in the expression of mesenchymal and epithelial markers contributing to the different migration behavior of these cells (Figures 2 and 3A–D).

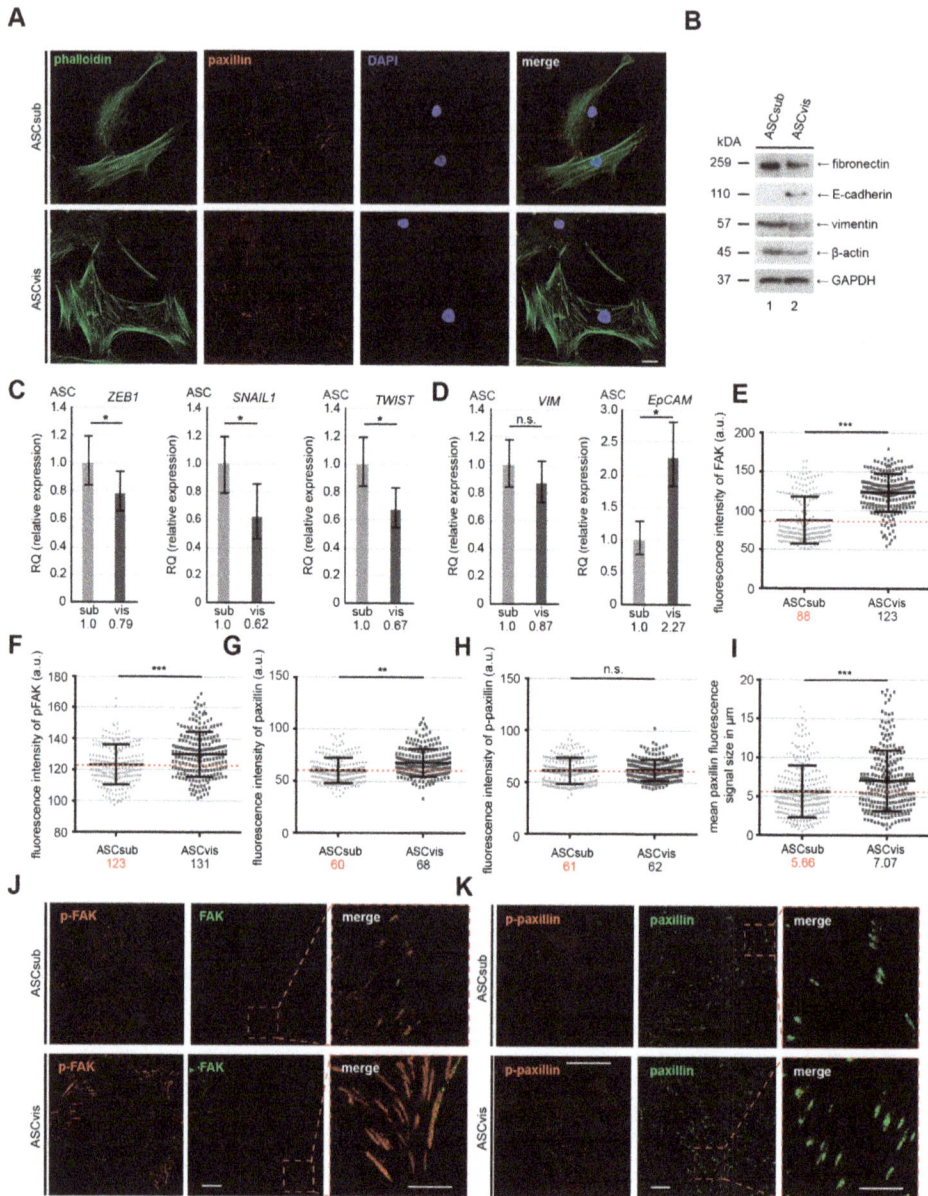

Figure 3. Subcutaneous ASCs show a typical mesenchymal-like phenotype compared to their visceral counterparts. (**A**) Immunofluorescence staining of ASCsub and ASCvis. ASCs were stained for phalloidin (green), paxillin (red) and DNA (blue) to underline their cell morphology. Examples are shown. Scale: 25 µm. (**B**) Cellular extracts from ASCs were prepared for Western blot analyses with antibodies against β-actin, E-cadherin, fibronectin and vimentin. Glyceraldehyde-3-phosphate dehydrogenase (GAPDH) served as loading control. (**C,D**) Gene levels of mesenchymal associated transcription factors and cytoskeleton proteins *ZEB1*, *SNAIL*, *TWIST*, *VIM*, and *EpCAM* are shown for subcutaneous and visceral ASCs. The results are from three experiments, presented as RQ with minimum and maximum range. RQ, relative quantification of gene expression. Student's t test, * $p < 0.05$. (**E–K**) The focal adhesion composition was analyzed by staining ASCs for focal adhesion

kinase (FAK) (green), p-FAK (red), and DNA (DAPI, blue), or for p-paxillin (red), paxillin (green) and DNA (DAPI, blue) for fluorescence microscopy. Quantification of the mean fluorescence intensity of FAK (**E**), p-FAK (**F**), paxillin (**G**) p-paxillin (**H**), and focal adhesion area (**I**) in ASCsub versus ASCvis (at least 200 FAs per staining). The results are based on three independent experiments and presented as scatter plot showing mean ± SEM. Unpaired Mann–Whitney *U*-test, ** $p < 0.01$, *** $p < 0.001$. a.u., arbitrary units. Representatives are depicted (**J,K**). Scale: 25 µm.

The FAs of both ASC types were analyzed in depth by immunofluorescence staining of focal adhesion kinase (FAK), phospho-FAK (p-FAK), paxillin, and p-paxillin (Figure 3E–K), the most important components of FAs, since the protein expression, phosphorylation status, and the FA composition are influenced by a variety of transcription factors, including *TWIST*, *SNAIL1*, and *ZEB1* [29,30]. Though showing no difference in p-paxillin signal, subcutaneous ASCs displayed significantly less mean fluorescence intensity of FAK (88 a.u.), p-FAK (123 a.u.), and paxillin (60 a.u.), in comparison with visceral ASCs (FAK (123 a.u.), p-FAK (131 a.u.), and paxillin (68 a.u.)) (Figure 3E–K). Furthermore, the size of FA correlates with its stability [31,32]. Indeed, the FA size was significantly enlarged in ASCvis (ASCvis; 7.07 µm), relative to ASCsub (5.66 µm) (Figure 3I).

More FA components (Figure 3E–H) and enlarged FA size (Figure 3I) indicate altered FA dynamics of visceral ASCs. We performed a nocodazole washout experiment to delineate this issue, in which MT depolymerization induced by nocodazole leads to stabilized FAs through stress fiber formation and the release from the nocodazole treatment triggers FA disassembly through rapid MT regrowth [33]. ASCs were subjected to nocodazole (10 µM), released for 0, 30, and 75 min., stained for p-FAK and paxillin, two important FA assembly factors, for microscopic evaluation (Figure 4A). Subcutaneous ASCs dynamically responded to the nocodazole release evidenced by rapidly decreased paxillin, p-FAK, and FA size at 30 min. Followed by efficiently recruiting these FA components, leading to enlarging FA size at 75 min. (Figure 4B–E, left panels). In line with the observations (Figure 3F,H,I), visceral ASCs showed high levels of paxillin and p-FAK and the large FAs, even after the cells were treated with nocodazole (Figure 4B–E, right panels, 0 h). Furthermore, despite disassembled FAs being triggered by the nocodazole release at 30 min., visceral ASCs had difficulty in reassembling their FAs at 75 min. by showing low p-FAK level and small FA size (Figure 4B–E, right panels). In sum, these results clearly suggest that visceral ASCs have stabilized FAs with a static turnover, whereas subcutaneous ASCs confer dynamic FAs, which contributes to their efficiently directed motility.

3.4. Visceral ASCs Have a Higher Osteogenic and Adipogenic Differentiation Capacity and Upregulated Levels of Stemness-Like Associated Genes

The differentiation capacity of ASCs that were isolated from different adipose tissue depots is the subject of controversial debates over the last decade, with multiple investigations reporting inconsistent results [5,6,11]. This could be ascribed to the usage of ASCs that were isolated from distinct donors with varied age, BMI, and gender, different isolation methods or varying ASC passages. We used matched ASCs from the same donor and in identical passage for differentiation experiments. We first analyzed multiple classical stemness/self-renewal associated genes, like myelocytomatosis proto-oncogene cellular homolog (*c-MYC*), SRY-box transcription factor 2 (*SOX2*), Krüppel-like factor 4 (*KLF4*), and *NANOG*, which are also known for their crucial role in osteogenic and adipogenic differentiation of ASCs [34–36]. In fact, ASCvis showed a significantly higher expression of stemness associated genes, like *c-MYC*, *SOX2*, *KLF4*, and *NANOG*, when compared to ASCsub (Figure 5A).

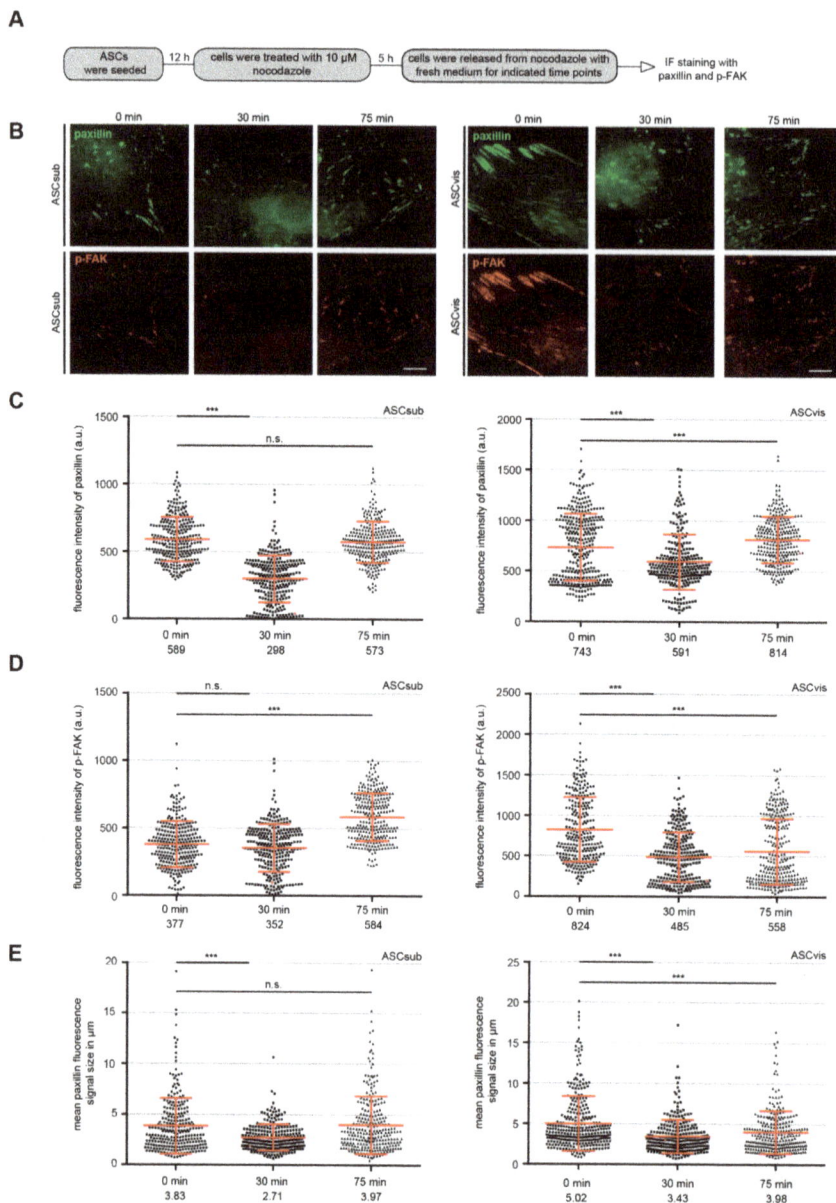

Figure 4. Subcutaneous ASCs dynamically disassemble and reassemble their FAs. (**A**) Schedule of the nocodazole washout assay. (**B**) ASCs were incubated for 5 h with 10 μM nocodazole followed by washout, where the microtubules (MTs) were allowed to regrow for 0, 30 and 75 min. Cells were stained for paxillin (green), p-FAK (red), and DNA (DAPI, blue). Representatives of FA disassembly/reassembly are shown. Scale: 15 μm. (**C**–**E**) Kinetics of FA disassembly during MT regrowth and FA reassembly after MT regrowth. Quantification of the mean fluorescence intensity of paxillin (**C**), p-FAK (**D**), and FA size (**E**) (270 FA per condition) is depicted. The results are based on three independent experiments and presented as scatter plots showing mean ± SEM. Unpaired Mann–Whitney U-test, ** $p < 0.01$, *** $p < 0.001$. a.u., arbitrary units.

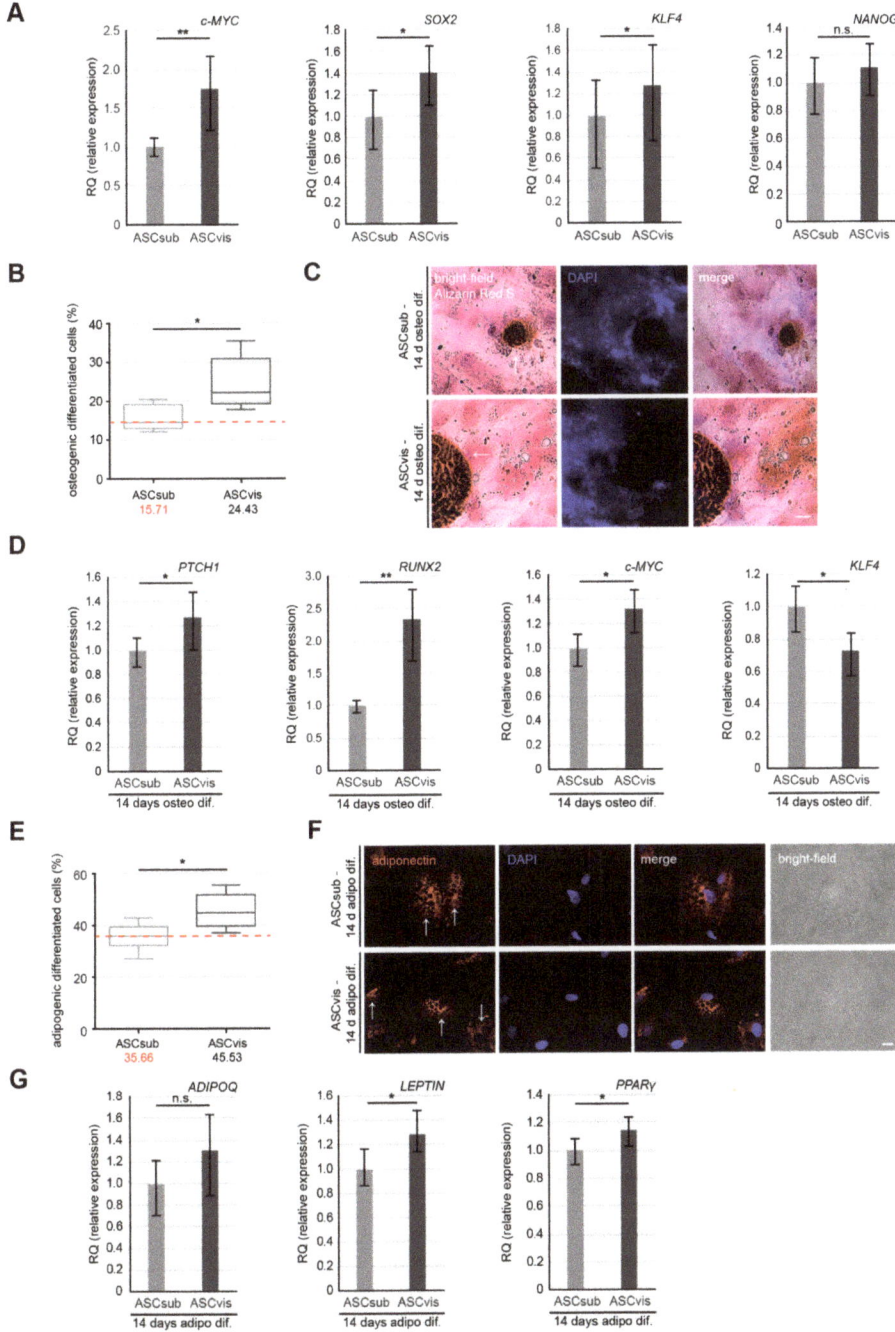

Figure 5. Visceral ASCs are superior in osteogenic and adipogenic differentiation compared to subcutaneous ASCs. (**A**) Gene levels of stemness/self-renewal associated genes *c-MYC*, *SOX2*, *KLF4*, and *NANOG* are shown for subcutaneous and visceral ASCs. The results are from three experiments, presented as RQ with minimum and maximum range. Student's t test, * $p < 0.05$, ** $p < 0.01$. (**B–D**) ASCsub and ASCvis cells were induced into osteogenic differentiation for up to 14 days. The percentage

of differentiated ASCs was evaluated by Alizarin Red S staining. (**B**) The quantification data are presented as median ± min/max whiskers (red dashed line indicates median value of ASCsub, $n = 300$ cells for each condition, pooled from three experiments). Student's t test, $* p < 0.05$. (**C**) Example images for Alizarin Red S staining are shown. Scale: 20 µm. (**D**) Expression levels of differentiation related genes *PTCH1* (1st graph), *RUNX2* (2nd graph), *KLF4* (3rd graph), and *c-MYC* (4th graph) in differentiated subcutaneous and visceral ASCs. The results are from three experiments and presented as RQ with minimum and maximum range. Student's t test, $* p < 0.05$, $** p < 0.01$. (**E–G**) Analyses of cells with lipid vacuoles after 14 days of adipogenic differentiation. (**E**) The quantification shows the percentage of cells differentiated into adipogenic-like cells. Results are presented as median ± min/max whiskers in visceral ASCs ($n = 200$ cells for each condition, pooled from three experiments) and the red dashed line illustrates the median value of ASCsub. Student's t test, $* p < 0.05$. (**F**) Representative images of cells displaying lipid vacuoles stained for adiponectin (red) and DNA (DAPI, blue). (**G**) Gene levels of *ADIPOQ, LEPTIN,* and *PPARγ* after adipogenic differentiation are shown for subcutaneous and visceral ASCs. The results are from three experiments, presented as RQ with minimum and maximum range. Student's t test, $* p < 0.05$.

ASCs were then differentiated to osteocytes or adipocytes for up to 14 days. The cells were stained with Alizarin Red S to visualize calcific deposition (osteogenic lineage) or adiponectin (adipogenic lineage). Relative to ASCvis (Figure 5C,F, lower panels), ASCsub showed lower numbers of positive cells that were stained with Alizarin Red S (Figure 5C, upper panel) or adiponectin (Figure 5F, upper panel). Further analysis revealed that, as compared to visceral ASCs with 24.4% osteogenic-like and 45.5% adipogenic-like cells, subcutaneous ASCs displayed 15.7% osteogenic-like and 35.6% adipogenic-like cells (Figure 5B,E). Total RNAs from these cells were also isolated for gene analysis. ASCvis showed enhanced levels of osteogenic related genes, including protein patched homolog 1 (*PTCH1*) and runt-related transcription factor (*RUNX2*) (Figure 5D, 1st and 2nd graph), as well as *c-MYC* (Figure 5D, 3rd graph). Interestingly, *KLF4*, which is a negative regulator for osteogenic differentiation, was upregulated in subcutaneous ASCs after differentiation (Figure 5D, 4th graph). Similar results were also obtained for adipogenic differentiation. Adiponectin (*ADIPOQ*), *LEPTIN*, and peroxisome proliferator activated receptor gamma (*PPARγ*), three adipogenic related genes, were increased in ASCvis upon differentiation (Figure 5G). These data strengthen the notion that visceral ASCs have an improved differentiation capability that is likely associated with a higher gene expression of stemness associated genes.

3.5. Subcutaneous ASCs are More Ciliated but Have A Less Active Sonic Hedgehog (Hh) Pathway

The primary cilium is a sensor organelle that is critical for responding to a variety of extra and intracellular stimuli as a central processing unit [37]. It is connected to many key functions of ASCs, like migration, secretion, and differentiation [38,39], and indispensable for the Hh signaling in mammals [40]. To compare the cilium size as well as the ciliated cell population between ASCsub and ASCvis, the cells were stained for acetylated α-tubulin, adenosine diphosphate ribosylation factor-like GTPase 13B (Arl13b), two typical cilium markers, and DNA followed by microscopic analysis (Figure 6A). The primary cilium size was comparable between both ASC subtypes with a mean cilium length of 4.61 µm in ASCsub and 4.60 µm in ASCvis (Figure 6A,B). While 28.6% of visceral ASCs were ciliated, the primary cilium was present in 43.9% of subcutaneous ASCs (Figure 6C). In line with less ciliated cells, the gene levels of Polo-like kinase 1 (*PLK1*), Polo-like kinase 4 (*PLK4*), and kinesin family member 2A (*KIF2A*), genes that are responsible for deciliation and here independent from their roles in mitosis, are upregulated in visceral ASCs (Figure 6D).

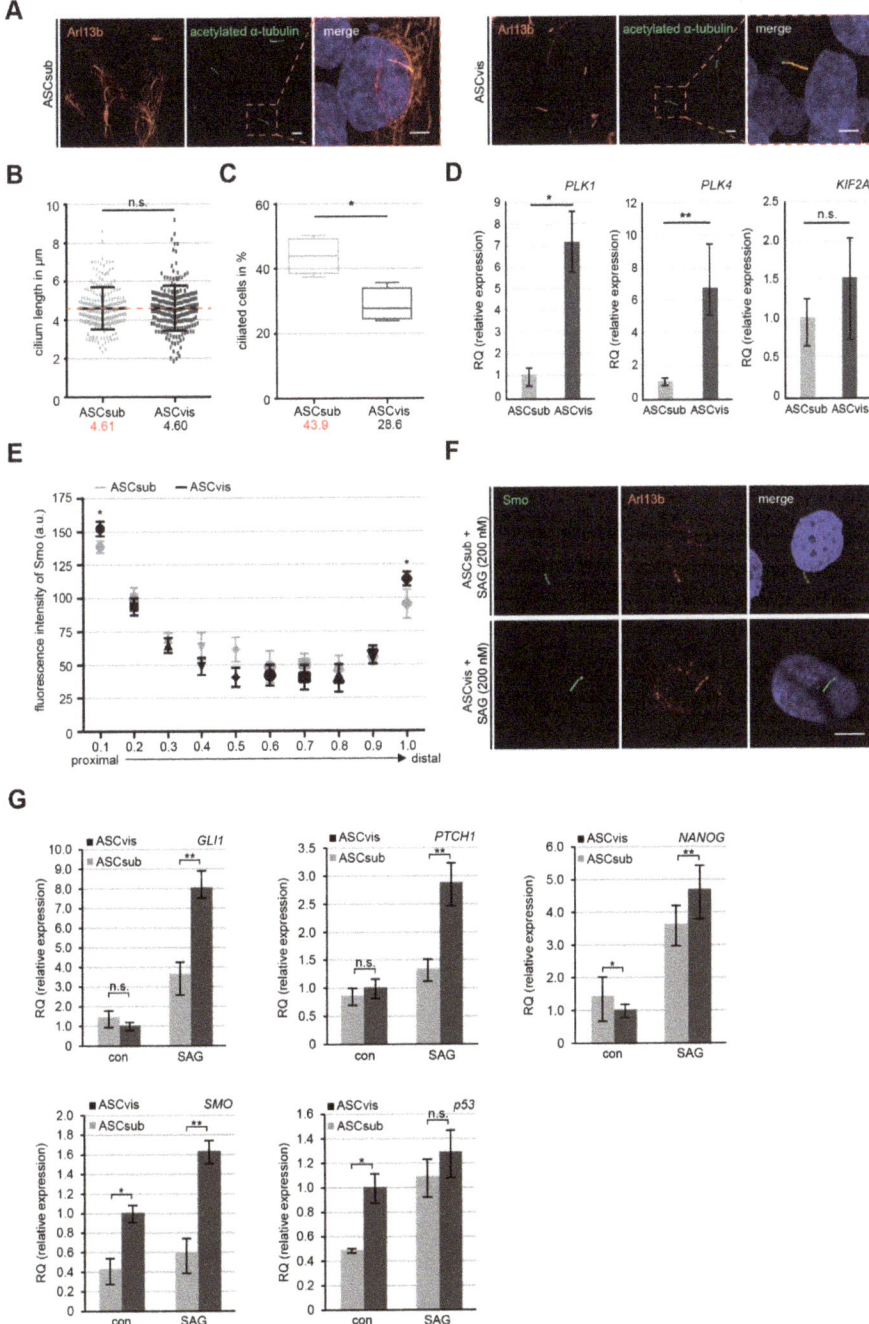

Figure 6. Visceral ASCs display high deciliation gene levels and enhanced activation of the sonic hedgehog (Hh) signaling pathway. (**A**) Primary cilia of ASCsub and ASCvis were stained for acetylated α-tubulin and Arl13b. Representatives are shown. Scale: 10 μm. Regions outlined in boxes are shown in a higher magnification. Inset scale: 10 μm. (**B**) The cilium length was evaluated. The results are based on six experiments using ASCs from six donors (*n* = 180 cilia for each group). (**C**) Ciliated ASCs

were evaluated and the results are presented as mean ± SEM (n = 600 cells, pooled from six experiments). Unpaired Mann–Whitney U-test, * $p < 0.05$. (**D**) The gene levels of deciliation regulators *PLK1*, *PLK4*, and *KIF2A*. The data are based on three experiments and presented as RQ with minimum and maximum range. Student's t test, * $p < 0.05$, ** $p < 0.01$. (**E–G**) Fluorescence intensities and expression levels of important genes related to the Hh pathway are shown for ASCs treated with SAG for 24 h. (**E**) Each point of the curve represents the mean fluorescence intensity (mean ± SEM) based on three experiments (n = 30 cilia). Unpaired Mann–Whitney U-test, * $p < 0.05$. (**F**) Representatives are shown for measurements of primary cilium staining of acetylated α-tubulin, Arl13b and Smoothened (Smo). Scale: 3 µm. (**G**) The gene levels of *GLI1*, *PTCH1*, *NANOG*, *SMO*, and *TP53* are shown for ASCs treated or non-treated with 200 nM SAG for 24 h. The results are from three experiments, merged as biological group, and presented as mean ± SEM. Student's t test, * $p < 0.05$, ** $p < 0.01$.

The Hh signaling pathway is exclusively mediated by the primary cilium and it is involved in the differentiation processes of multiple types of various stem/mesenchymal stem cells, including ASCs [38,41]. The activation of the Hh pathway is a signaling cascade recruiting Smoothened (Smo) and glioma-associated oncogene homolog 1–3 (Gli1-3) to the primary cilium, which leads to an accumulation of these proteins on the proximal base and distal tip of the cilium [42]. ASCs were treated with 200 nM of SAG, a smoothened agonist, for 16 h, to compare the activation and response of this pathway between both subtypes. The treated ASCs were stained for Arl13b, Smo, and pericentrin for microscopy. Line scan analysis of fluorescent Smo was performed from the proximal base to the distal tip of cilia (Figure 6F). Subcutaneous ASCs demonstrated a significantly lowered intensity of Smo on the proximal as well as the distal part of the primary cilium when compared to visceral ASCs (Figure 6E), which suggests the hampered recruitment of Smo to the cilium in ASCsub. Furthermore, gene analysis revealed a significantly lower expression of Hh related genes *GLI1*, *PTCH1*, *SMO*, and two downstream targets *TP53* and *NANOG* after 24 h SAG stimulation in subcutaneous ASCs relative to visceral ASCs (Figure 6G). The less active Hh signaling could be an additional explanation for the reduced adipogenic/osteogenic differentiation capacity of subcutaneous ASCs.

3.6. Visceral ASCs Secrete More Inflammatory Cytokines

MSCs, especially ASCs, are well known as a source of many secreted cytokines, chemokines, and growth factors regulating diverse cell-cell communications [43]. As reported previously, we analyzed the secretion of multiple factors from ASCsub and ASCvis by using a cytokine array demonstrating the secretion of various inflammation cytokines [13]. To corroborate these results, the concentrations of interleukin 6 (IL-6), interleukin 8 (IL-8), and tumor necrosis factor α (TNFα) were measured in the supernatant of both ASC subtypes by enzyme-linked immunosorbent assay (ELISA). Subcutaneous ASCs secreted significantly less of all three inflammatory cytokines, with 186 pg/mL of IL-6, 676 pg/mL of IL-8, and 111 pg/mL of TNFα when compared to 236 pg/mL of IL-6, 761 pg/mL of IL-8, and 194 pg/mL of TNFα secreted by ASCvis (Figure 7A). In support of these observations, the gene levels of *IL-6*, *IL-8*, *IL-10*, and *TNFα* were higher in visceral ASCs as compared to subcutaneous ASCs (Figure 7B).

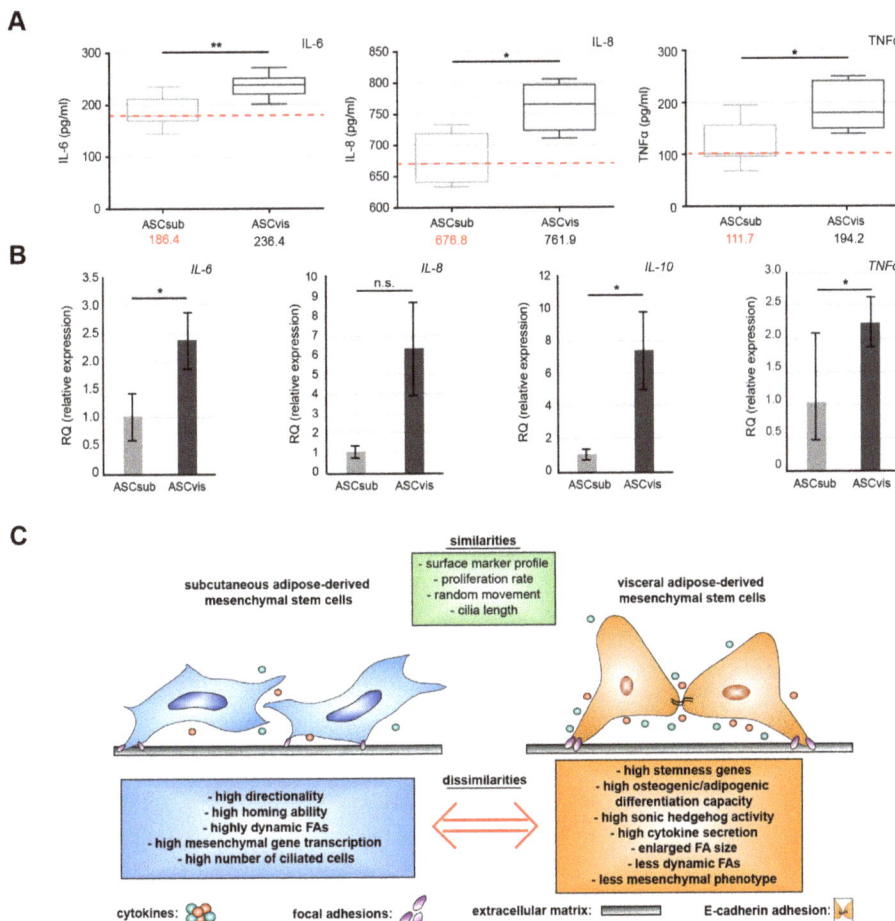

Figure 7. Visceral ASCs secrete more pro-inflammatory cytokines. (**A**) The supernatants of subcutaneous and visceral ASCs in the third passage were collected after 72 h culture and used for evaluation of IL-6 (left), IL-8 (middle) and TNF-α (right) by enzyme-linked immunosorbent assay (ELISA). The results are from four experiments and presented as median ± min/max whiskers in box plots. Student's t test, * $p < 0.05$, ** $p < 0.01$. (**B**) The gene levels of *IL-6, IL-8, IL-10,* and *TNFα*. The data are based on three experiments and presented as RQ with minimum and maximum range. Student's t test, * $p < 0.05$. (**C**) Schematic illustration of the proposed similarities and dissimilarities between both ASC subtypes. The key dissimilarities between subcutaneous and visceral ASCs are their migration mode, differentiation capacity, and cytokine secretion, which affect a variety of different pathways, like the Hh signaling on the primary cilium.

4. Discussion

ASCs have gained high attention as a promising tool for novel cell-based therapies in the field of regenerative medicine, supported by multiple encouraging preclinical studies in a variety of human diseases [44,45]. However, the diversity among ASCs that were isolated from different adipose tissue depots affects their biological functions and features [5,6,11]. In this work, we have isolated ASCs from subcutaneous and visceral adipose tissue of the same donors and systematically characterized multiple features of these paired ASCs in detail.

The results show that both subcutaneous and visceral ASCs display relatively comparable percentages of cells positive for cell surface markers, which are characteristic for MSCs [25]. Cell viability, cell cycle distribution, and mitotic cell population are also similar between subcutaneous and visceral ASCs, which is in agreement with the results from several groups [46–48] and yet inconsistent with the data from other studies [11,49–51]. This discrepancy generally results from non-matched donors and varied methodology for ASC isolation/culture. It is observed in many studies that subcutaneous and visceral ASCs were derived from donors without further description of related clinical information, like age, gender, and BMI, or from other species [46–50,52]. These heterogeneous data underscore the requirement of matched donor collectives and standardized protocols. Although it is reported that the proliferation rate of ASCs is hardly changed by the reproductive status [53], we do not exclude the possibility that pregnancy related hormones influence some of ASC features.

One key feature of mesenchymal stem cells is their homing ability toward damaged tissue and to serve in these areas as a reservoir for growth factors and regenerative promoters [54]. We showed that, relative to visceral ASCs, subcutaneous ASCs have a more directed mode of motility, evidenced by single-cell tracking, and especially homing assays, in which ASCs move toward different cell lines, like MCF-7, MDA-MB231, or themselves. Moreover, subcutaneous ASCs display a classical mesenchymal phenotype with a spindle-like form and a small cell body, whereas visceral ASCs show a large cell body and some likeness of an "apical-basal polarity" [55]. In line with these findings, well-known mesenchymal markers, like fibronectin and vimentin, as well as genes of mesenchymal related transcription factors, including *SNAIL*, *SLUG*, *TWIST*, and *ZEB1*, were low in visceral ASCs. This could contribute to the decreased directional movement of visceral ASCs, since an increased mesenchymal phenotype correlates with an enhanced directional motility, as reported for multiple cell lines during the process of the epithelial-to-mesenchymal transition (EMT) [56,57]. The analyses of important FA proteins illustrate a more complex pattern: FAK, p-FAK, and paxillin were significantly higher in visceral ASCs, which is often associated with efficient cellular migration [58]. However, FA size is related to the migration rate and the residence time of FAK and paxillin [31,32]. Indeed, visceral ASCs displayed highly enlarged FAs, as shown in cells switching from an epithelial to mesenchymal phenotype [30], which implies an accumulation of these proteins mediated by a slower FA turnover rate in visceral ASCs. This assumption was further corroborated by the data from the nocodazole washout assay, illustrating more dynamic FAs in subcutaneous ASCs with a higher rate of FA disassembly and reassembly after the nocodazole release as compared to visceral ASCs.

In conclusion, we show that subcutaneous ASCs conduct a more directional movement that is associated with an efficient FA turnover than visceral ASCs, though both subtypes move with comparable rates. This difference could be likely ascribed to their different origins [59] with distinct biological functions. An enhanced homing ability might be important to execute the protective and cell renewal functions of the subcutaneous AT [6], whereas the visceral AT is important in controlling metabolism and inflammatory signals [5], which are less dependent on the homing/migration ability of these cells.

In agreement with this notion, visceral ASCs secreted high levels of different chemokines/cytokines that are involved in autocrine and paracrine regulation. Among these cytokines, IL-6, IL-8, and TNFα were highly secreted by visceral ASCs, which is in line with the results that were derived from a recent report [60]. This substantial secretion of inflammatory cytokines is likely associated with their impact on the surrounding cells and microenvironment, which was previously shown in breast cancer cell lines MCF-7, MDA-MB-231, and non-tumorigenic breast epithelial cells, like MCF-10A [13,61].

Another characteristic property of ASCs is their capacity to differentiate into multiple cell types, including osteocytes and adipocytes [8]. We found that visceral ASCs have an increased differentiation potential toward the osteogenic and adipogenic lineage as compared to subcutaneous ASCs. This could be ascribed to an enhanced gene expression of stemness/self-renewal associated genes *c-MYC*, *KLF4*, *NANOG*, and *SOX2*, which are reported to be essential for the differentiation of MSCs/ASCs [35,36,62,63]. Especially, *c-MYC* has been shown to be crucial for the initiation of the adipogenic differentiation by regulating key genes, like fatty acid-binding protein 4 (*FABP4*), *PPARγ*, *ADIPOQ*, and *LEPTIN* in ASCs [63]. These results are not consistent with data from other studies, showing that subcutaneous ASCs are more competent in differentiation [50,64], again indicating the inconsistent results in this field. Again, this might be attributable to species differences and non-matched donors. Additionally, we are not able to exclude the impact of donors' reproductive state, which might enhance this capability of visceral ASCs, although *Ng* et al. have reported no significant differences between isolated ASCs from pregnant, premenopausal, and menopausal donors [53].

Interestingly, an increased number of subcutaneous ASCs were ciliated, which could be associated with their motility, as primary cilia are especially involved in directional migration [65]. However, relative to visceral ASCs, subcutaneous ASCs displayed less activation of the sonic Hh pathway upon stimulation, which is associated with less expression of its downstream targets. The Hh pathway is important for differentiation, since a report showed that the removal of the primary cilia and its associated Hh signaling leads to an increased ASC proliferation and decreased Runx2, alkaline phosphatase, and bone morphogenetic protein-2 mRNA (BMP2) expression, finally reducing their osteogenic differentiation potential [39]. Moreover, we have recently reported that the impaired differentiation capacity of obese ASCs is rescuable through the restoration of the cilium length and the sonic Hh pathway [16]. These data suggest that the less active Hh pathway in subcutaneous ASCs could be linked to their lower differentiation ability.

5. Conclusions

This work demonstrates that the ASCs isolated from subcutaneous and visceral AT share some characteristics, including their cell surface marker profile, cell viability, and cell cycle distribution, but they differ in multiple key aspects, like motility, FA dynamics, secretion of inflammatory cytokines, the expression of stemness related genes, differentiation capability, and primary cilia associated signaling (Figure 7E). These data may be of help for cell-based therapeutic strategies in a wide spectrum of diseases. Heterogeneous results in differentiation and proliferation emphasize the necessity for a standardization of donor selection and matched donor collectives, ASC isolation, characterization, and experimental protocols. Particularly, the donor age and BMI are reported to have great influence on the proliferation and differentiation ability of ASCs. Further investigations are required for studying the interactions of ASCs with their surrounding cells, like immune cells and fibroblasts, and to define their biological functions and molecular mechanisms in vivo via animal models.

Author Contributions: Conceptualization, A.R. and J.Y.; Data curation, A.R., A.F., S.R., N.-N.K., Samira C.H. and Babek Khan Safdar; Funding acquisition, A.R., C.S., F.L. and J.Y.; Investigation, A.R., A.F., S.R., N.-N.K., S.C.H. and B.K.S.; Methodology, A.R., A.F., S.R., N.-N.K., S.C.H. and B.K.S.; Project administration, A.R.; Resources, K.F., C.M., C.S., F.L. and J.Y.; Supervision, J.Y.; Visualization, A.R.; Writing—original draft, A.R.; Writing—review & editing, A.R., C.S., F.L. and J.Y.

Funding: This research project was funded by the Deutsche Forschungsgemeinschaft (DFG, German Research Foundation, project number 413992926) and by a young investigator grant in the Frankfurt Research Promotion Program (FFF) of the Faculty of Medicine of the Goethe University.

Acknowledgments: We are grateful to our patients and our clinical team for making this study possible.

Conflicts of Interest: The authors declare no conflict of interest. The funders had no role in the design of the study; in the collection, analyses, or interpretation of data; in the writing of the manuscript, or in the decision to publish the results.

References

1. Luong, Q.; Huang, J.; Lee, K.Y. Deciphering White Adipose Tissue Heterogeneity. *Biology* **2019**, *8*, 23. [CrossRef] [PubMed]
2. Natarajan, S.K.; Rasineni, K.; Ganesan, M.; Feng, D.; McVicker, B.L.; McNiven, M.A.; Osna, N.A.; Mott, J.L.; Casey, C.A.; Kharbanda, K.K. Structure, Function And Metabolism Of Hepatic And Adipose Tissue Lipid Droplets: Implications In Alcoholic Liver Disease. *Curr. Mol. Pharmacol.* **2017**, *10*, 237–248. [CrossRef] [PubMed]

3. McNamara, J.; Huber, K. Metabolic and Endocrine Role of Adipose Tissue During Lactation. *Annu. Rev. Anim. Biosci.* **2018**, *6*, 177–195. [CrossRef] [PubMed]
4. Tchkonia, T.; Thomou, T.; Zhu, Y.; Karagiannides, I.; Pothoulakis, C.; Jensen, M.D.; Kirkland, J.L. Mechanisms and metabolic implications of regional differences among fat depots. *Cell Metab.* **2013**, *17*, 644–656. [CrossRef] [PubMed]
5. Ibrahim, M.M. Subcutaneous and visceral adipose tissue: Structural and functional differences. *Obes. Rev.* **2010**, *11*, 11–18. [CrossRef]
6. Schoettl, T.; Fischer, I.P.; Ussar, S. Heterogeneity of adipose tissue in development and metabolic function. *J. Exp. Boil.* **2018**, *221*, jeb162958. [CrossRef]
7. Girousse, A.; Gil-Ortega, M.; Bourlier, V.; Bergeaud, C.; Sastourné-Arrey, Q.; Moro, C.; Barreau, C.; Guissard, C.; Vion, J.; Arnaud, E.; et al. The Release of Adipose Stromal Cells from Subcutaneous Adipose Tissue Regulates Ectopic Intramuscular Adipocyte Deposition. *Cell Rep.* **2019**, *27*, 323–333. [CrossRef]
8. Louwen, F.; Ritter, A.; Kreis, N.N.; Yuan, J. Insight into the development of obesity: Functional alterations of adipose-derived mesenchymal stem cells. *Obes. Rev.* **2018**, *19*, 888–904. [CrossRef]
9. Strong, A.L.; Burow, M.E.; Gimble, J.M.; Bunnell, B.A. Concise review: The obesity cancer paradigm: Exploration of the interactions and crosstalk with adipose stem cells. *Stem Cells* **2015**, *33*, 318–326. [CrossRef]
10. Patrikoski, M.; Mannerstrom, B.; Miettinen, S. Perspectives for Clinical Translation of Adipose Stromal/Stem Cells. *Stem Cells Int.* **2019**, *2019*, 5858247. [CrossRef]
11. Silva, K.R.; Baptista, L.S. Adipose-derived stromal/stem cells from different adipose depots in obesity development. *World J. Stem Cells* **2019**, *11*, 147–166. [CrossRef] [PubMed]
12. Si, Z.Z.; Wang, X.; Sun, C.H.; Kang, Y.C.; Xu, J.K.; Wang, X.D.; Hui, Y. Adipose-derived stem cells: Sources, potency, and implications for regenerative therapies. *Biomed. Pharm.* **2019**, *114*, 108765. [CrossRef] [PubMed]
13. Ritter, A.; Friemel, A.; Fornoff, F.; Adjan, M.; Solbach, C.; Yuan, J.; Louwen, F. Characterization of adipose-derived stem cells from subcutaneous and visceral adipose tissues and their function in breast cancer cells. *Oncotarget* **2015**, *6*, 34475–34493. [CrossRef] [PubMed]
14. Ritter, A.; Friemel, A.; Kreis, N.N.; Louwen, F.; Yuan, J. Impact of Polo-like kinase 1 inhibitors on human adipose tissue-derived mesenchymal stem cells. *Oncotarget* **2016**, *7*, 84271–84285. [CrossRef]
15. Ritter, A.; Friemel, A.; Kreis, N.N.; Hoock, S.C.; Roth, S.; Kielland-Kaisen, U.; Bruggmann, D.; Solbach, C.; Louwen, F.; Yuan, J. Primary Cilia Are Dysfunctional in Obese Adipose-Derived Mesenchymal Stem Cells. *Stem Cell Rep.* **2018**, *10*, 583–599. [CrossRef]
16. Ritter, A.; Kreis, N.N.; Roth, S.; Friemel, A.; Jennewein, L.; Eichbaum, C.; Solbach, C.; Louwen, F.; Yuan, J. Restoration of primary cilia in obese adipose-derived mesenchymal stem cells by inhibiting Aurora A or extracellular signal-regulated kinase. *Stem Cell Res. Ther.* **2019**, *10*, 255. [CrossRef]
17. Kreis, N.N.; Friemel, A.; Zimmer, B.; Roth, S.; Rieger, M.A.; Rolle, U.; Louwen, F.; Yuan, J.P. Mitotic p21(Cip1/CDKN1A) is regulated by cyclin-dependent kinase 1 phosphorylation. *Oncotarget* **2016**, *7*, 50215–50228. [CrossRef]
18. He, M.; Subramanian, R.; Bangs, F.; Omelchenko, T.; Liem, K.F., Jr.; Kapoor, T.M.; Anderson, K.V. The kinesin-4 protein Kif7 regulates mammalian Hedgehog signalling by organizing the cilium tip compartment. *Nat. Cell Biol.* **2014**, *16*, 663–672. [CrossRef]
19. Hoock, S.C.; Ritter, A.; Steinhauser, K.; Roth, S.; Behrends, C.; Oswald, F.; Solbach, C.; Louwen, F.; Kreis, N.N.; Yuan, J. RITA modulates cell migration and invasion by affecting focal adhesion dynamics. *Mol. Oncol.* **2019**, *13*, 2121–2141. [CrossRef]
20. Kreis, N.N.; Louwen, F.; Zimmer, B.; Yuan, J. Loss of p21Cip1/CDKN1A renders cancer cells susceptible to Polo-like kinase 1 inhibition. *Oncotarget* **2015**, *6*, 6611–6626. [CrossRef]
21. Muschol-Steinmetz, C.; Jasmer, B.; Kreis, N.N.; Steinhauser, K.; Ritter, A.; Rolle, U.; Yuan, J.; Louwen, F. B-cell lymphoma 6 promotes proliferation and survival of trophoblastic cells. *Cell Cycle* **2016**, *15*, 827–839. [CrossRef] [PubMed]
22. Steinhauser, K.; Kloble, P.; Kreis, N.N.; Ritter, A.; Friemel, A.; Roth, S.; Reichel, J.M.; Michaelis, J.; Rieger, M.A.; Louwen, F.; et al. Deficiency of RITA results in multiple mitotic defects by affecting microtubule dynamics. *Oncogene* **2017**, *36*, 2146–2159. [CrossRef] [PubMed]
23. Muschol-Steinmetz, C.; Friemel, A.; Kreis, N.N.; Reinhard, J.; Yuan, J.; Louwen, F. Function of survivin in trophoblastic cells of the placenta. *PLoS ONE* **2013**, *8*, e73337. [CrossRef] [PubMed]

24. Wu, J.; Ivanov, A.I.; Fisher, P.B.; Fu, Z. Polo-like kinase 1 induces epithelial-to-mesenchymal transition and promotes epithelial cell motility by activating CRAF/ERK signaling. *Elife* **2016**, *5*, e10734. [CrossRef]
25. Dominici, M.; Le Blanc, K.; Mueller, I.; Slaper-Cortenbach, I.; Marini, F.; Krause, D.; Deans, R.; Keating, A.; Prockop, D.; Horwitz, E. Minimal criteria for defining multipotent mesenchymal stromal cells. The International Society for Cellular Therapy position statement. *Cytotherapy* **2006**, *8*, 315–317. [CrossRef]
26. Mildmay-White, A.; Khan, W. Cell Surface Markers on Adipose-Derived Stem Cells: A Systematic Review. *Curr. Stem Cell Res. Ther.* **2017**, *12*, 484–492. [CrossRef]
27. De Becker, A.; Riet, I.V. Homing and migration of mesenchymal stromal cells: How to improve the efficacy of cell therapy? *World J. Stem Cells* **2016**, *8*, 73–87. [CrossRef]
28. Scioli, M.G.; Storti, G.; D'Amico, F.; Gentile, P.; Kim, B.S.; Cervelli, V.; Orlandi, A. Adipose-Derived Stem Cells in Cancer Progression: New Perspectives and Opportunities. *Int. J. Mol. Sci.* **2019**, *20*, 3296. [CrossRef]
29. Goodwin, J.M.; Svensson, R.U.; Lou, H.J.; Winslow, M.M.; Turk, B.E.; Shaw, R.J. An AMPK-independent signaling pathway downstream of the LKB1 tumor suppressor controls Snail1 and metastatic potential. *Mol. Cell* **2014**, *55*, 436–450. [CrossRef]
30. Mekhdjian, A.H.; Kai, F.B.; Rubashkin, M.G.; Prahl, L.S.; Przybyla, L.M.; McGregor, A.L.; Bell, E.S.; Barnes, J.M.; DuFort, C.C.; Ou, G.Q.; et al. Integrin-mediated traction force enhances paxillin molecular associations and adhesion dynamics that increase the invasiveness of tumor cells into a three-dimensional extracellular matrix. *Mol. Biol. Cell* **2017**, *28*, 1467–1488. [CrossRef]
31. Kim, D.H.; Wirtz, D. Focal Adhesion Size Uniquely Predicts Cell Migration. *Biophys. J.* **2013**, *104*, 319a. [CrossRef]
32. Le Devedec, S.E.; Geverts, B.; de Bont, H.; Yan, K.; Verbeek, F.J.; Houtsmuller, A.B.; van de Water, B. The residence time of focal adhesion kinase (FAK) and paxillin at focal adhesions in renal epithelial cells is determined by adhesion size, strength and life cycle status. *J. Cell Sci.* **2012**, *125*, 4498–4506. [CrossRef] [PubMed]
33. Ezratty, E.J.; Partridge, M.A.; Gundersen, G.G. Microtubule-induced focal adhesion disassembly is mediated by dynamin and focal adhesion kinase. *Nat. Cell Biol.* **2005**, *7*, 581. [CrossRef] [PubMed]
34. Hu, C.; Zhao, L.; Li, L. Current understanding of adipose-derived mesenchymal stem cell-based therapies in liver diseases. *Stem Cell Res. Ther.* **2019**, *10*, 199. [CrossRef]
35. Han, S.M.; Han, S.H.; Coh, Y.R.; Jang, G.; Chan Ra, J.; Kang, S.K.; Lee, H.W.; Youn, H.Y. Enhanced proliferation and differentiation of Oct4—And Sox2—Overexpressing human adipose tissue mesenchymal stem cells. *Exp. Mol. Med.* **2014**, *46*, e101. [CrossRef]
36. Park, S.B.; Seo, K.W.; So, A.Y.; Seo, M.S.; Yu, K.R.; Kang, S.K.; Kang, K.S. SOX2 has a crucial role in the lineage determination and proliferation of mesenchymal stem cells through Dickkopf-1 and c-MYC. *Cell Death Differ.* **2012**, *19*, 534–545. [CrossRef]
37. Malicki, J.J.; Johnson, C.A. The Cilium: Cellular Antenna and Central Processing Unit. *Trends Cell Biol.* **2017**, *27*, 126–140. [CrossRef]
38. Ritter, A.; Louwen, F.; Yuan, J. Deficient primary cilia in obese adipose-derived mesenchymal stem cells: Obesity, a secondary ciliopathy? *Obes. Rev.* **2018**, *19*, 1317–1328. [CrossRef]
39. Bodle, J.C.; Rubenstein, C.D.; Phillips, M.E.; Bernacki, S.H.; Qi, J.; Banes, A.J.; Loboa, E.G. Primary cilia: The chemical antenna regulating human adipose-derived stem cell osteogenesis. *PLoS ONE* **2013**, *8*, e62554. [CrossRef]
40. Pak, E.; Segal, R.A. Hedgehog Signal Transduction: Key Players, Oncogenic Drivers, and Cancer Therapy. *Dev. Cell* **2016**, *38*, 333–344. [CrossRef]
41. Jia, Y.; Wang, Y.; Xie, J. The Hedgehog pathway: Role in cell differentiation, polarity and proliferation. *Arch. Toxicol.* **2015**, *89*, 179–191. [CrossRef] [PubMed]
42. Briscoe, J.; Therond, P.P. The mechanisms of Hedgehog signalling and its roles in development and disease. *Nat. Rev. Mol. Cell Biol.* **2013**, *14*, 416–429. [CrossRef] [PubMed]
43. Dubey, N.K.; Mishra, V.K.; Dubey, R.; Deng, Y.-H.; Tsai, F.-C.; Deng, W.-P. Revisiting the Advances in Isolation, Characterization and Secretome of Adipose-Derived Stromal/Stem Cells. *Int. J. Mol. Sci.* **2018**, *19*, 2200. [CrossRef] [PubMed]
44. Sabol, R.A.; Bowles, A.C.; A.; Wise, R.; Pashos, N.; Bunnell, B.A. Therapeutic Potential of Adipose Stem Cells. In *Advances in Experimental Medicine and Biology*; Springer: New York, NY, USA, 2018; pp. 1–11. [CrossRef]

45. Hong, S.J.; Traktuev, D.O.; March, K.L. Therapeutic potential of adipose-derived stem cells in vascular growth and tissue repair. *Curr. Opin. Organ Transplant.* **2010**, *15*, 86–91. [CrossRef] [PubMed]
46. Toyoda, M.; Matsubara, Y.; Lin, K.; Sugimachi, K.; Furue, M. Characterization and comparison of adipose tissue-derived cells from human subcutaneous and omental adipose tissues. *Cell Biochem. Funct.* **2009**, *27*, 440–447. [CrossRef] [PubMed]
47. Tchkonia, T.; Tchoukalova, Y.D.; Giorgadze, N.; Pirtskhalava, T.; Karagiannides, I.; Forse, R.A.; Koo, A.; Stevenson, M.; Chinnappan, D.; Cartwright, A.; et al. Abundance of two human preadipocyte subtypes with distinct capacities for replication, adipogenesis, and apoptosis varies among fat depots. *Am. J. Physiol. Metab.* **2005**, *288*, E267–E277. [CrossRef] [PubMed]
48. Shahparaki, A.; Grunder, L.; Sorisky, A. Comparison of human abdominal subcutaneous versus omental preadipocyte differentiation in primary culture. *Metabolism* **2002**, *51*, 1211–1215. [CrossRef]
49. Baglioni, S.; Cantini, G.; Poli, G.; Francalanci, M.; Squecco, R.; Di Franco, A.; Borgogni, E.; Frontera, S.; Nesi, G.; Liotta, F.; et al. Functional differences in visceral and subcutaneous fat pads originate from differences in the adipose stem cell. *PLoS ONE* **2012**, *7*, e36569. [CrossRef]
50. Tang, Y.; Pan, Z.; Zou, Y.; He, Y.; Yang, P.; Tang, Q.-Q.; Yin, F. A comparative assessment of adipose-derived stem cells from subcutaneous and visceral fat as a potential cell source for knee osteoarthritis treatment. *J. Cell. Mol. Med.* **2017**, *21*, 2153–2162. [CrossRef]
51. Kim, B.; Lee, B.; Kim, M.-K.; Gong, S.P.; Park, N.H.; Chung, H.H.; Kim, H.S.; No, J.H.; Park, W.Y.; Park, A.K.; et al. Gene expression profiles of human subcutaneous and visceral adipose-derived stem cells. *Cell Biochem. Funct.* **2016**, *34*, 563–571. [CrossRef]
52. Macotela, Y.; Emanuelli, B.; Mori, M.A.; Gesta, S.; Schulz, T.J.; Tseng, Y.-H.; Kahn, C.R. Intrinsic Differences in Adipocyte Precursor Cells from Different White Fat Depots. *Diabetes* **2012**, *61*, 1691–1699. [CrossRef] [PubMed]
53. Ng, L.; Yip, S.; Wong, H.; Yam, G.H.; Liu, Y.; Lui, W.; Wang, C.; Choy, K. Adipose-derived stem cells from pregnant women show higher proliferation rate unrelated to estrogen. *Hum. Reprod.* **2009**, *24*, 1164–1170. [CrossRef] [PubMed]
54. Ullah, M.; Liu, D.D.; Thakor, A.S. Mesenchymal Stromal Cell Homing: Mechanisms and Strategies for Improvement. *iScience* **2019**, *15*, 421–438. [CrossRef] [PubMed]
55. Lamouille, S.; Xu, J.; Derynck, R. Molecular mechanisms of epithelial–mesenchymal transition. *Nat. Rev. Mol. Cell Boil.* **2014**, *15*, 178–196. [CrossRef] [PubMed]
56. Saunders, L.R.; McClay, D.R. Sub-circuits of a gene regulatory network control a developmental epithelial-mesenchymal transition. *Development* **2014**, *141*, 1503–1513. [CrossRef] [PubMed]
57. Campbell, K.; Casanova, J. A common framework for EMT and collective cell migration. *Development* **2016**, *143*, 4291–4300. [CrossRef] [PubMed]
58. Sieg, D.J.; Hauck, C.R.; Schlaepfer, D.D. Required role of focal adhesion kinase (FAK) for integrin-stimulated cell migration. *J. Cell Sci.* **1999**, *112*, 2677–2691.
59. Chau, Y.-Y.; Bandiera, R.; Serrels, A.; Martínez-Estrada, O.M.; Qing, W.; Lee, M.; Slight, J.; Thornburn, A.; Berry, R.; Mc Haffie, S.; et al. Visceral and subcutaneous fat have different origins and evidence supports a mesothelial source. *Nat. Cell Biol.* **2014**, *16*, 367–375. [CrossRef]
60. Silva, K.R.; Côrtes, I.; Liechocki, S.; Carneiro, J.R.I.; Souza, A.A.P.; Borojevic, R.; Maya-Monteiro, C.M.; Baptista, L.S. Characterization of stromal vascular fraction and adipose stem cells from subcutaneous, preperitoneal and visceral morbidly obese human adipose tissue depots. *PLoS ONE* **2017**, *12*, e0174115. [CrossRef]
61. Schweizer, R.; Tsuji, W.; Gorantla, V.S.; Marra, K.G.; Rubin, J.P.; Plock, J.A. The Role of Adipose-Derived Stem Cells in Breast Cancer Progression and Metastasis. *Stem Cells Int.* **2015**, *17*. [CrossRef]
62. Pitrone, M.; Pizzolanti, G.; Coppola, A.; Tomasello, L.; Martorana, S.; Pantuso, G.; Giordano, C. Knockdown of NANOG Reduces Cell Proliferation and Induces G0/G1 Cell Cycle Arrest in Human Adipose Stem Cells. *Int. J. Mol. Sci.* **2019**, *20*, 2580. [CrossRef] [PubMed]
63. Deisenroth, C.; Black, M.B.; Pendse, S.; Pluta, L.; Witherspoon, S.M.; McMullen, P.D.; Thomas, R.S. MYC Is an Early Response Regulator of Human Adipogenesis in Adipose Stem Cells. *PLoS ONE* **2014**, *9*, e114133. [CrossRef] [PubMed]

64. Joe, A.W.; Yi, L.; Even, Y.; Vogl, A.W.; Rossi, F.M. Depot-specific differences in adipogenic progenitor abundance and proliferative response to high-fat diet. *Stem Cells* **2009**, *27*, 2563–2570. [CrossRef] [PubMed]
65. Jones, T.J.; Adapala, R.K.; Geldenhuys, W.J.; Bursley, C.; Aboualaiwi, W.A.; Nauli, S.M.; Thodeti, C.K. Primary Cilia Regulates the Directional Migration and Barrier Integrity of Endothelial Cells Through the Modulation of Hsp27 Dependent Actin Cytoskeletal Organization. *J. Cell Physiol.* **2012**, *227*, 70–76. [CrossRef] [PubMed]

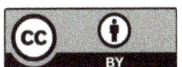

© 2019 by the authors. Licensee MDPI, Basel, Switzerland. This article is an open access article distributed under the terms and conditions of the Creative Commons Attribution (CC BY) license (http://creativecommons.org/licenses/by/4.0/).

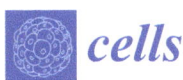

Article

Stem Cells Derived from Lipoma and Adipose Tissue—Similar Mesenchymal Phenotype but Different Differentiation Capacity Governed by Distinct Molecular Signature

Sanja Stojanović [1,*], Stevo Najman [1] and Aleksandra Korać [2]

1 Department of Biology and Human Genetics and Department for Cell and Tissue Engineering, Faculty of Medicine, University of Niš, 18000 Niš, Serbia; stevo.najman@medfak.ni.ac.rs
2 Faculty of Biology, University of Belgrade, 11000 Belgrade, Serbia; aleksandra.korac@bio.bg.ac.rs
* Correspondence: s.sanja88@gmail.com or sanja.stojanovic@medfak.ni.ac.rs; Tel.: +38-11-8422-6644 (ext. 126)

Received: 28 October 2018; Accepted: 6 December 2018; Published: 8 December 2018

Abstract: Lipomas are benign adipose tissue tumors of unknown etiology, which can vary in size, number, body localization and cell populations within the tissue. Lipoma-derived stem cells (LDSCs) are proposed as a potential tool in regenerative medicine and tissue engineering due to their similar characteristics with adipose-derived stem cells (ADSCs) reported so far. Our study is among the first giving detailed insights into the molecular signature and differences in the differentiation capacity of LDSCs in vitro compared to ADSCs. Mesenchymal stem cell phenotype was analyzed by gene expression and flow cytometric analysis of stem cell markers. Adipogenesis and osteogenesis were analyzed by microscopic analysis, cytochemical and immunocytochemical staining, gene and protein expression analyses. We showed that both LDSCs and ADSCs were mesenchymal stem cells with similar phenotype and stemness state but different molecular basis for potential differentiation. Adipogenesis-related genes expression pattern and presence of more mature adipocytes in ADSCs than in LDSCs after 21 days of adipogenic differentiation, indicated that differentiation capacity of LDSCs was significantly lower compared to ADSCs. Analysis of osteogenesis-related markers after 16 days of osteogenic differentiation revealed that both types of cells had characteristic osteoblast-like phenotype, but were at different stages of osteogenesis. Differences observed between LDSCs and ADSCs are probably due to the distinct molecular signature and their commitment in the tissue that governs their different capacity and fate during adipogenic and osteogenic induction in vitro despite their similar mesenchymal phenotype.

Keywords: lipomas; adipose tissue; stem cells; adipogenesis; osteogenesis

1. Introduction

Adipose-derived stem cells (ADSCs) are adult mesenchymal stem cells (MSCs) originated from adipose tissue that show a great morphological and functional similarity with MSCs from bone marrow but with additional advantages [1]. ADSCs can be isolated from abundant and easily accessible adipose tissue in large quantities with a minimal invasive procedure either from liposuction aspirates or adipose tissue biopsies [2] and have properties that make them good candidates for regenerative medicine applications [3]. The use of ADSCs in tissue engineering and regenerative medicine is very promising due to their self-renewal potential, proliferation capacity and great potential to differentiate into numerous cell types particularly adipocytes, osteoblasts, chondrocytes and endothelial cells [4–7]. It is reported that ADSCs can be successfully differentiated into the cells of all three germ lines which means that they can be considered as pluripotent and makes them a good candidate for wide range applications in the field of biomedical sciences [4].

Lipomas are benign tumors of adipose tissue and represent one of the most common soft tissue neoplasms of mesenchymal origin [8,9]. Lipomas can be solitary, multiple generalized lipomatosis and multiple symmetric, usually slowly growing, diffused or encapsulated, can vary in size and shape and show great heterogeneity in cell populations presented within the tissue [10,11]. The occurrence of lipomas in all body parts has been reported, mostly in subcutaneous depots but also in other tissues, organs and body cavities. Both male and female can be affected and all ages although they usually appear in the middle age [9,12]. Several studies reported that lipoma tissue is a good source of stem cells that might be used for regenerative medicine purposes, naming lipoma "useless tissue useful in the application of regenerative medicine and tissue engineering" [13]. Isolation and characterization of MSCs from lipoma, so called lipoma-derived stem cells (LDSCs) was reported and it has been shown that those cells are very similar to ones isolated from normal adipose tissue [14]. It has been shown that LDSCs can proliferate in a similar manner as ADSCs, express characteristic mesenchymal stem cell markers and can differentiate into adipocytes, osteoblasts and chondrocytes like ADSCs [13,15,16]. There are, however, only few publications and studies that dealt with some of the LDSCs properties. In almost all publications authors showed that LDSCs have the same potential to differentiate into osteoblasts and adipocytes as ADSCs with very few reports on different proliferation potential and characteristics of LDSCs compared to ADSCs [17]. Also, there are reports about formation of bone and cartilaginous structures within lipoma tissue and its ossification in various parts of the body [18], with considerations that stem cells from lipoma tissue may be responsible for those processes [19].

Bearing in mind that lipomas are adipose tissue tumors with insufficiently clarified etiology and pathogenesis, and that transformations of lipoma tissue into hard tissue structures can occur, which implies the role of LDSCs, as well as potential use of LDSCs in regenerative purposes reported so far and lack of detailed comparison with ADSCs; the request and the need for further investigation on molecular and cellular features of LDSCs arises, as potential cause of lipoma formation and their possible application in regenerative medicine, as well as detailed comparison with ADSCs from normal adipose tissue. To the best of our knowledge, our study is among the first giving detailed insights into the molecular signature of LDSCs, with the first data on adipogenic- and osteogenic-related markers' expression and comparison with ADSCs, as well as showing that LDSCs and ADSCs have different characteristics particularly in the differentiation capacity in vitro. Here we presented the cellular and molecular features and comparison of those two types of MSCs with special emphasis on adipogenic and osteogenic differentiation capacity.

2. Materials and Methods

2.1. Patients

Lipoma tissue samples were obtained at surgical clinics of the Clinical Center Niš, Serbia after surgical removal of solitary subcutaneous lipomas that were clinically and pathologically diagnosed as lipoma and distinguished from other adipose tissue neoplasms. Subcutaneous adipose tissue samples were obtained from non-cancer patients during other surgeries. All patients gave their informed written consent and the study was approved by the Local Ethical Committee of the Faculty of Medicine, University of Niš, Serbia (approvals no. 01-6481-15 and 12-6316-2/4). Tissue sample biopsies from 14 patients were analyzed, among them 8 lipomas and 6 normal adipose tissue samples. Average age of patients with lipoma was 48.3 ± 8.3 while average age of non-lipoma patients was 49.5 ± 11.1. In the group of patients with lipoma, 5 were female and 3 were male, while in the non-lipoma group of patients 4 were female and 2 were male. Lipomas and adipose tissue samples were taken from several subcutaneous body depots: upper arm, back, neck, abdomen, hip and thigh. Body mass index (BMI) for all patients was less than 30, indicated non-obese patients.

2.2. Isolation and Cultivation of Mesenchymal Stem Cells

Both lipoma-derived stem cells (LDSCs) and adipose-derived stem cells (ADSCs) were isolated by enzymatic digestion of tissue samples, respectively. Tissue samples were washed, cut into small pieces and placed in 0.1% collagenase type I solution (StemCell Technologies, Vancouver, CO, Canada), in a water bath at 37 °C for 45 min. Tissue homogenates were then vortex and filtered and cell culture media was added to stop collagenase. Stromal vascular fraction (SVF) of cells was obtained by centrifugation for 15 min at 1500 rpm, collected from the bottom of the tube and seeded in 25 cm^2 cell culture flask (Greiner Bio One, Kremsmünster, Austria) in standard cell culture medium (DM) that contained Dulbecco's Modified Eagle's medium (DMEM), 10% fetal bovine serum (FBS), 2 mM stable glutamine and 1% antibiotic-antimycotic solution (all purchased from Capricorn Scientific, Ebsdorfergrund, Germany). Cells were washed and media was changed 16–18 h after isolation to remove non-attached cells. After reaching the 70–80% confluency, first cell passage was performed (P1), which enabled purification of mesenchymal stem cells. Cells were cultured in standard cell culture conditions which mean temperature of 37 °C and humidified atmosphere with the presence of 5% CO_2. Medium was changed every three days.

2.3. Differentiation of Cells

For differentiation assays, cells at passage 2 (P2) were used. Cells were passaged by using 0.25 U/mL dispase in DMEM/F-12 (StemCell Technologies, Vancouver, CO, Canada) and 0.05% trypsin-EDTA solution (Capricorn Scientific, Ebsdorfergrund, Germany), centrifuged and cell number was determined by Trypan blue dye exclusion assay on Countess™ automated cell counter (Thermo Scientific, Waltham, MA, USA). For adipogenic differentiation assay, 5000 cells per cm^2 were seeded onto sterile glass coverslips in 24-well culture plates (Greiner Bio One, Kremsmünster, Austria) and left to attach overnight. Medium in which cells were seeded was then replaced with adipocyte differentiation media (AM) which was purchased from Gibco® (Carlsbad, CA, USA), (StemPro™ Adipogenesis Differentiation Kit) or standard cell culture media (DM). Cells were cultured in AM and DM media up to 21 days. Media were changed every 3 to 4 days. For osteogenic differentiation assay, 3000 cells per cm^2 were seeded onto sterile glass coverslips in 24-well culture plates and left to attach overnight. Medium in which cells were seeded was then replaced with osteogenic differentiation media (OS) or standard cell culture media (DM). Osteogenic differentiation media was prepared by adding 0.1 µM of dexamethasone (D4902, Sigma, St. Louis, MO, USA), 50 µM L-ascorbic acid 2-phosphate (49752, Sigma) and 2 mM β-Glycerophosphate (AppliChem, Darmstadt, Germany) to the DM medium. Cells were cultured in OS and DM media up to 16 days. Media were changed every 3 to 4 days in both assays and cells were cultured in standard cell culture conditions.

2.4. Light Microscopy

Cells after isolation, during differentiation studies and after staining were monitored on inverted light microscope (Observer Z1, Carl Zeiss, Oberkochen, Germany), under phase contrast and bright field. The images were acquired using the camera AxioCam HR (Carl Zeiss, Germany) and the software ZEN 2 blue edition (Carl Zeiss, Germany).

2.5. Flow Cytometry

Expression of mesenchymal stem cell surface marker CD105 was analyzed on both LDSCs and ADSCs, respectively, at P2 (before differentiation assays). After trypsinization, centrifugation and washing, cells were stained for 15 min with PE conjugated monoclonal mouse anti-CD105 human antibody (Clone 43A4E1, Miltenyi Biotec, Bergisch Gladbach, Germany) at 4 °C. After washing steps, cells were re-suspended in a buffer and analyzed on BD LSRFortessa™ cell analyzer with BD FACSDiva™ software v8 (BD Biosciences, Heidelberg, Germany). A total of minimum 100,000 cells were usually acquired for each sample.

2.6. RNA Isolation and Reverse Transcription

LDSCs and ADSCs at passage 2 (day 0 in differentiation assay), at day 21 in adipogenic differentiation assay and days 8 and 16 in osteogenic differentiation assay were placed in RNAlater® (Ambion, Life Technologies, Carlsbad, CA, USA) and stored at −80°C until RNA purification step. The total RNA was isolated from the cells using RNeasy Mini Kit (Qiagen, Venlo, The Netherlands) according to the manufacturer's instructions. DNase I RNase-free set (Qiagen) was used for on-column digestion of residual genomic DNA, according to the manufacturer's instructions. The RNA concentration was determined immediately after isolation using Qubit™ RNA HS Assay Kit (Thermo Scientific, Waltham, MA, USA) on Qubit® 2.0 fluorimeter (Invitrogen, Thermo Scientific, Waltham, MA, USA), according to the manufacturer's instructions. Total RNA was reversely transcribed into single-stranded cDNA using High-capacity cDNA Reverse Transcription Kit (Applied Biosystems®, Foster City, CA, USA), according to the manufacturer's instructions, with 100 ng per reaction per sample. Reverse transcription was performed in the PCR thermal cycler SureCycler8800 (Agilent Technologies, Santa Clara, CA, USA). The protocol conditions were: 10 min at 25 °C, 120 min at 37 °C, 5 min at 85°C and cooling at 4 °C. The synthesized cDNA was stored at −80 °C and was later used as a template for qPCR to determine the relative gene expression.

2.7. Real Time PCR

Quantitative real time PCR reactions were performed by real time thermal cycler Stratagene Mx3005P (Agilent Technologies, Santa Clara, CA, USA). The qPCR reactions were prepared by using SYBR Fast Universal 2x qPCR Master Mix (Kapa Biosystems, Wilmington, MA, USA), according to the manufacturer's instruction. ROX was used as a reference dye. Pre-designed primer sets (QuantiTect primer assay kits) were purchased from Qiagen, The Netherlands. Primer kits, consisted of both forward and reverse primers, were used for the following genes: *GAPDH* (QT00079247), *CD44* (QT00073549), *POU5F1* (QT00210840), *BGLAP* (QT00232771), *RUNX2* (QT00998102), *DLK1* (QT00093128), *PPARG* (QT00029841), *LEP* (QT00030261), and *ADIPOQ* (QT00014091). The protocol conditions were: (1) enzyme activation: 3 min at 95 °C (1 cycle); (2) denaturation: 3 s at 95 °C and annealing/extension (with data acquisition): 30 s at 60 °C (40 cycles). The specific binding of primers was confirmed by melting curve analysis and specific length product visualization on electrophoresis gel. The expression level of each target gene was normalized to the glyceraldehyde-3-phosphate dehydrogenase housekeeping gene expression (*GAPDH*) in the same sample. The relative gene expression data analysis was performed by the relative quantification method $2^{-\Delta\Delta Ct}$ as described by Livak and Schmittgen [20]. Human XpressRef Universal Total RNA (338112, Qiagen) was used as calibrator for all qPCR reactions.

2.8. Oil Red O Staining

To assess the mature adipocytes' formation after 21 days of adipogenic differentiation, the presence of lipid droplets was analyzed by Oil Red O staining. LDSCs and ADSCs cells were fixed in 10% neutral buffered formalin (NBF), washed, incubated for 3 min in 60% isopropanol and then Oil Red O solution was applied for 15 min. After washing, cells were counterstained with Mayer's hematoxylin (Bio-Optica, Milan, Italy) for 1 min and imaged. Quantification of lipid droplets was performed by dissolving the Oil red O dye in 100% isopropanol and measuring absorbance at 450 nm on multichannel spectrophotometer (Multiskan Ascent plate reader, ThermoLab Systems, Helsinki, Finland).

2.9. Cytochemical Staining for Calcium Deposits

For the detection of calcium deposits in cells underwent osteogenic differentiation, Alizarin red S (ARS) and Von Kossa staining was performed. After 16 days of osteogenic differentiation, LDSCs and ADSCs were fixed in 10% NBF. Alizarin red S (A5533, Sigma-Aldrich, St. Louis, MO, USA) staining solution at concentration 2% was applied to the cells and incubated for 45 min at room temperature

(RT) in the dark. Cells were then washed and analyzed under the microscope. Quantification of inorganic deposits was performed by dissolving ARS in 10% acetic acid solution and absorbance measurement at 405 nm on plate reader. For Von Kossa staining, 2% silver nitrate solution was applied to the fixed cells and exposed to the UV light for 30 min at RT. After washing cells were treated with 5% sodium thiosulfate solution for 5 min at RT, counterstained with Nuclear Fast Red Solution (N069.1, Carl Roth, Karlsruhe, Germany) for 5 min and mounted with DPX mounting medium (06522, Sigma).

2.10. Immunocytochemistry

Immunoexpression of adiponectin in LDSCs and ADSCs differentiated for 21 day toward adipocytes was analyzed by immunocytochemical staining. Cells were fixed in 10% NBF for 15 min, washed and endogenous peroxide and protein block were applied. Anti-adiponectin antibody ([19F1], ab22554, Abcam, Cambridge, UK) was applied on cells at dilution 1:400 and incubated over night at +4 °C. For visualization, rabbit specific HRP/DAB (ABC) detection IHC kit (ab64261, Abcam, Cambridge, UK) was used according to the manufacturer's protocol. Cells were counterstained with Mayer's hematoxylin and mounted with VectaMount Permanent Mounting Medium (Vector Laboratories, Peterborough, UK).

2.11. ELISA Assays

Measurement of secretion products in cell culture media of LDSCs and ADSCs differentiated into adipocytes and osteoblasts was performed by ELISA assays. Level of osteoprotegerin, as osteoblast marker, was analyzed at day 16 of osteogenic differentiation while level of leptin, as mature adipocyte marker, was analyzed at day 21 of adipogenic differentiation in cell culture supernatant. Both leptin and osteoprotegerin measurements were performed using 72 h conditioned media. Human Osteoprotegerin ELISA Kit (ab100617) was purchased from Abcam, UK while Human Leptin Quantikine ELISA Kit (DLP00) was purchased from RnD systems (Minneapolis, MN, USA). Both ELISAs were performed according to the manufacturer's instructions, respectively. Values are expressed as pg of leptin or osteoprotegerin per ml.

2.12. Statistical Analysis

Results of real time PCR analyses and ELISA assays are presented as scatterplots with median using the templates published by Weissgerber et al. [21]. All the results are statistically processed and for all samples median as well as mean values were calculated. Mean values are presented with standard deviation (SD). Data were analyzed by one-way ANOVA or Mann–Whitney U-test to compare and determine statistically significant differences between the samples. The value of $p < 0.05$ was considered as significant.

3. Results

3.1. Analysis of Mesenchymal Stem Cell Phenotype

In Figure 1 the morphology of LDSCs (a,b) and ADSCs (c,d) is presented. There were no differences in morphology between LDSCs and ADSCs either at day 3 after isolation (Figure 1a,c) or at passage 1 day 4 (Figure 1b,d).

Flow cytometric analysis (Figure 2a–d) showed high expression of surface stem cell marker CD105 in both LDSCs (Figure 2a) and ADSCs (Figure 2c) at passage 2, just before differentiation assays. Non-specific antibody binding was excluded by using isotype control (Figure 2b,d).

Real time PCR analysis of *CD44* and *POU5F1* stem cell markers' expression (Figure 2e,f) confirmed that both LDSCs and ADSCs express these genes at passage 2. Slightly higher expression of *CD44* in ADSCs compared to LDSCs (Figure 2e) was not statistically significant ($p = 0.1$).

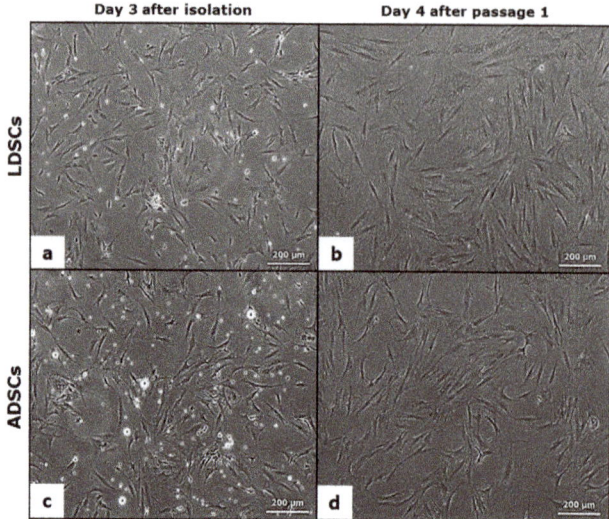

Figure 1. Morphology of lipoma-derived stem cells (LDSCs) (**a,b**) and adipose-derived stem cells (ADSCs) (**c,d**) cultures; Images were acquired at day 3 after isolation (**a,c**) and at day 4 after passage 1 (**b,d**); phase contrast with objective magnification 10×; cells are spindle-like in shape which is typical for mesenchymal stem cells.

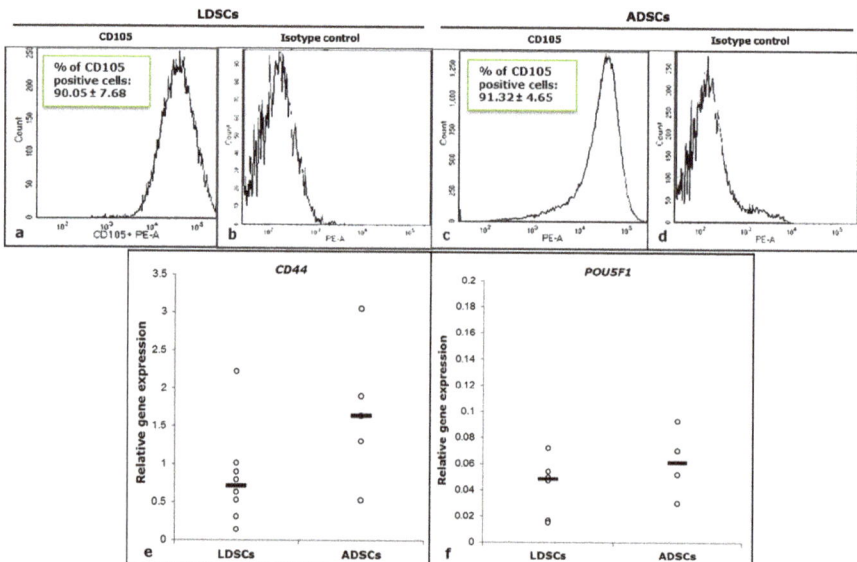

Figure 2. Flow cytometric analysis of CD105 cell surface marker expression in LDSCs (**a**) and ADSCs (**c**) at passage 2 (representative histograms per each group of samples with % of CD105 positive cells presented as mean ± SD, n (LDSCs) = 6 and n (ADSCs) = 4); corresponding isotype controls (**b,d**); Relative expression of *CD44* (**e**) and *POU5F1* (**f**) genes in LDSCs and ADSCs at passage 2 (day 0 in differentiation assays), normalized to *GAPDH*, presented as scatterplots with median; sample size for *CD44*: n (LDSCs) = 8 and n (ADSCs) = 5, for *POU5F1*: n (LDSCs) = 6 and n (ADSCs) = 4.

We also analyzed expression levels of genes characteristically expressed during osteogenesis (*RUNX2* and *BGLAP*) and adipogenesis (*ADIPOQ, LEP, PPARG* and *DLK1*) in cells at passage 2, day 0 in differentiation studies (Figure 3). Differences in expression levels of all examined genes were noticed between LDSCs and ADSCs, but statistically significant only for *RUNX2* and *BGLAP*. *RUNX2* expression was higher in LDSCs compared to ADSCs while *BGLAP* expression was higher in ADSCs compared to LDSCs ($p < 0.05$).

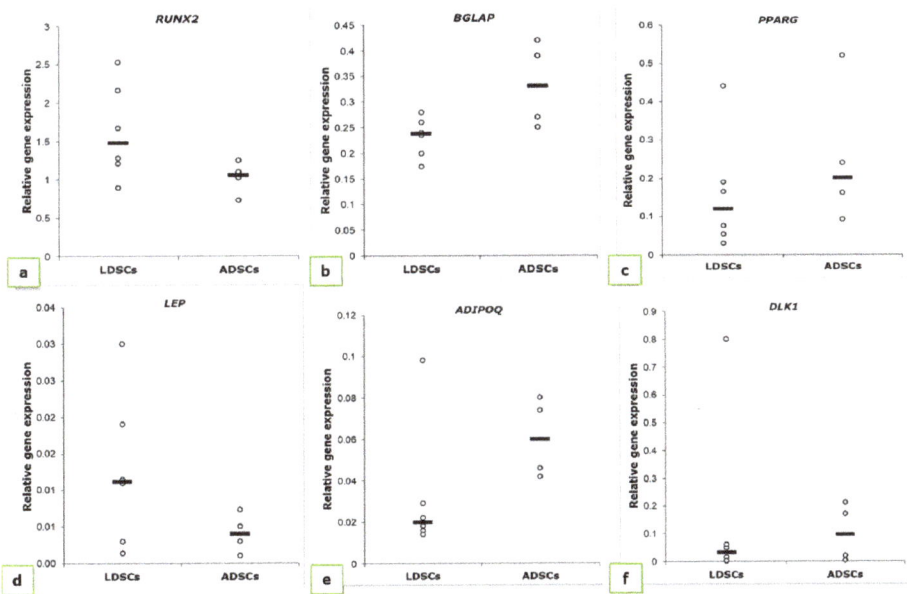

Figure 3. Relative expression of *RUNX2* (**a**), *BGLAP* (**b**), *PPARG* (**c**), *LEP* (**d**), *ADIPOQ* (**e**) and *DLK1* (**f**) genes in LDSCs and ADSCs at passage 2 (day 0 in differentiation assays), normalized to *GAPDH*; significant difference between cells was noticed for *RUNX2* and *BGLAP* expression ($p < 0.05$); scatterplots with median; n (LDSCs) = 6 and n (ADSCs) = 4 for all genes.

3.2. Adipogenic Differentiation

Adipogenic differentiation of both LDSCs and ADSCs was analyzed after 21 days of cultivation in adipogenic medium (AM). As control, cells were cultivated in standard medium (DM) under the same conditions. Characteristic adipocyte-like phenotype and the presence of lipid droplets were noticed in both LDSCs (Figure 4a,b) and ADSCs (Figure 4e,f) after 21 days of differentiation. However, lipid droplets were noticeably significantly more present in the ADSCs (Figure 4e,f) compared to LDSCs (Figure 4a,b) which indicates higher adipogenic potential of ADSCs compared to LDSCs. Further, changes in the morphology, from mesenchymal to epithelial-like, characteristic for adipocytes, were noticed in both ADSCs and LDSCs culture. Cells cultivated in medium DM retained their mesenchymal-like and fibroblastic-like shape, very similar in both LDSCs (Figure 4c,d) and ADSCs (Figure 4g,h).

After 21 days of adipogenic differentiation, presence of lipids was confirmed by Oil red O staining (Figure 5). Significantly more lipids were accumulated in ADSCs culture (Figure 5e,f) than LDSCs culture (Figure 5a,b), as confirmed by quantification of Oil red O dye (Figure 5i), indicating higher adipogenic differentiation potential of ADSCs. This was confirmed by adiponectin immunostaining after 21 days of adipogenic differentiation of ADSCs and LDSCs (Figure 6). Although both ADSCs and LDSCs were positive for adiponectin, much stronger staining was observed in ADSCs (Figure 6a,c).

Neither LDSCs nor ADSCs cultivated in DM medium were positive for adiponectin excluding possibility of spontaneous adipogenesis (Figure 6b,d). Non-specific staining was not present, indicated by control staining omitting primary antibody (Figure 6e,f).

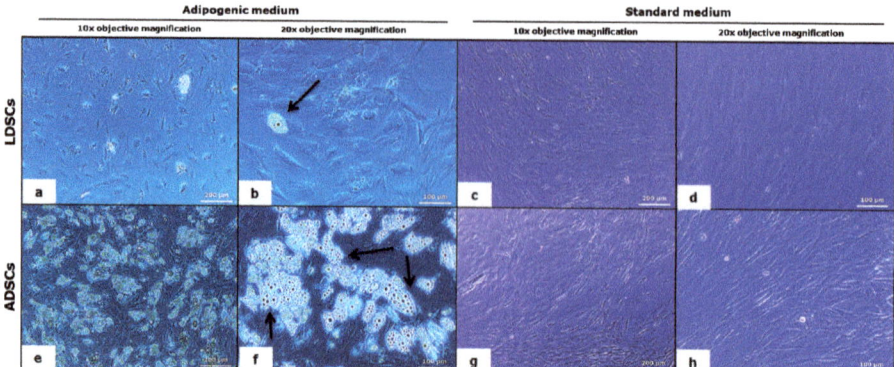

Figure 4. Light microscopic analysis of adipocytes' formation after 21 day of adipogenic differentiation; LDSCs in adipogenic medium (AM) (**a**,**b**), LDSCs in standard medium (DM) (**c**,**d**), ADSCs in AM medium (**e**,**f**) and ADSCs in DM medium (**g**,**h**); phase contrast with objective magnification 10× (**a**,**c**,**e**,**g**) and 20× (**b**,**d**,**f**,**h**); arrows indicate mature adipocytes.

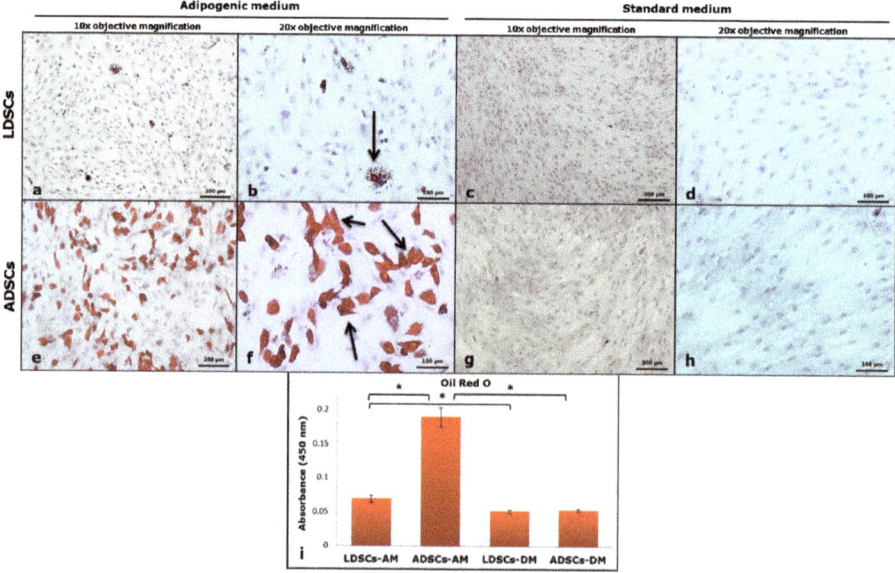

Figure 5. Oil red O staining of cells after 21 day of adipogenic differentiation; LDSCs in adipogenic medium (AM) (**a**,**b**), LDSCs in standard medium (DM) (**c**,**d**), ADSCs in AM medium (**e**,**f**) and ADSCs in DM medium (**g**,**h**); bright field with objective magnification 10× (**a**,**c**,**e**,**g**) and 20× (**b**,**d**,**f**,**h**); arrows indicate accumulation of lipids in cells; quantitative measurement of Oil red O dye (**i**), presented as mean ± SD, n = 4 for all groups; (*) $p < 0.05$.

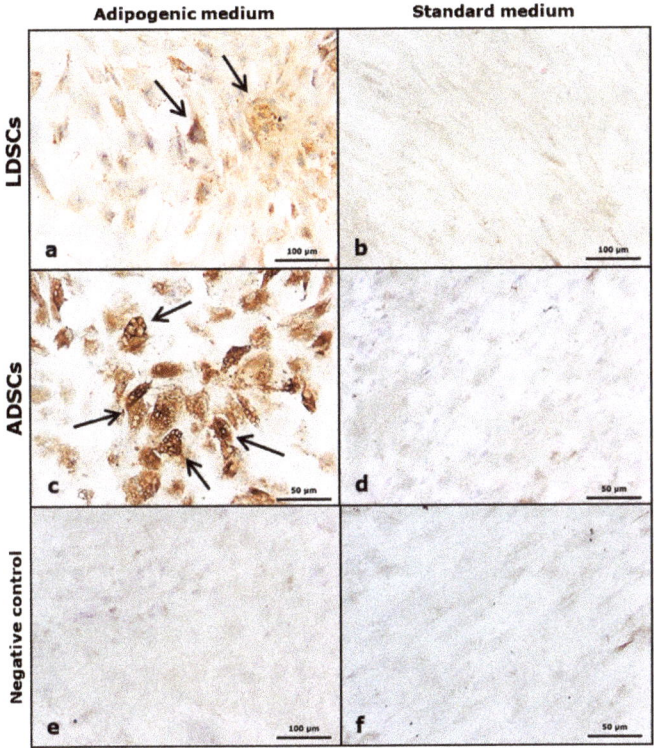

Figure 6. Immunoexpression of adiponectin in cells after 21 day of adipogenic differentiation; LDSCs in adipogenic medium (AM) (**a**), LDSCs in standard medium (DM) (**b**), ADSCs in AM medium (**c**) and ADSCs in DM medium (**d**); cells stained without primary antibody (non-specific background staining control – negative control) in AM medium (**e**) and in DM medium (**f**); bright field with objective magnification 20×; arrows indicate positive adiponectin immunostaining (brown).

After 21 days of adipogenic differentiation, leptin concentration was measured in cell culture supernatant, by ELISA assay (Figure 7). Significantly higher concentration of leptin was observed in ADSCs in AM than in DM medium ($p < 0.05$), but no significant difference in leptin secretion was observed in LDSCs during differentiation. Leptin concentration was higher, but not statistically significant, in ADSCs than in LDSCs cultured in AM medium.

We performed quantitative real time PCR to determine the expression levels of adipogenesis-related genes: adiponectin (*ADIPOQ*), leptin (*LEP*), PPAR-gamma (*PPARG*) and Pref-1 (*DLK1*), after 21 days of adipogenic differentiation (Figure 8, Table 1). As expected, expression of mature adipocytes' markers *ADIPOQ*, *LEP* and *PPARG* increased in differentiated ADSCs (Figure 8a–c; Table 1) statistically significant ($p < 0.05$) while expression of *DLK1*, characteristic marker of pre-adipocytes, decreased (Figure 8d; Table 1). Expression levels of *ADIPOQ* and *LEP* slightly increased in LDSCs during differentiation ($p < 0.05$ only for *ADIPOQ*), but at much lower extent than in ADSCs. No significant changes in *PPARG* expression were observed in LDSCs (Figure 8c; Table 1) while *DLK1* expression significantly increased in LDSCs during differentiation (Figure 8d; Table 1). Cells cultivated in DM media did not show significant increase in adipogenic genes expression (Figure 8, Table 1).

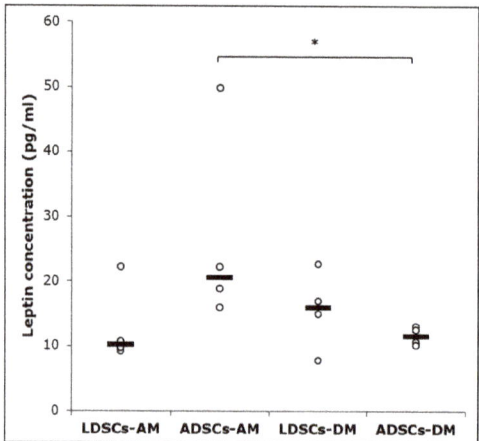

Figure 7. Leptin concentration in cell culture supernatant of LDSCs and ADSCs measured by ELISA at day 21 of adipogenic differentiation; scatterplots with median; n = 4 for all groups; (*) $p < 0.05$.

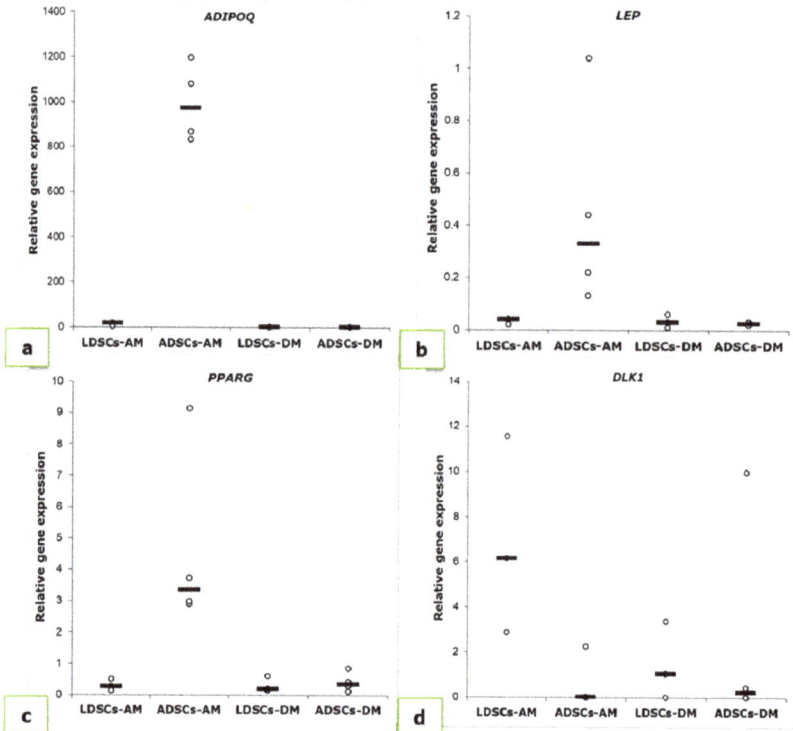

Figure 8. Relative expression levels ($2^{-\Delta\Delta Ct}$) of genes for adiponectin (*ADIPOQ*) (**a**), leptin (*LEP*) (**b**), PPAR-gamma (*PPARG*) (**c**) and Pref-1 (*DLK1*) (**d**), measured in LDSCs and ADSCs at day 21 of adipogenic differentiation and normalized to *GAPDH*; scatterplots with median; n = 4 for all groups and genes.

Table 1. Relative expression of *ADIPOQ*, *LEP*, *PPARG* and *DLK1* in LDSCs and ADSCs at day 21 of adipogenic differentiation, normalized to *GAPDH* and compared to the cells at P2 (day 0). Results are expressed as mean values ± SD. Asterisks represent statistical significance compared to P2 (day 0).

Cell Type	*ADIPOQ*			*LEP*		
	P2 (Day 0)	21 Day		P2 (Day 0)	21 Day	
		AM	DM		AM	DM
LDSCs	0.033 ± 0.033	12.530 ± 7.31 *	0.400 ± 0.35	0.0130 ± 0.011	0.03 ± 0.012 *	0.030 ± 0.025
ADSCs	0.061 ± 0.019	993.84 ± 174.09 ***	0.515 ± 0.45	0.0041 ± 0.003	0.46 ± 0.41 ***	0.025 ± 0.006 **
	PPARG			*DLK1*		
	P2 (Day 0)	21 Day		P2 (Day 0)	21 Day	
		AM	DM		AM	DM
LDSCs	0.159 ± 0.151	0.30 ± 0.187	0.32 ± 0.247	0.32 ± 0.725	6.86 ± 4.38 *	1.50 ± 1.73
ADSCs	0.250 ± 0.188	4.92 ± 3.50 *	0.42 ± 0.315	0.10 ± 0.105	0.57 ± 1.13	2.61 ± 4.92

* $p < 0.05$, ** $p < 0.01$, *** $p < 0.001$.

3.3. Osteogenic Differentiation

Osteogenic differentiation of both LDSCs and ADSCs was analyzed after 8 and 16 days of cultivation of cells in OS medium. As control, cells were cultivated in medium DM under the same conditions. Characteristic osteoblast-like phenotype and accumulation of inorganic material were noticed at day 16 in both LDSCs and ADSCs cultured in OS medium, as observed by light microscopy (Figure 9a,c). The cells cultivated in medium DM retained their mesenchymal-like and fibroblastic-like shape, very similar in both LDSCs (Figure 9b) and ADSCs (Figure 9d).

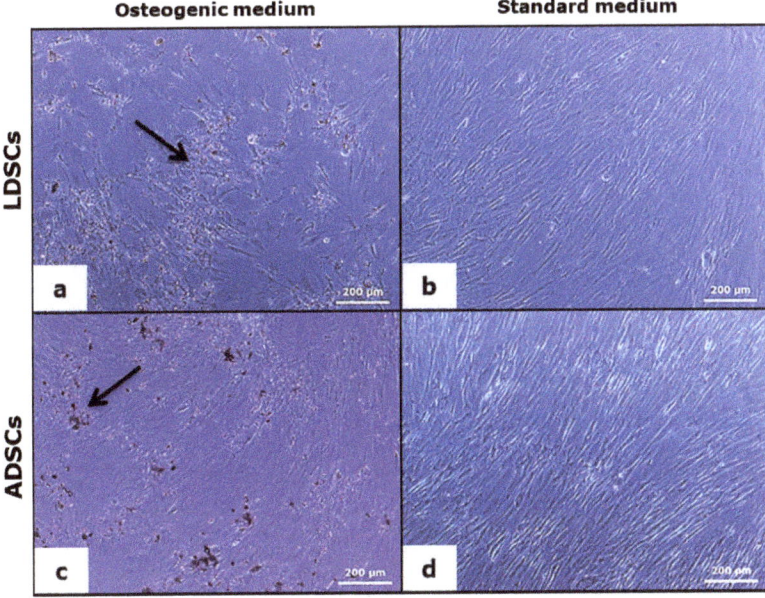

Figure 9. Light microscopic analysis of osteoblasts' formation after 16 days of osteogenic differentiation; LDSCs in osteogenic medium (OS) (**a**) LDSCs in standard medium (DM) (**b**) ADSCs in OS medium (**c**) and ADSCs in DM medium (**d**); phase contrast with objective magnification 10×; arrows indicate inorganic material deposition.

Inorganic deposits were stained by Von Kossa and Alizarin red S staining methods (Figure 10). Dark grey/black deposits in LDSCs (Figure 10a) and ADSCs (Figure 10e), indicating positive Von Kossa staining, and red colored deposits, indicating positive ARS staining, in LDSCs (Figure 10c) and ADSCs (Figure 10g) were noticed after 16 days in OS media. No colored deposits were observed in DM media neither in LDSCs nor ADSCs, after Von Kossa (Figure 10b,f) and ARS staining (Figure 10d,h).

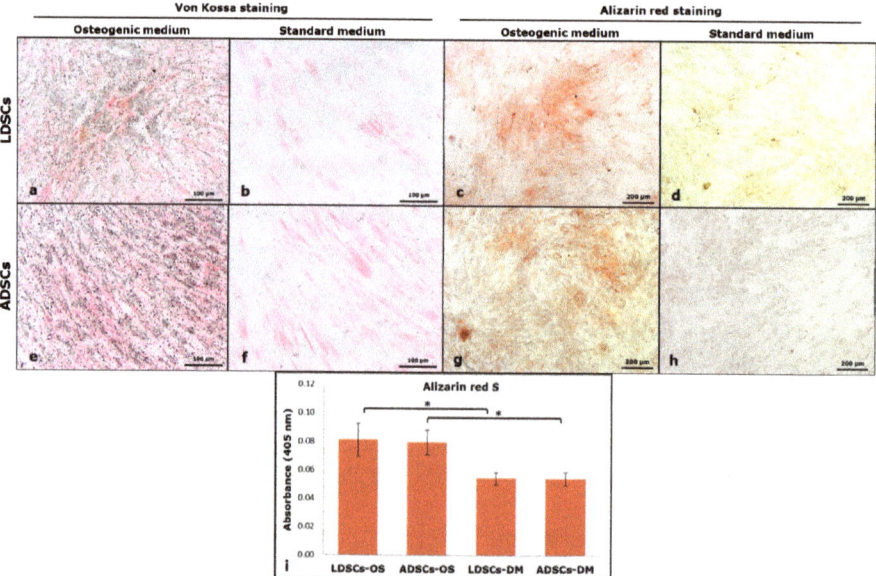

Figure 10. Von Kossa staining of cells at day 16 of osteogenic differentiation; LDSCs in osteogenic medium (OS) (**a**) LDSCs in standard medium (DM) (**b**) ADSCs in OS medium (**e**) and ADSCs in DM medium (**f**); dark grey/black deposits' color in (**a**) and (**e**) indicates positive staining; Alizarin red S staining of cells at day 16 of osteogenic differentiation; LDSCs in OS medium (**c**) LDSCs in DM medium (**d**) ADSCs in OS medium (**g**) and ADSCs in DM medium (**h**); red deposits' color in (**c**) and (**g**) indicates positive Alizarin red S (ARS)staining; All images were acquired at bright field with objective magnification 10×; quantitative measurement of ARS dye (**i**), presented as mean ± SD, n (LDSCs) = 5 and n (ADSCs) = 4 for all groups; (*) $p < 0.05$.

After 16 days of osteogenic differentiation, osteoprotegerin (OPG) concentration was measured in cell culture supernatant by ELISA (Figure 11). Significantly higher concentration of OPG ($p < 0.05$) was observed in ADSCs cultured in OS medium than in standard DM medium, and ADSCs than in LDSCs cultured in OS medium. No statistical significance was found between LDSCs cultured in OS compared to DM medium.

Relative expression levels of osteogenesis-related genes: runt related transcription factor 2 (*RUNX2*) and osteocalcin (*BGLAP*) were measured at two time points during osteogenic differentiation, 8 and 16 days (Figure 12, Table 2). After 8 days, the increase in *RUNX2* expression was observed in both LDSCs and ADSCs, but more pronounced in ADSCs than in LDSCs (Table 2). After 16 days of differentiation, *RUNX2* expression pattern has changed so that expression was higher in LDSCs cultured in OS than in DM medium, while lower in ADSCs cultured in OS than in DM medium (Figure 12b, Table 2). *BGLAP* expression slightly increased during differentiation and it was significantly higher in ADSCs than in LDSCs at both time points.

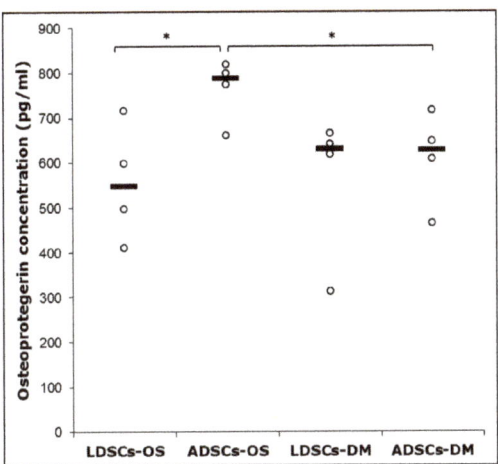

Figure 11. Osteoprotegerin concentration in cell culture supernatant of LDSCs and ADSCs, measured by ELISA at day 16 of osteogenic differentiation; scatterplots with median; n = 4 for all groups; (*) $p < 0.05$.

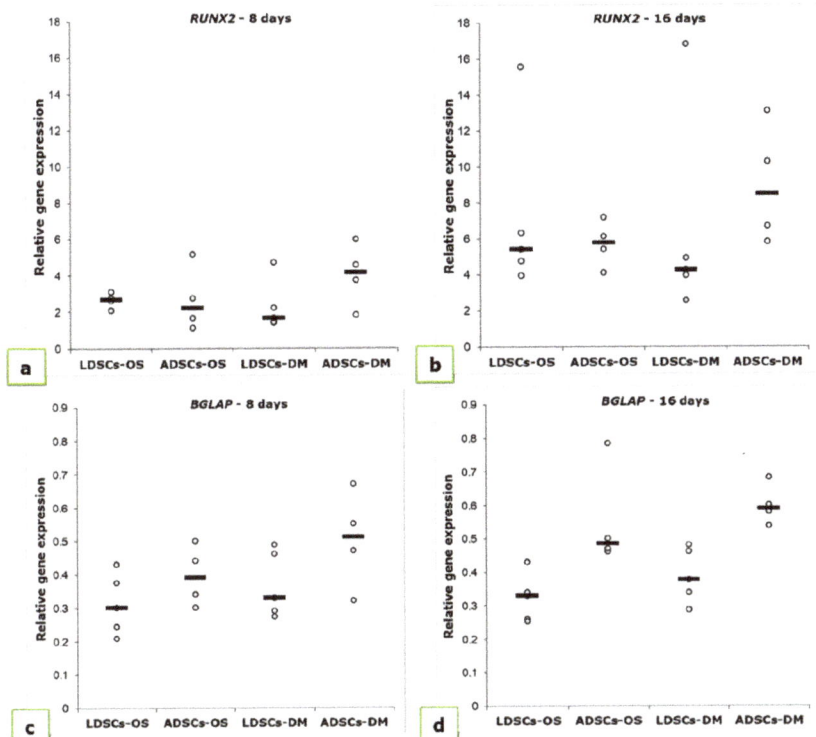

Figure 12. Relative expression levels ($2^{-\Delta\Delta Ct}$) of *RUNX2* (**a**,**b**) and *BGLAP* (**c**,**d**) measured in LDSCs and ADSCs at day 8 (**a**,**c**) and day 16 (**b**,**d**) of osteogenic differentiation and normalized to *GAPDH*; scatterplots with median; n (LDSCs) = 5 and n (ADSCs) = 4 for all groups.

Table 2. Relative expression of *RUNX2* and *BGLAP* in LDSCs and ADSCs at days 8 and 16 of osteogenic differentiation, normalized to *GAPDH* and compared to the cells at P2 (day 0). Results are expressed as mean values ± SD. Asterisks represent statistical significance compared to P2 (day 0).

Cell Type	RUNX2				
	P2 (Day 0)	8 Days		16 Days	
		OS	DM	OS	DM
LDSCs	1.620 ± 0.622	2.156 ± 1.133	2.27 ± 1.390	7.194 ± 4.76 *	6.478 ± 5.83
ADSCs	1.013 ± 0.214	2.670 ± 1.799	4.01 ± 1.747 *	5.685 ± 1.29 ***	8.960 ± 3.35 **
	BGLAP				
	P2 (Day 0)	8 Days		16 Days	
		OS	DM	OS	DM
LDSCs	0.23 ± 0.039	0.312 ± 0.091 *	0.368 ± 0.099 *	0.323 ± 0.072 *	0.388 ± 0.081 **
ADSCs	0.33 ± 0.085	0.395 ± 0.091	0.503 ± 0.147	0.554 ± 0.155 *	0.600 ± 0.062 **

* $p < 0.05$, ** $p < 0.01$, *** $p < 0.001$.

4. Discussion

Our study is among the first giving detailed analysis of stem cells isolated from lipoma and comparison with stem cells isolated from normal adipose tissue. The distinct signature of these cells governs the capacity for adipogenic and osteogenic differentiation which we analyzed on cellular and molecular levels.

Lipomas, used in our study, were located subcutaneously at different body locations. To compare cells isolated from lipoma with the cells isolated from normal adipose tissue, we used samples of subcutaneous adipose tissue from different body depots as well. It was reported that there is no statistically significant evidence of depot-related effects on proliferation and differentiation potential of ADSCs, while difference was noticed in apoptosis susceptibility and lipolysis [22]. Other study has shown that subcutaneous ADSCs, compared with ADSCs from other depots, have greater differentiation potential and recommend them as optimal choice for angiogenic and osteogenic regeneration [23]. Regarding the impact of donor age on the properties of ADSCs, results found in published data are diverse. Some studies showed that there are age-related differences in proliferation of ADSCs and lipid accumulation during adipogenic differentiation, with decrease in proliferation rate and increased lipid accumulation during aging [22]. Others reported that growth kinetics, osteogenic and chondrogenic differentiation potentials of ADSCs were adversely affected by increased donor age while adipogenic differentiation potential was maintained during aging [24]. On the other side, it is reported that the use of adipose stem cells for bone tissue engineering is not limited by the donor's age as shown by osteogenic differentiation of ADSCs isolated from differently aged patients, on the scaffold-free 3D osteogenic graft intended for the treatment of bone defects [25]. In our study, both groups of patients were of similar age (average age of patients with lipoma was 48.3 ± 8.3 while average age of non-lipoma patients was 49.5 ± 11.1) which means that differences in the properties of LDSCs and ADSCs could not be affected by the differences in patients' age.

Mesenchymal stem cells isolated from adipose tissue show a spindle-cell-like bipolar morphology which is typical for mesenchymal stem cells [23,26]. It has been shown that subcutaneous ADSCs are more homogenous in morphology with less variations in cell diameter up to passage 12, compared to other adipose tissue depots [23]. In our study, the morphology of LDSCs and ADSCs was very similar and typical mesenchymal-like, without significant differences observed between LDSCs and ADSCs after isolation as well as after cell passage (Figure 1). Although, some authors reported that ADSCs have consistent morphology while LDSCs did not [17], several studies showed that morphology of LDSCs is very much alike ADSCs and there were no morphological differences between those two cell types after long-term culture [13,14].

To be considered as stem cells, cells should fulfil some phenotypic criteria and to express so called stemness-related markers which include panel of both intracellular and surface molecules. Oct4, the most commonly examined intracellular marker, is a transcriptional factor encoded by the *POU5F1* gene. It is expressed in embryonic stem cells [27] and also in adult human stem cells [28], and is essential for pluripotency, self-renewal, proliferation and survival of mesenchymal stem cells [29]. Expression level of Oct4 in cells is reported to define the balance between differentiation and de-differentiation in stem cells [30]. In our study, both LDSCs and ADSCs expressed *POU5F1* with no statistically significant difference in expression level when compared (Figure 2f). There is a lack of data in the literature on Oct4 expression in LDSCs, however, there are some reports on expression of *POU5F1* in lipoma tissue, and it has been shown that this gene is up-regulated in lipoma compared to the normal adipose tissue [31].

CD44 is a transmembrane glycoprotein which is very important for cell differentiation and functions as a receptor for hyaluronic acid that is involved in cell–cell and cell-matrix interactions, mediates cell adhesion and migration, and interacts with other ligands, such as osteopontin, collagen, and matrix metalloproteinases (MMPs). Numerous studies have shown that CD44, as well as *CD44* gene, is expressed in ADSCs and is considered as one of the highly expressed positive stem cell markers in ADSCs [4,23,32,33]. In a very few studies dealing with LDSCs, it was shown that CD44 is expressed in LDSCs and there is no difference in expression level between LDSCs and ADSCs [17]. Zavan et al. [31] showed that *CD44* is up-regulated in lipoma tissue compared to normal adipose tissue. In our study, both ADSCs and LDCSs express the *CD44* (Figure 2e) although LDSCs slightly less but not significantly. The lower *CD44* expression in LDSCs may be the consequence of hypermethylation of the *CD44* gene which is the case in tumor development [34]. This finding could be taken into consideration to explain weaker differentiation potential of LDSCs as shown later.

Endoglin (ENG) or CD105 is a type I membrane glycoprotein and is a part of the TGF beta receptor complex. It is highly expressed in ADSCs and MSCs in general, and represents one of the commonly used positive markers for their characterization [4,23,32,33,35]. In our study both LDSCs and ADSCs expressed high levels of CD105 as evaluated by flow cytometry (Figure 2a,c). There are opposite findings in literature about expression of CD105 in LDSCs. Some authors reported that expression of CD105 is similar in LDSCs and ADSCs as analyzed by flow cytometry [17], which is in accordance with our results, while others reported low CD105 expression in LDSCs [15]. This opposite finding of Tremp et al. [15] is probably due to the different type of lipoma used, lack of comparative measurement of its expression in normal ADSCs and analysis in SVF cells while our cells were characterized at passage 2. Chang et al. [36] analyzed, by flow cytometry, the expression of CD105 in cells isolated from two different types of lipoma and showed that all cells highly express CD105 (greater than 90%) with no difference between different types of lipoma samples. It has been shown that expression of CD105, and other stem cells surface markers, is low in SVF cells, but increases during cultivation and passages while isolated SVF has high expression levels of pluripotency (embryonic stem cell) markers, which decrease with cultivation and passages [37,38]. This is one of the main reasons why we used cells at passage 2 for further differentiation studies since they expressed both pluripotency markers (Oct4) as well as stem cell surface markers CD44 and CD105, at this point (Figure 2).

The ADSCs at passage 2 or 3 uniformly express stem cell markers and are morphologically a homogeneous population [26,39]. This finding is confirmed in our study as well, showing that both LDSCs and ADSCs express stem cell markers and are morphologically homogeneous at passage 2. Our results of stemness-related markers' analysis suggest that both LDSCs and ADSCs in our study were mesenchymal stem cells, which means that both had similar phenotype and stemness state before differentiation. Senescence (or aging) of cells represents an irreversible process during which stem cells lose their stemness-related phenotype and differentiation potential, and occurs in long-term cell culture and at late cell passages [40–42]. ADSCs are shown to enter into senescence after passage 10 [41] and at lower extent than stem cells of other origin [42]. We used cells at early passage (P2) for differentiation studies thus avoiding the influence of cell senescence on differentiation potential.

Our results are among the first presenting detailed analysis of molecular signature of LDSCs in comparison with ADSCs, which were examined at the same time and under the same conditions. To the best of our knowledge, there are no data on expression of adipogenic- and osteogenic-related markers in stem cells isolated from lipoma tissue. We analyzed relative expression levels of genes *ADIPOQ*, *LEP*, *PPARG*, *DLK1*, *RUNX2* and *BGLAP* in LDSCs and ADSCs at passage 2, before differentiation started (Figure 3). These results are of great importance for analysis of differentiation capacity of those cells and differences between them, since these results gave us information about the basal levels of mRNA from genes that we examined during adipogenic and osteogenic differentiation. We showed that there are slight differences in all analyzed genes, however, statistically significant difference between LDSCs and ADSCs was observed for *RUNX2* and *BGLAP* only. This could explain the differences in the osteogenic differentiation dynamics between LDSCs and ADSCs noticed in our study. There is one report on adiponectin and PPAR-γ expression in sorted LDSCs (distinguished CD34+ cells) evaluated by immunocytochemical staining, and it has been shown that adiponectin expression was lower in CD34+ cultured cells from lipoma compared to CD34+ isolated from normal adipose tissue with no difference in the expression of PPAR-γ [31]. This finding correlates with our results of gene expression analysis (Figure 3c,e). Although there are no studies on gene expression in isolated cells some research groups investigated the differences in expression of *ADIPOQ*, *LEP* and *PPARG*, *RUNX2* and *BGLAP* in lipoma tissue and compared it with normal adipose tissue [14,31]. It has been shown that, in tissue samples, expression of *LEP* was higher while expression of *ADIPOQ* was lower in lipoma compared to normal adipose tissue, which is the expression pattern characteristic for obesity [14]. The same pattern of *LEP* and *ADIPOQ* gene expression was observed in our study in isolated cells (Figure 3d,e). Suga et al. [14], in the same study, showed that expression of *PPARG* in lipoma was not distinctly different from that in normal adipose tissue. Our results showed that *PPARG* is more expressed in ADSCs compared to LDSCs, but not statistically significant, probably due to heterogeneity among samples (Figure 3c). In the study by Zavan et al. [31], authors showed that expression of *LEP*, *ADIPOQ* and *PPARG* genes is up-regulated while *RUNX2* was less expressed in lipoma compared to normal adipose tissue, which is, except *LEP*, different from the findings in previous study, and our results on isolated cells.

Stem cells isolated from adipose tissue have great ability to differentiate into adipocytes and therefore are promising tool in soft tissue engineering and regenerative medicine [43]. We induced both LDSCs and ADSCs into adipocytes by cultivation in adipogenic medium for 21 day. Microscopic analysis of cells (Figure 4), Oil red O staining of lipid droplets (Figure 5), adiponectin immunoexpression (Figure 6) and leptin concentration measurement in media after 21 day (Figure 7) showed that adipogenesis in LDSCs was restricted and that LDSCs have weaker capacity to differentiate into adipocytes compared to ADSCs. These findings on cellular and protein expression levels were confirmed at gene expression level as well. Adiponectin and leptin are adipokines secreted by mature adipocytes and are commonly used as markers of adipocytes [44]. In our study, *ADIPOQ*, *LEP* and *PPARG* were significantly less expressed in LDSCs compared to ADSCs in AM medium (Figure 8) with no significant difference in *LEP* and *PPARG* expression between LDSCs cultured in different media like for ADSCs. Pref-1 is a preadipocyte marker encoded by *DLK1* gene, whose expression decreases during adipogenesis with its high expression in preadipocytes and very low or absent expression in mature adipocytes [45–48]. For mature adipocytes' formation, decreased Pref-1 level is necessary. It has been shown that Pref-1 expression is high in ADSCs before differentiation while 14 days of adipogenic differentiation it is almost non-detectable [48]. Our results showed that *DLK1* is significantly more expressed in LDSCs cultured in AM medium for 21 day compared to ADSCs in the same medium ($p < 0.05$) (Figure 8d). Regarding ADSCs, *DLK1* expression was decreased in AM medium compared to DM medium which is in accordance with the dynamics of Pref-1 expression during adipogenesis. High levels of *DLK1* could be related with lower degree of LDSCs differentiation into adipocytes in our study. There are only few publications reported adipogenic differentiation of LDSCs. Suga et al. [14] reported that there were no differences in the capacity for adipogenic differentiation of LDSCs compared to ADSCs, at passage 1, as evaluated by lipid droplets staining and quantification. By the same analyses employed, other studies revealed that high lipid content was observed in differentiated LDSCs [15] and that cells were differentiated into adipocytes successfully, similar to ADSCs [16], but no comparative results with normal ADSCs were shown in those two studies. The ability of LDSCs to differentiate into adipocytes at early as well as late passages was reported to be similar as of ADSCs, evaluated by lipid droplets presence and staining [13]. Our results are more complex since we assessed the adipogenic differentiation potential of both LDSCs and ADSCs at different levels and by different methods. This study is, according to our knowledge, the first dealing with the adipogenic differentiation of LDSCs by analyzing the markers of this process on several levels—cellular, molecular and gene, but in the same time comparing that with ADSCs isolated from normal tissue. According to the adipogenesis-related gene expression signature as well as phenotypic changes and protein levels in LDSCs and ADSCs after 21 day of adipogenic differentiation, compared to the cells at day 0 (passage 2), we can conclude that adipogenesis was not complete in LDSCs and differentiation capacity of LDSCs compared to ADSCs was significantly lower.

Adipose-derived stem cells have a great potential to differentiate into osteoblasts and therefore represent a promising tool in bone tissue engineering for making bone grafts with different biomaterials to regenerate and repair the bone defects [23,49,50]. It has been shown that stem cells from subcutaneous adipose tissue show good osteogenic differentiation potential at passage 2 [23], that we also used in our study. After 16 days of osteogenic differentiation, phenotypic changes in both LDSCs and ADSCs cultured in OS medium were observed so that cells became more epithelial-like and less fibroblastic-like, and accumulation of inorganic matrix components was noticed (Figure 9), slightly more in ADSCs culture. No significant difference was found in ARS staining between LDSCs and ADSCs but slightly darker Von Kossa staining was observed in ADSCs.

Osteoprotegerin (OPG) is secreted by osteoblasts, is a marker of their functional state since it is important for regulation of osteoblast-osteoclast homeostasis [51], promotes pre-osteoblasts and matrix maturation [52] and its secretion is up-regulated during osteogenic differentiation in vitro [53]. In our study, significant difference in osteoprotegerin (OPG) secretion, measured by ELISA, between LDSCs and ADSCs cultured in OS medium for 16 days, was noticed with higher OPG concentration found in ADSCs compared to LDSCs (Figure 11).

Differences between LDSCs and ADSCs in osteogenic differentiation capacity were also observed at gene expression level in our study. *RUNX2* expression increased in both cell cultures during differentiation so it was higher in ADSCs than in LDSCs at day 8 and higher in LDSCs than ADSCs at day 16 (Figure 12a,b; Table 2). RUNX2 is a transcription factor involved in osteogenesis and is essential for osteoblast differentiation [54–56]. RUNX2 promotes osteoblast differentiation at an early stage, by inducing the expression of genes for bone matrix proteins such as osteopontin, osteocalcin, collagen type 1, etc., but also its high expression can inhibit osteoblast differentiation at a late stage [54,57]. In order to achieve osteoblast maturation, it is necessary that RUNX2 is initially upregulated to induce the expression of bone matrix proteins, but its expression should then decrease to enable the process of differentiation into mature osteoblasts to be continued. However, if RUNX2 is constantly upregulated, then osteoblasts maturation cannot be achieved. In our study, *RUNX2* is upregulated in LDSCs after 16 days, compared to ADSCs, which could be one of the reasons for lower expression of *BGLAP* in LDSCs compared to ADSCs. It was reported that OPG was overexpressed in pre-osteoblasts when RUNX2 was downregulated while osteoblast differentiation was arrested in RUNX2 overexpressing cells [52]. Our results are similar with these findings, since LDSCs have higher expression of *RUNX2* but lower expression of OPG, compared to ADSCs at day 16 of osteogenic differentiation where *RUNX2* expression was down-regulated and OPG was up-regulated. Osteocalcin is a protein secreted by mature osteoblasts and plays important role in bone calcification and mineralization of MSCs during osteogenic differentiation [58,59]. It was reported that *BGLAP* expression begins to increase after 14 days of osteogenic differentiation of MSCs [58,59]. In our study, *BGLAP* expression increased during differentiation in both cultures and it was higher in differentiated ADSCs than LDSCs after

16 days (Figure 12c,d; Table 2). Both LDSCs and ADSCs in our study had characteristic osteoblast-like phenotype after 16 days of osteogenic induction but, based on osteogenic genes' expression dynamics, osteogenesis was at different stages in those cells and one of the reasons could be higher *RUNX2* expression in LDSCs at passage 2 (Figure 3a).

There are very few publications with data about osteogenic differentiation of stem cells isolated from lipoma tissue. Makiguchi et al. [16] showed that ADSCs isolated from lipoma tissue can differentiate into osteoblasts after 21 days in OS media, as evaluated by alkaline phosphatase activity and calcium concentration measurement. It was also reported by Lin et al. [13] that LDSCs can be successfully differentiated into osteoblasts, but only Von Kossa staining of calcium deposits was performed in this study. No other markers or details on osteogenic differentiation of these cells were reported. However, there are numerous reports on lipoma tissue ossification observed in different parts of the body [8,16,18,19,60–63] and this phenomenon could be explained by the existence of stem cells in lipoma tissue that may differentiate into osteoblasts and chondrocytes.

Upregulated expression of *RUNX2* in LDSCs, in our study, could be also considered as a reason why adipogenic differentiation of LDSCs was at lower extent since it has been shown by other authors that overexpression of RUNX2 inhibits adipogenesis [55,64,65]. Taking this finding together with the previously considered higher *RUNX2* expression before differentiation, at day 0 (passage 2) in LDSCs compared to ADSCs, it is a significant indication that *RUNX2* expression, together with *DLK1* expression pattern, is an important mechanism for suppressing LDSCs differentiation capabilities. On the other side, higher expression of *RUNX2* in LDSCs may suggest potential osteogenic capacity of those cells, which could be one of the possible mechanisms of bone and cartilaginous structures' formation in the cases of aforementioned osteolipoma, since higher expression of RUNX2 is necessary at an early stage of both osteogenesis and chondrogenesis.

5. Conclusions

Our study is among the first that provides detailed analysis of stem cells isolated from lipoma and comparison with the stem cells isolated from normal adipose tissue, on cellular and molecular levels. Results of our study suggest that both LDSCs and ADSCs were mesenchymal stem cells with similar phenotype and stemness state for potential differentiation. According to analyzes of adipogenesis-related markers at cellular and molecular level and microscopic analysis after 21 day of adipogenic differentiation we can conclude that differentiation capacity of LDSCs compared to ADSCs was significantly lower. Analysis of osteogenesis-related markers revealed that both types of cells had characteristic osteoblast-like phenotype after 16 days of osteogenic induction but were at different stages of osteogenesis. Differences between LDSCs and ADSCs, after isolation from the tissue, are probably due to the distinct molecular signature and their commitment in the tissue that will governs their different capacity and fate during adipogenic and osteogenic induction in vitro. These results provide new insights into the cellular and molecular basis of lipoma etiopathogenesis and imply that the potential use of LDSCs in tissue engineering and regenerative medicine should be re-considered or at least other ways of using these cells for regeneration purposes should be discussed.

Author Contributions: Conceptualization, S.S. and S.N.; methodology, S.S. and S.N.; validation, S.S. and S.N.; formal analysis, S.S.; investigation, S.S.; resources, S.N.; writing—original draft preparation, S.S.; writing—review and editing, S.N., A.K. and S.S.; visualization, S.S.; supervision, S.N. and A.K.; project administration, S.N.; funding acquisition, S.N. and A.K.

Funding: This research was funded by the Ministry of Education, Science and Technological development, of the Republic of Serbia (Grants No. III 41017 and OI 173055).

Acknowledgments: Authors would like to thank the doctors and staff at the surgical clinics of the Clinical Center Niš, Serbia for their help with tissue samples collection.

Conflicts of Interest: The authors declare no conflict of interest. The funders had no role in the design of the study; in the collection, analyses, or interpretation of data; in the writing of the manuscript, or in the decision to publish the results.

References

1. Mizuno, H.; Tobita, M.; Uysal, A.C. Concise review: Adipose-derived stem cells as a novel tool for future regenerative medicine. *Stem Cells* **2012**, *30*, 804–810. [CrossRef]
2. Bunnell, B.A.; Flaat, M.; Gagliardi, C.; Patel, B.; Ripoll, C. Adipose-derived stem cells: Isolation, expansion and differentiation. *Methods* **2008**, *45*, 115–120. [CrossRef] [PubMed]
3. Gimble, J.M.; Katz, A.J.; Bunnell, B.A. Adipose-derived stem cells for regenerative medicine. *Circ. Res.* **2007**, *100*, 1249–1260. [CrossRef]
4. Baer, P.C.; Geiger, H. Adipose-derived mesenchymal stromal/ stem cells: Tissue localization, characterization, and heterogeneity. *Stem Cells Int.* **2012**, *2012*. [CrossRef] [PubMed]
5. Cvetković, V.J.; Najdanović, J.G.; Vukelić-Nikolić, M.Đ.; Stojanović, S.; Najman, S.J. Osteogenic potential of in vitro osteo-induced adipose-derived mesenchymal stem cells combined with platelet-rich plasma in an ectopic model. *Int. Orthop.* **2015**, *39*, 2173–2180. [CrossRef] [PubMed]
6. Najdanović, J.G.; Cvetković, V.J.; Stojanović, S.; Vukelić-Nikolić, M.Đ.; Stanisavljević, M.N.; Živković, J.M.; Najman, S.J. The influence of adipose-derived stem cells induced into endothelial cells on ectopic vasculogenesis and osteogenesis. *Cell. Mol. Bioeng.* **2015**, *8*, 577–590. [CrossRef]
7. Najman, S.J.; Cvetković, V.J.; Najdanović, J.G.; Stojanović, S.; Vukelić-Nikolić, M.Đ.; Vučković, I.; Petrović, D. Ectopic osteogenic capacity of freshly isolated adipose-derived stromal vascular fraction cells supported with platelet-rich plasma: A simulation of intraoperative procedure. *J. Cranio Maxillofac. Surg.* **2016**, *44*, 1750–1760. [CrossRef] [PubMed]
8. Omonte, S.V.; de Andrade, B.A.; Leal, R.M.; Capistrano, H.M.; Souza, P.E.; Horta, M.C. Osteolipoma: A rare tumor in the oral cavity. *Oral Surg. Oral Med. Oral Pathol. Oral Radiol.* **2016**, *122*, e8–e13. [CrossRef]
9. Mohammed, U.; Samaila, M.O.; Abubakar, M. Pattern of adipose tissue tumors in Ahmadu Bello University Teaching Hospital, Zaria, Nigeria. *Ann. Niger. Med.* **2014**, *8*, 8–10. [CrossRef]
10. Mentzel, T.; Fletcher, C.D. Lipomatous tumours of soft tissues: An update. *Virchows Arch.* **1995**, *427*, 353–363. [CrossRef]
11. Marques, M.C.; Garcia, H. Lipomatous Tumors. In *Imaging of Soft Tissue Tumors*; De Schepper, A.M., Parizel, P.M., Ramon, F., De Beuckeleer, L., Vandevenne, J.E., Eds.; Springer: Berlin Heidelberg, Germany, 1997; pp. 191–207. ISBN 978-3-662-07859-4.
12. Ingari, J.V.; Faillace, J.J. Benign tumors of fibrous tissue and adipose tissue in the hand. *Hand Clin.* **2004**, *20*, 243–248. [CrossRef] [PubMed]
13. Lin, T.M.; Chang, H.W.; Wang, K.H.; Kao, A.P.; Chang, C.C.; Wen, C.H.; Lai, C.S.; Lin, S.D. Isolation and identification of mesenchymal stem cells from human lipoma tissue. *Biochem. Biophys. Res. Commun.* **2007**, *361*, 883–889. [CrossRef] [PubMed]
14. Suga, H.; Eto, H.; Inoue, K.; Aoi, N.; Kato, H.; Araki, J.; Higashino, T.; Yoshimura, K. Cellular and molecular features of lipoma tissue: Comparison with normal adipose tissue. *Br. J. Dermatol.* **2009**, *161*, 819–825. [CrossRef] [PubMed]
15. Tremp, M.; Menzi, N.; Tchang, L.; di Summa, P.G.; Schaefer, D.J.; Kalbermatten, D.F. Adipose-derived stromal cells from lipomas: Isolation, characterisation and review of the literature. *Pathobiology* **2016**, *83*, 258–266. [CrossRef] [PubMed]
16. Makiguchi, T.; Terashi, H.; Hashikawa, K.; Yokoo, S.; Kusaka, J. Osteolipoma in the glabella: Pathogenesis associated with mesenchymal lipoma-derived stem cells. *J. Craniofac. Surg.* **2013**, *24*, 1310–1313. [CrossRef] [PubMed]
17. Qian, Y.W.; Gao, J.H.; Lu, F.; Zheng, X.D. The differences between adipose tissue derived stem cells and lipoma mesenchymal stem cells incharacteristics. *Zhonghua Zheng Xing Wai Ke Za Zhi* **2010**, *26*, 125–132. (In Chinese) [PubMed]
18. Val-Bernal, J.F.; Val, D.; Garijo, M.F.; Vega, A.; González-Vela, M.C. Subcutaneous ossifying lipoma: Case report and review of the literature. *J. Cutan. Pathol.* **2007**, *34*, 788–792. [CrossRef]
19. Sunohara, M.; Ozawa, T.; Morimoto, K.; Tateishi, C.; Ishii, M. Lipoma with bone and cartilage components in the left axilla of a middle-aged woman. *Aesthet. Plast. Surg.* **2012**, *36*, 1164–1167. [CrossRef]
20. Livak, K.J.; Schmittgen, T.D. Analysis of Relative Gene Expression Data Using Real-Time Quantitative PCR and the $2^{-\Delta\Delta CT}$ Method. *Methods* **2001**, *25*, 402–408. [CrossRef]

21. Weissgerber, T.L.; Milic, N.M.; Winham, S.J.; Garovic, V.D. Beyond bar and line graphs: Time for a new data presentation paradigm. *PLoS Biol.* **2015**, *13*, e1002128. [CrossRef]
22. Schipper, B.M.; Marra, K.G.; Zhang, W.; Donnenberg, A.D.; Rubin, J.P. Regional anatomic and age effects on cell function of human adipose-derived stem cells. *Ann. Plast. Surg.* **2008**, *60*, 538–544. [CrossRef] [PubMed]
23. Jung, S.; Kleineidam, B.; Kleinheinz, J. Regenerative potential of human adipose-derived stromal cells of various origins. *J. Cranio Maxillofac. Surg.* **2015**, *43*, 2144–2151. [CrossRef] [PubMed]
24. Choudhery, M.S.; Badowski, M.; Muise, A.; Pierce, J.; Harris, D.T. Donor age negatively impacts adipose tissue-derived mesenchymal stem cell expansion and differentiation. *J. Transl. Med.* **2014**, *12*. [CrossRef] [PubMed]
25. Dufrane, D. Impact of age on human adipose stem cells for bone tissue engineering. *Cell Transplant.* **2017**, *26*, 1496–1504. [CrossRef] [PubMed]
26. Baer, P.C. Adipose-derived mesenchymal stromal/stem cells: An update on their phenotype in vivo and in vitro. *World J. Stem Cells* **2014**, *6*, 256–265. [CrossRef] [PubMed]
27. Nichols, J.; Zevnik, B.; Anastassiadis, K.; Niwa, H.; Klewe-Nebenius, D.; Chambers, I.; Schöler, H.; Smith, A. Formation of pluripotent stem cells in the mammalian embryo depends on the POU transcription factor Oct4. *Cell* **1998**, *95*, 379–391. [CrossRef]
28. Tai, M.H.; Chang, C.C.; Kiupel, M.; Webster, J.D.; Olson, L.K.; Trosko, J.E. Oct4 expression in adult human stem cells: Evidence in support of the stem cell theory of carcinogenesis. *Carcinogenesis* **2005**, *26*, 495–502. [CrossRef]
29. Han, S.M.; Han, S.H.; Coh, Y.R.; Jang, G.; Chan Ra, J.; Kang, S.K.; Lee, H.W.; Youn, H.Y. Enhanced proliferation and differentiation of Oct4- and Sox2-overexpressing human adipose tissue mesenchymal stem cells. *Exp. Mol. Med.* **2014**, *46*. [CrossRef]
30. Niwa, H.; Miyazaki, J.-i.; Smith, A.G. Quantitative expression of Oct-3/4 defines differentiation, dedifferentiation or self-renewal of ES cells. *Nat. Genet.* **2000**, *24*, 372–376. [CrossRef]
31. Zavan, B.; De Francesco, F.; D'Andrea, F.; Ferroni, L.; Gardin, C.; Salzillo, R.; Nicoletti, G.; Ferraro, G.A. Persistence of CD34 stem marker in human lipoma: Searching for cancer stem cells. *Int. J. Biol. Sci.* **2015**, *11*, 1127–1139. [CrossRef]
32. Ranera, B.; Lyahyai, J.; Romero, A.; Vázquez, F.J.; Remacha, A.R.; Bernal, M.L.; Zaragoza, P.; Rodellar, C.; Martín-Burriel, I. Immunophenotype and gene expression profiles of cell surface markers of mesenchymal stem cells derived from equine bone marrow and adipose tissue. *Vet. Immunol. Immunopathol.* **2011**, *144*, 147–154. [CrossRef]
33. Watson, J.E.; Patel, N.A.; Carter, G.; Moor, A.; Patel, R.; Ghansah, T.; Mathur, A.; Murr, M.M.; Bickford, P.; Gould, L.J.; et al. Comparison of markers and functional attributes of human adipose-derived stem cells and dedifferentiated adipocyte cells from subcutaneous fat of an obese diabetic donor. *Adv. Wound Care* **2014**, *3*, 219–228. [CrossRef] [PubMed]
34. Yan, P.; Mühlethaler, A.; Bourloud, K.B.; Beck, M.N.; Gross, N. Hypermethylation-mediated regulation of CD44 gene expression in human neuroblastoma. *Gene. Chromosom. Cancer* **2003**, *36*, 129–138. [CrossRef] [PubMed]
35. Lin, C.S.; Xin, Z.C.; Dai, J.; Lue, T.F. Commonly used mesenchymal stem cell markers and tracking labels: limitations and challenges. *Histol. Histopathol.* **2013**, *28*, 1109–1116. [CrossRef]
36. Chang, H.; Park, S.O.; Jin, U.S.; Hong, K.Y. Characterization of two distinct lipomas: A comparative analysis from surgical perspective. *J. Plast. Surg. Hand Surg.* **2018**, *52*, 178–184. [CrossRef] [PubMed]
37. Varma, M.J.; Breuls, R.G.; Schouten, T.E.; Jurgens, W.J.; Bontkes, H.J.; Schuurhuis, G.J.; van Ham, S.M.; van Milligen, F.J. Phenotypical and functional characterization of freshly isolated adipose tissue-derived stem cells. *Stem Cells Dev.* **2007**, *16*, 91–104. [CrossRef] [PubMed]
38. Taha, M.F.; Javeri, A.; Rohban, S.; Mowla, S.J. Upregulation of pluripotency markers in adipose tissue-derived stem cells by miR-302 and leukemia inhibitory factor. *Biomed. Res. Int.* **2014**, *2014*. [CrossRef] [PubMed]
39. Gronthos, S.; Franklin, D.M.; Leddy, H.A.; Robey, P.G.; Storms, R.W.; Gimble, J.M. Surface protein characterization of human adipose tissue-derived stromal cells. *J. Cell. Physiol.* **2001**, *189*, 54–63. [CrossRef]
40. Legzdina, D.; Romanauska, A.; Nikulshin, S.; Kozlovska, T.; Berzins, U. Characterization of senescence of culture-expanded human adipose-derived mesenchymal stem cells. *Int. J. Stem Cells* **2016**, *9*, 124–136. [CrossRef]

41. Truong, N.C.; Bui, K.H.T.; Van Pham, P. Characterization of senescence of human adipose-derived stem cells after long-term expansion. In *Advances in Experimental Medicine and Biology*; Cohen, I.R., Lajtha, A., Lambris, J.D., Paoletti, R., Rezaei, N., Eds.; Springer: New York, NY, USA, 2018; pp. 1–20. ISSN 0065-2598.
42. Kern, S.; Eichler, H.; Stoeve, J.; Klüter, H.; Bieback, K. Comparative analysis of mesenchymal stem cells from bone marrow, umbilical cord blood, or adipose tissue. *Stem Cells* **2006**, *24*, 1294–1301. [CrossRef]
43. Locke, M.; Windsor, J.; Dunbar, P.R. Human adipose-derived stem cells: Isolation, characterization and applications in surgery. *ANZ J. Surg.* **2009**, *79*, 235–244. [CrossRef] [PubMed]
44. Fantuzzi, G. Adipose tissue, adipokines, and inflammation. *J. Allergy Clin. Immunol.* **2005**, *115*, 911–919. [CrossRef]
45. Sul, H.S. Minireview: Pref-1: Role in adipogenesis and mesenchymal cell fate. *Mol. Endocrinol.* **2009**, *23*, 1717–1725. [CrossRef] [PubMed]
46. Wang, Y.; Hudak, C.; Sul, H.S. Role of preadipocyte factor 1 in adipocyte differentiation. *Clin. Lipidol.* **2010**, *5*, 109–115. [CrossRef]
47. Hudak, C.S.; Sul, H.S. Pref-1, a gatekeeper of adipogenesis. *Front. Endocrinol.* **2013**, *4*. [CrossRef] [PubMed]
48. Mitterberger, M.C.; Lechner, S.; Mattesich, M.; Kaiser, A.; Probst, D.; Wenger, N.; Pierer, G.; Zwerschke, W. DLK1(PREF1) is a negative regulator of adipogenesis in $CD105^+/CD90^+/CD34^+/CD31^-/FABP4^-$ adipose-derived stromal cells from subcutaneous abdominal fat pats of adult women. *Stem Cell Res.* **2012**, *9*, 35–48. [CrossRef] [PubMed]
49. Ciuffi, S.; Zonefrati, R.; Brandi, M.L. Adipose stem cells for bone tissue repair. *Clin. Cases Miner. Bone Metab.* **2017**, *14*, 217–226. [CrossRef]
50. Bhattacharya, I.; Ghayor, C.; Weber, F.E. The use of adipose tissue-derived progenitors in bone tissue engineering—A review. *Transfus. Med. Hemother.* **2016**, *43*, 336–343. [CrossRef]
51. Udagawa, N.; Takahashi, N.; Yasuda, H.; Mizuno, A.; Itoh, K.; Ueno, Y.; Shinki, T.; Gillespie, M.T.; Martin, T.J.; Higashio, K.; et al. Osteoprotegerin produced by osteoblasts is an important regulator in osteoclast development and function. *Endocrinology* **2000**, *141*, 3478–3484. [CrossRef]
52. Yu, H.; de Vos, P.; Ren, Y. Overexpression of osteoprotegerin promotes preosteoblast differentiation to mature osteoblasts. *Angle Orthodont.* **2011**, *81*, 100–106. [CrossRef]
53. Zajdel, A.; Kałucka, M.; Kokoszka-Mikołaj, E.; Wilczok, A. Osteogenic differentiation of human mesenchymal stem cells from adipose tissue and Wharton's jelly of the umbilical cord. *Acta Biochim. Pol.* **2017**, *64*, 365–369. [CrossRef] [PubMed]
54. Komori, T. Runx2, a multifunctional transcription factor in skeletal development. *J. Cell. Biochem.* **2002**, *87*, 1–8. [CrossRef] [PubMed]
55. Komori, T. Regulation of skeletal development by the Runx family of transcription factors. *J. Cell. Biochem.* **2005**, *95*, 445–453. [CrossRef] [PubMed]
56. Katagiri, T.; Takahashi, N. Regulatory mechanisms of osteoblast and osteoclast differentiation. *Oral Dis.* **2002**, *8*, 147–159. [CrossRef] [PubMed]
57. Komori, T. Regulation of bone development and maintenance by Runx2. *Front. Biosci.* **2008**, *13*, 898–903. [CrossRef] [PubMed]
58. Tsao, Y.T.; Huang, Y.J.; Wu, H.H.; Liu, Y.A.; Liu, Y.S.; Lee, O.K. Osteocalcin mediates biomineralization during osteogenic maturation in human mesenchymal stromal cells. *Int. J. Mol. Sci.* **2017**, *18*. [CrossRef] [PubMed]
59. Wang, L.; Li, Z.Y.; Wang, Y.P.; Wu, Z.H.; Yu, B. Dynamic expression profiles of marker genes in osteogenic differentiation of human bone marrow-derived mesenchymal stem cells. *Chin. Med. Sci. J.* **2015**, *30*, 108–113. [CrossRef]
60. Firth, N.A.; Allsobrook, O.; Patel, M. Osteolipoma of the buccal mucosa: A case report. *Aust. Dent. J.* **2017**, *62*, 378–381. [CrossRef]
61. Demiralp, B.; Alderete, J.F.; Kose, O.; Ozcan, A.; Cicek, I.; Basbozkurt, M. Osteolipoma independent of bone tissue: A case report. *Cases J.* **2009**, *2*. [CrossRef]
62. Raghunath, V.; Manjunatha, B.S. Osteolipoma of floor of the mouth. *BMJ Case Rep.* **2015**, *2015*. [CrossRef]
63. Kwan Ip, N.S.; Lau, H.W.; Wong, W.Y.; Yuen, M.K. Osteolipoma in the Forearm. *J. Clin. Imaging Sci.* **2018**, *8*. [CrossRef] [PubMed]

64. Rosen, E.D.; MacDougald, O.A. Adipocyte differentiation from the inside out. *Nat. Rev. Mol. Cell Biol.* **2006**, *7*, 885–896. [CrossRef] [PubMed]
65. Enomoto, H.; Furuichi, T.; Zanma, A.; Yamana, K.; Yoshida, C.; Sumitani, S.; Yamamoto, H.; Enomoto-Iwamoto, M.; Iwamoto, M.; Komori, T. Runx2 deficiency in chondrocytes causes adipogenic changes in vitro. *J. Cell Sci.* **2004**, *117*, 417–425. [CrossRef] [PubMed]

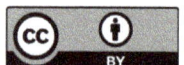
© 2018 by the authors. Licensee MDPI, Basel, Switzerland. This article is an open access article distributed under the terms and conditions of the Creative Commons Attribution (CC BY) license (http://creativecommons.org/licenses/by/4.0/).

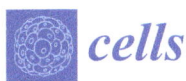

Article

Isolation, Characterization, Differentiation and Immunomodulatory Capacity of Mesenchymal Stromal/Stem Cells from Human Perirenal Adipose Tissue

Patrick C. Baer [1,*,†], Benjamin Koch [1,†], Elena Hickmann [1], Ralf Schubert [2], Jindrich Cinatl Jr. [3], Ingeborg A. Hauser [1] and Helmut Geiger [1]

1. Division of Nephrology, Department of Internal Medicine III, University Hospital, Goethe University, 60596 Frankfurt/M., Germany; b.koch@med.uni-frankfurt.de (B.K.); elena.hickmann@gmx.de (E.H.); ingeborg.hauser@kgu.de (I.A.H.); h.geiger@em.uni-frankfurt.de (H.G.)
2. Division of Allergology, Pneumology and Cystic Fibrosis, Department for Children and Adolescents, University Hospital, Goethe University, 60596 Frankfurt/M., Germany; ralf.schubert@kgu.de
3. Institute of Medical Virology, University Hospital, Goethe University, 60596 Frankfurt/M., Germany; cinatl@em.uni-frankfurt.de
* Correspondence: patrick.baer@kgu.de or p.baer@em.uni-frankfurt.de; Tel.: +49-69-6301-5554; Fax: +49-69-6301-4749
† These authors contributed equally to this paper.

Received: 12 October 2019; Accepted: 29 October 2019; Published: 29 October 2019

Abstract: Mesenchymal stromal/stem cells (MSCs) are immature multipotent cells, which represent a rare population in the perivascular niche within nearly all tissues. The most abundant source to isolate MSCs is adipose tissue. Currently, perirenal adipose tissue is rarely described as the source of MSCs. MSCs were isolated from perirenal adipose tissue (prASCs) from patients undergoing tumor nephrectomies, cultured and characterized by flow cytometry and their differentiation potential into adipocytes, chondrocytes, osteoblasts and epithelial cells. Furthermore, prASCs were stimulated with lipopolysaccharide (LPS), lipoteichoic acid (LTA) or a mixture of cytokines (cytomix). In addition, prASC susceptibility to human cytomegalovirus (HCMV) was investigated. The expression of inflammatory readouts was estimated by qPCR and immunoassay. HCMV infection was analyzed by qPCR and immunostaining. Characterization of cultured prASCs shows the cells meet the criteria of MSCs and prASCs can undergo trilineage differentiation. Cultured prASCs can be induced to differentiate into epithelial cells, shown by cytokeratin 18 expression. Stimulation of prASCs with LPS or cytomix suggests the cells are capable of initiating an inflammation-like response upon stimulation with LPS or cytokines, whereas, LTA did not induce a significant effect on the readouts (ICAM-1, IL-6, TNFα, MCP-1 mRNA and IL-6 protein). HCMV broadly infects prASCs, showing a viral load dependent cytopathological effect (CPE). Our current study summarizes the isolation and culture of prASCs, clearly characterizes the cells, and demonstrates their immunomodulatory potential and high permissiveness for HCMV.

Keywords: mesenchymal stromal/stem cells; perirenal; adipose tissue; fat; characterization; stimulation; lipopolysaccharide; cytokines; cytomegalovirus

1. Introduction

Mesenchymal stromal/stem cells (MSCs) are immature multipotent stromal cells, which represent a rare population in the perivascular niche within fully specialized tissues throughout the whole body [1]. The cells can be isolated from nearly all adult tissues, for example, adipose tissue, solid organs and bone marrow [2,3], and proliferated in vitro. Cultured MSCs release a broad range of growth factors, cytokines, and chemokines [4,5] in the culture supernatant that may improve regeneration in injured cells, organs or tissue. Therefore, MSCs are an optimal source for tissue regeneration support therapies after tissue injury. The organ-protective effects of MSCs, their conditioned medium or extracellular vesicles have been investigated in the last decade, demonstrating that either infused stem cells or their derivates facilitated tissue and organ regeneration predominantly by released regeneration-promoting factors. Furthermore, MSCs have immunological properties, including anti-inflammatory, immunoregulatory and immunosuppressive capacities [6,7], and are, therefore, active immunomodulators during inflammation and sepsis. This immunomodulatory activity has been attributed to the secretion of soluble factors. The MSCs were shown to interact with a variety of immune cells, including CD4 and CD8 T cells, natural killer cells, B cells, monocytes and dendritic cells [8]. The MSCs have also been shown to express Toll-like receptors (TLRs), the major molecules linking innate and adaptive immunity [9]. The TLRs act as sensors for invading pathogens broadly distributed on immune cells and are involved in the pathogenesis of chronic inflammatory and infectious diseases [10].

Recent data have suggested that adipose tissue located in different anatomical locations of the body appear to have distinct cellular compositions and diverse functions [11–13]. In humans, fat depot-specific differences are clinically relevant owing to the observation that increased abdominal white fat is associated with insulin resistance, while subcutaneous white adipose tissue exerts a protective effect against metabolic syndrome [11]. Para- and perirenal adipose tissue is a fat pad located in the retroperitoneal space. Perirenal fat is separated from pararenal fat by the renal fascia, and surrounds each kidney [14]. It is a collection of adipose tissue located superficial to the renal cortex and is part of the visceral fat, which can be divided into perirenal, gonadal, epicardial, retroperitoneal, omental and mesenteric fat depots [15]. They are composed mainly of white adipose cells that store energy and produce soluble inflammatory cytokines [14,16]. Perirenal fat shares the same developmental origin as typical visceral fat [14]. However, each white adipose tissue depot can be described as a separate mini-organ [15], and perirenal fat and typical visceral fat are different in histology, physiology and functions [14]. The vascularization of perirenal adipose tissue grows from branches of the abdominal aorta, which also supplies blood to the kidney cortex. Therefore, effects on renal cells through soluble factor released by cells from the perirenal adipose tissue are possible [16]. Renal adipose tissue has been linked recently to effects on kidney function and blood hypertension [17] and a neuronal link from perirenal adipose tissue to multiple central nervous system's regions has been shown in animal data [18]. Perirenal tissue is rarely analyzed for viral infections, however MSC from selected organs other than perirenal tissue show susceptibility and permissiveness for human cytomegalovirus (HCMV) infection [19,20]

The object of this study was to describe the isolation and culture of human perirenal adipose-derived stromal/stem cells (prASCs) in detail and to characterize cultured cells and their differentiation potential into adipocytes, chondrocytes, osteoblasts and epithelial cells. The present study further investigated the immunomodulatory potential of prASCs after stimulation with lipopolysaccharide (LPS), lipoteichoic acid (LTA), a mixture of cytokines (cytomix), or infection with HCMV. Whereas, few studies used human prASCs in vitro [21–23], there is currently no other study which fully described the isolation, characterization, differentiation and immunomodulatory potential of human prASCs as well as their susceptibility to HCMV.

2. Materials and Methods

2.1. Perirenal Adipose Tissue

Human perirenal adipose tissue was obtained from patients undergoing tumor nephrectomies. This study was approved by the ethics committee of the clinic of the Goethe University, Frankfurt (UGO 03/10, Amendment).

2.2. Cell Isolation and Culture

Human MSCs were isolated from perirenal adipose tissue from 15 different donors. The tissue was minced by using two scalpels and disintegrated as small as possible for cell isolation. The minced tissue was then digested at 37 °C with collagenase (1 mg/mL; CellSystems, Troisdorf, Germany) and continuous agitation for 60 min. Cells were then separated from the remaining fibrous material and the floating adipocytes by centrifugation at 300× g. The pelleted cells were collected, and the procedure was repeated twice. The sedimented cells were washed with phosphate-buffered saline (PBS) and filtered through a 125-μm plastic mesh (Millipore, Schwalbach, Germany). Erythrocyte contamination, if required, was reduced by density gradient centrifugation with Bicoll (Biochrom, Berlin, Germany), because high erythrocyte contamination was found to decrease ASCs adherence and proliferation markedly. It was observed in previous experiments, that a preceding density gradient separation provided a better yield of adipose-derived stromal/stem cells (ASCs) than treatment with an erythrocyte lysing buffer [24]. Finally, the cells were plated for initial cell culture and cultured at 37 °C in an atmosphere of 5% CO_2 in humid air. Dulbecco's modified Eagle's medium (DMEM; Sigma, Taufkirchen, Germany) was used with a physiologic glucose concentration (100 mg/dl) supplemented with 10% fetal bovine serum (FBS; Biochrom, Berlin, Germany) as the standard culture medium. Primary isolated cells were intensively washed with PBS after 18–24 h of initial plating to remove debris and non-adherent cells. The medium was then replaced every three to four days. Subconfluent cells were passaged by trypsinization. In all experiments we used cultured prASCs in early passages (between 2 and 5).

2.3. Cell Characterizations Using Flow Cytometry and Immunofluorescence Staining

Cell morphology was examined by phase contrast microscopy. Flow cytometric analysis was used to show the characteristic marker expression of cultured prASCs. Cells were detached from the cell culture plastic and stained with directly labeled antibodies (CD73-PerCP-eFluo710 (eBioscience, San Diego, CA, USA), CD90-FITC (BD Bioscience, Heidelberg, Germany), CD105-PE, CD29-FITC and CD45-PE (all from Immunotools, Friesoythe, Germany)). The labeled prASCs were then measured using a flow cytometer (BD Biosciences, Heidelberg, Germany). All experiments included negative controls with corresponding isotype controls. Cells were gated by forward and sideward scatter to eliminate debris.

Cells were cultured on chamber slides (Nunc Lab-Tech®), rinsed three times with PBS and fixed with ice-cold methanol/acetone (1:1) for 5 min for immunofluorescence staining. Unspecific binding sites were blocked with PBS containing 5% normal goat serum for 20 min. Primary antibody (anti-vimentin or anti-cytokeratin 18 (CK-18); both from ExBio, Vestec, Czech Republic) was applied after washing and incubated for 45 min at 37 °C with gentle shaking. Afterwards, cells were washed and incubated with a Cy^3-conjugated secondary monoclonal antibody for 45 min at 37 °C. All dilutions of antibodies were made in PBS containing 1% goat serum. 4,6-diamidino-2-phenylindole dihydrochloride (DAPI; 0.5 μg/mL) was added to the secondary antibody solution for nuclear staining. Controls of nonspecific fluorescence were performed on fixed cells processed without the primary antibody. The cells were washed and covered in Moviol. The slides were stored at 4 °C and analyzed with a fluorescence microscope (Zeiss, Heidelberg, Germany).

2.4. Induction of Cell Differentiation

The trilineage differentiation potential of cultured prASCs was induced by incubation in differentiation media for 14 days, followed by the verification of differentiation by standard staining methods (Oil Red O, Alcian Blue, and Alizarin staining, respectively), as further described. Media were changed every three to four days.

Adipogenic differentiation was induced in adipogenic medium containing high glucose content (4.5 g/L), insulin (1.74 μM, Novo Nordisk), dexamethasone (0.1 μM, Ratiopharm), isobutyl-methylxanthin (0.5 mM, Sigma), indomethacine (200 µM, Fluka), and 10% FBS. Oil Red O (Sigma) staining revealed the accumulation of lipid droplets in intracellular vacuoles indicating adipogenic differentiation.

The chondrogenic differentiation of prASCs was induced in chondrogenic medium containing ascorbic acid (50 nM; Merck), insulin (6.25 µg/mL, Novo Nordisk), transforming growth factor β (10 ng/mL, Peprotech) and 1% FBS. The chondrogenic phenotype was assessed by Alcian Blue 8GX staining (Fluka).

Osteogenic differentiation of prASCs was induced in osteogenic medium containing ascorbic acid (50 µM; Merck), glycerophosphate (10 mM, Sigma), dexamethasone (1 µM, Ratiopharm), recombinant bone morphogenic protein-2 (100 ng/mL, Immunotools, Friesoythe) and 15% FBS. After 14 days of incubation, the osteogenic phenotype was assessed by staining according to Alizarin Red S staining (Fluka).

The cells were incubated with all-trans retinoid acid (ATRA; Sigma) at a final concentration of 5 µM for epithelial differentiation. This concentration was determined by taking a pattern of our previous studies and testing with proliferation and vitality assays [25,26]. A stock solution of ATRA dissolved in dimethyl sulfoxide at 10 mM was kept at −80 °C. The ATRA was dissolved in DMEM substituted with 10% FBS for cell culture. The equivalent volume of solvent (dimethyl sulfoxide) without ATRA was used in control samples. Epithelial differentiation medium was replaced every three to four days during a total incubation period of 14 days, followed by analysis of the epithelial differentiation by expression of CK-18 using qPCR, Western blotting and immunofluorescence staining

2.5. Stimulation with LPS, LTA, and Cytokines

Cells were grown in 24-well culture plates (for IL-6 measurements in the supernatant) or small cell culture flasks (25 cm^2 for PCR analyses) to subconfluence. Cells were then washed with PBS and treated with TLR-4 ligand LPS (LPS-EB ultrapure from E. coli 0111: B4; 10, 100, 1000 ng/mL; Invivogen, San Diego, USA, Cat. No. tlrl-3pelps), TLR-2 ligand LTA (from Staphylococcus aureus; 1000 ng/mL; Invivogen, Cat. No. tlrl-slta), or cytomix (IFNγ, 200 U/mL; IL-1β, 25 U/mL, and TNFα, 10 ng/mL) diluted in DMEM with 10% FBS. The RNA was isolated after 4 h of stimulation, and supernatants were harvested after 48 h for IL-6 quantification. Therefore, supernatants were collected, centrifuged at 300× g for 5 min and assessed for the cytokine by an immunoassay or stored at −20 °C for later measurement.

2.6. HCMV Infection

prASCs were infected with HCMV patient isolate Hi91 [27] at a multiplicity of infection (MOI) of 0.05, 0.5, 1 and 4. Expression of HCMV-specific late antigen was detected 96 h post-infection by immunoperoxidase staining using monoclonal antibodies directed against gB/gpUL55-encoded antigen (kindly provided by K. Radsak, Institut für Virologie, Marburg, Germany) as previously described [28]. Other samples were used for extraction of total RNA and cDNA synthesis. Changes in gene expression of selected targets were quantified by qPCR in triplicate measurements.

2.7. Cell Viability Assays

Cell viability of prASCs was determined by by two viability assays, a photometric assay using 2,3-Bis-(2-Methoxy-4-Nitro-5-Sulfophenyl)-2H-Tetrazolium-5-Carboxanilide (XTT), as described previously [29], and a fluorescent-based assay using calcein-acetoxymethyl (calcein-AM, Biolegend, San Diego, USA), to determine any possible cytotoxic effects during the stimulations. In brief, 5000 cells/well were seeded in 96-well plates. We measured each stimulation in quintuplicate for each biological replicate. One day after seeding, the prASCs were stimulated for 96 h as described above. The XTT reagent was then added to the wells, as described by the manufacturer (AppliChem, Darmstadt, Germany), and incubated at 37 °C for 4 h. Absorbance was measured in an Apollo LB911 microplate reader (Berthold, Bad Wildbad, Germany) at 492 vs. 650 nm. Data are expressed as arbitrary units and calculated as a percent in relation to the control. For the fluorescence assay, cells were washed and calcein-AM (1 µM) was added incubated at 37 °C for 30 min. Then, fluorescence was measured immediately using a fluorescence reader (BMG Fluostar, Ortenberg, Germany) with excitation and emission wavelengths of 485 and 515 nm. Cells incubated in buffer without calcein-AM were used as background controls. Data are expressed as arbitrary fluorescence units.

2.8. PCR

We performed a single-step RNA isolation protocol using Nucleozol (Macherey-Nagel, Düren, Germany) to extract RNA from cultured prASCs. Then, cDNAs were synthesized from isolated RNA for 30 min at 37 °C using 1 µg RNA, 50 µM random hexamers, 1 mM deoxynucleotide-tripheosphate mix, 50 units of reverse transcriptase (Fermentas, St. Leon-Rot, Germany) in 10× PCR buffer, 1 mM β-mercaptoethanol and 5 mM MgCl$_2$. A Hot FIREPol EvaGreen Mix Plus was used (Solis Biodyne, Tartu, Estonia) for the master mix; the primer mix and RNAse-free water were added. Quantitative PCR (qPCR) was carried out in 96-well plates using the following conditions: Twelve minutes at 95 °C for enzyme activation, 15 s at 95 °C for denaturation, 20 s at 63 °C for annealing and 30 s at 72 °C for elongation (40 cycles). Finally, a melting curve analysis was executed. The quantification of the PCR fragment was performed using the ABI Prism® 7900HT Fast Real-Time PCR System with a Sequence Detection System SDS 2.4.1 (Thermo Fisher Scientific). Relative quantification was assessed by the ΔΔCT method [30], using β-actin as a calibrator, and levels of target gene expression were estimated by $2^{-\Delta\Delta Ct}$. In selected experiments, PCR products were separated by agarose gel electrophoresis (2%) and observed under UV illumination. Primer pairs were synthesized by Thermo Fisher Scientific (Germany) and are listed in Table 1.

Table 1. Primer used for qPCR analyses.

Gene	Primer Forward	Primer Reverse	Product Length (bp)	NCBI Reference Sequence
CK-18	CAC AGT CTG CTG AGG TTG GA	CAA GCT GGC CTT CAG ATT TC	110	NM_000224
ICAM-1	CAGTGACTGTCACTCGAGATCT	CCTCTTGGCTTAGTCATGTGAC	500	NM_000201.3
IL-6	AAAGATGGCTGAAAAAGATGGATGC	ACAGCTCTGGCTTGTTCCTCACTAC	150	NM_000600.4
MCP-1	CCCCAGTCACCTGCTGTTAT	AGATCTCCTTGGCCACAATG	135	NM_002982.4
TNFα	CGGGACGTGGAGCTGGCCGAGGAG	CACCAGCTGGTTATCTCTCAGCTC	354	NM_000594.4
TLR-2	GCCCATTGCTCTTTCACTGCTT	ATGACCCCCAAGACCCACAC	96	NM_003264.4
TLR-4	CCCGACAACCTCCCCTTCTC	GGGCTAAACTCTGGATGGGGT	211	NM_003266
UL83	GCAGCCACGGGATCGTACT	GGCTTTTACCTCACACGAGCATT	159	NC_006273
β-actin	ACT GGA ACG GTG AAG GGT GAC	AGA GAA GTG GGG TGG CTT TT	169	NM_001101

2.9. Western Blot

The cells were processed for Western blotting, as described previously [31]. In brief, the cells were lysed using 10 mM Tris pH 7.4, 0.1% SDS, 0.1% Tween20, 0.5% TritonX100, 150 mM NaCl, 10 mM EDTA, 1 M urea, 10 mM NEM, 4 mM benzamidine and 1 mM PMSF and collected by scraping. After centrifugation, the pellet was suspended in Laemmli's buffer and heated at 95 °C for 5 min prior to electrophoresis on a 10% SDS polyacrylamide gel. The protein content was determined by a standard assay and an equal volume of protein was loaded into each lane. The separated proteins were transferred electrophoretically to Immobilon transfer membrane (Millipore). Membranes were blocked for 2 h. Immunoblotting was performed by incubating with antibodies against CK-18 (resulting in a 45 kDa band, ExBio, Vestec, Czech Republic) or β-Actin (resulting in a 42 kDa band, Sigma Aldrich), followed by a secondary antibody (horseradish peroxidase-conjugated anti-mouse or anti-rabbit IgG; Amersham Pharmacia). Protein bands were made visible using the Peqlab Fusion FX system (VWR, Darmstadt, Germany) followed by densitometric evaluation using ImageJ 1.8.0 (NIH, www.nih.gov).

2.10. Immunoassay

Interleukin-6 was quantified using a commercially available enzyme-linked immunosorbent assay kit (ELISA) (Immunotools, Friesoythe, Germany). In brief, the wells of 96-well microtiter plates were coated with an anti-human IL-6 antibody overnight at room temperature (RT). Nonspecific binding sites were blocked with PBS/2% BSA/0.05% Tween20 for 1 h. The plates were then washed with PBS/0.05% Tween and the standard (8–500 pg/mL), and the samples were added for 2 h at RT. All samples were diluted in assay buffer (1:25) and run in duplicate. The plates were washed and incubated with biotinylated anti-IL-6 for 2 h at RT, washed again and incubated with horseradish-peroxidasestreptavidin for 30 min. After washing, TMB was added for 5–20 min and the substrate reaction was stopped and measured (450 vs. 620 nm). The data are presented as ng/mL of IL-6 in the supernatant.

2.11. Statistical Analysis

The data are expressed as mean ± standard deviation (SD). Analysis of variance with Dunnett's Multiple Comparison Test or Student's t-test were used for statistical analysis. p values < 0.05 were considered significant.

3. Results

3.1. Isolation and Characterization of prASCs

We used an average of 75 g of perirenal adipose tissue to isolate prASCs, yielding 6.9×10^8 cells seeded in total, corresponding to approximately 9.2×10^6 primary isolated cells per gram tissue. Nevertheless, only some of these cells adhere to cell culture plastic and proliferate. Approximately 80–90% of the isolated cells do not adhere and were aspirated with the first washing after 24 h. Adhered primary cells cultured in a 75 cm^2 cell culture flask need up to seven days to reach subconfluence (~80–85%), the situation where the cells were subcultured for the first time. At this time, an average of 3.75×10^5 cells were grown in the 75 cm^2 cell culture flask (corresponding to 5000 cells/cm^2 growth area).

Cultured prASCs displayed a spindle-shaped fibroblastoid morphology (Figure 1A). Primary isolated cells are morphologically more heterogeneous than cultures after passaging. Nevertheless, cultured cells became morphologically increasingly homogeneous in higher passages. Contaminations with cells of epithelial morphology or pre-adipocytes were not detectable in the culture at passage 2. In addition, immunofluorescence staining in passage 2 revealed that all the cells cultured (100%) expressed vimentin (Figure 1B), also showing a very homogeneous cell culture of mesenchymal origin. There were no vimentin-negative cells detectable in any staining done.

The cells were also characterized by flow cytometric analysis utilizing characteristic markers for MSCs in vitro. Cultured prASCs expressed CD29, CD73, CD 90 and CD105 but did not express CD45 (Figure 1C). Furthermore, cultured prASCs were positive for CD44 and CD166 and did not express the endothelial markers CD31 and C11b, which are expressed on the surface of many leukocytes, including monocytes, granulocytes and macrophages (data not shown).

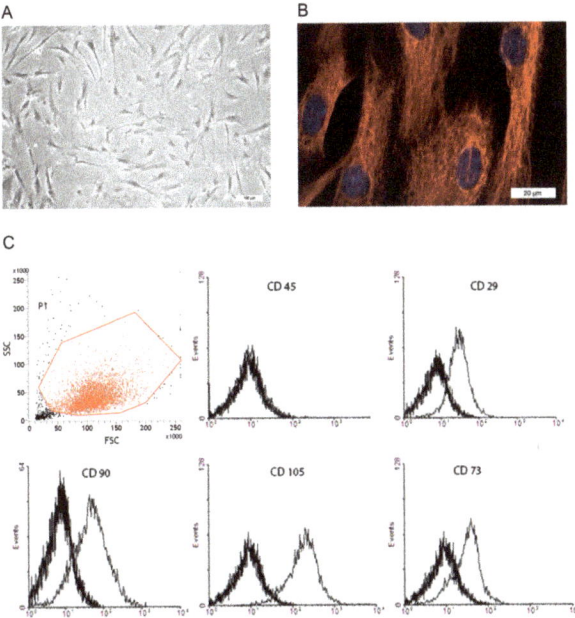

Figure 1. Characterization of human perirenal mesenchymal stromal/stem cells (prASCs) in vitro. (**A**) Characteristic phase contrast microscopy of prASCs in passage 2 (bar: 100 µm); (**B**) Immunofluorescence staining of intermediate filament vimentin, nuclei were counterstained with DAPI (bar: 20 µm); (**C**) Representative flow cytometric overlay histograms of characteristic marker expression (CD73, CD90, CD105, CD29) and of CD45, a pan leukocyte marker which is not expressed on MSCs. Thick black histograms represent isotype controls. A dot plot shows the forward and sideward scatter analysis with the gating strategy to eliminate debris.

3.2. Differentiation of prASCs

We investigated the differentiation potential of prASCs into adipocytes, chondrocytes, osteoblasts and epithelial cells. We used the differentiation media described in the case of trilineage differentiation of cultured prASCs. After 14 days of incubation, the verification of differentiation was done by standard staining methods (Oil Red O, Alcian Blue and Alizarin staining, respectively). Incubation of undifferentiated prASCs for 14 days under adipogenic conditions induced the de novo formation of cytoplasmatic lipid droplets, a characteristic of pre-adipocytes, stained by Oil Red O staining (Figure 2B). Chondrogenic-induced prASCs exhibit an intense blue color following Alcian Blue 8GX staining (Figure 2D), indicative of cartilage extracellular matrix accumulation. Induction of osteogenic differentiation of the cells for 14 days resulted in the deposition of mineralized nodules that stained red by Alizarin Red S staining (Figure 2F), characteristic for osteoblasts. Cells cultured in osteogenic induction medium changed from an elongated mesenchymal appearance to a multilateral form with a tightly packed multilayer.

Control cells cultured in standard medium were not stained by Oil Red O (Figure 2A), Alcian Blue 8GX (Figure 2C) or Alizarin Red staining (Figure 2E).

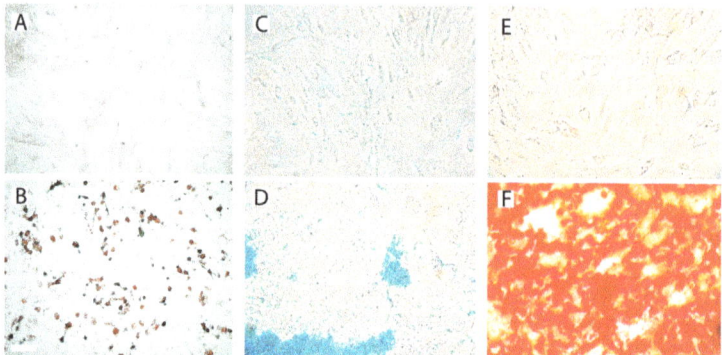

Figure 2. Trilineage differentiation of cultured prASCs. Differentiation into adipocytes, chondrocytes and osteoblasts was induced by adipogenic (**B**), chondrogenic (**D**) and osteogenic (**F**) medium for 14 days. Control cells were cultured in standard culture medium for 14 days (**A,C,E**) After 14 days of incubation in either standard or differentiation medium, cultures were stained with Oil Red O (**A,B**), Alcian Blue 8GX (**C,D**) or Alizarin Red S (**E,F**) (bar: 100 µm).

In addition to their trilineage differentiation potential, prASCs were also able to differentiate into the epithelial lineage. In order to elucidate the influence of ATRA on prASCs differentiation, expression of CK-18, an early epithelial marker, was evaluated by qPCR analysis (Figure 3A), immunofluorescence staining (Figure 3B) and Western blotting (Figure 3C,D). After incubation with ATRA for 14 days, the expression of CK-18 mRNA was 6.2-fold induced compared to unstimulated control cells (Figure 3A). Immunofluorescence staining revealed that approximately 45% of the cells were CK-18 positive (Figure 3B), and Western blot analysis also clearly showed the significant induction of CK-18 protein in epithelial-induced prASCs (Figure 3C) (densitometric analysis calculated in percent: control (standard medium) = 100% (background signal); ATRA = 286% (Figure 3D)).

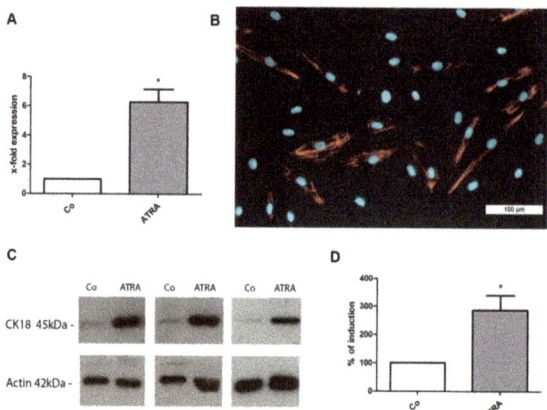

Figure 3. Induction of epithelial differentiation. (**A**) Analysis of cytokeratin 18 (CK-18) induction by qPCR. The expression levels in each experiment were normalized using β-actin as a housekeeping gene and are expressed relative to the unstimulated control using the ΔΔCT method (n = 6; * $p < 0.05$); (**B**) Characteristic immunofluorescence staining of CK-18 after epithelial differentiation with ATRA (14 days). Nuclei were stained with DAPI (bar: 100 µm); (**C**) Characteristic Western blots. Expression of CK-18 (45 kDa) and β-actin (42 kDa) of the unstimulated control cells (Co) and after incubation with ATRA (5 µM) for 14 days; (**D**) Densitometric evaluation of CK-18 induction in relation to undifferentiated controls (= 100%) (n = 5; * $p < 0.05$).

3.3. Stimulation with LPS, LTA and Cytokines

We added increasing concentrations of LPS, a major component of the outer membrane of Gram-negative bacteria, to the cell supernatant and evaluated the response by qPCR and an immunoassay to test the responsiveness of prASCs to pro-inflammatory stimuli. In addition, we stimulated the cells with LTA, a key cell wall component of Gram-positive bacteria and potent stimulator of TLR-2. A mixture of pro-inflammatory cytokines (cytomix: IFNγ, 200 U/mL; IL-1β, 25 U/mL; and TNFα, 10 ng/mL) was used as a positive stimulation control. In particular, prASCs produced a set of inflammatory mediators in response to the bacterial or cytokine stimulation. The mRNA expression of ICAM-1, MCP-1, TNFα and IL-6 was upregulated in response to the TLR-4 agonist LPS (Figure 4A–D). The cytomix induced a significantly higher induction of ICAM-1, MCP-1 and IL-6 than stimulation with LPS, whereas there were no significant differences in the induction of TNFα mRNA expression. We also detected no significant differences between the different stimulation doses of LPS. On the other hand, LTA induced no significant effect on the cytokines analyzed, whereas TLR-2 was shown to be expressed (Figure 4E). Total mRNA was isolated from the prASCs in passage 2 cultured in standard medium to determine the constitutive expression of the relevant receptors for the bacterial infections (TLR-2 for LTA and TLR-4 for LPS). Both receptors were found to be expressed, whereas TLR-2 only showed a weak but specific signal at 96 bp.

Furthermore, qPCR analysis revealed that some mRNAs were constitutively expressed in vitro. IL-6 and MCP-1 mRNA were highly detectable in the unstimulated control (CT values approximately 22 and 28, respectively (water: undetectable)), and ICAM-1 was slightly expressed compared with the unstimulated control (CT value approximately 30 (water: 37)). On the other hand, TNFα mRNA was not detected in the unstimulated prASCs.

At the protein level, IL-6 is constitutively released by prASCs (8.9 ± 1.5 ng/mL; mean $\pm$ SD, $n = 4$). When the cells were stimulated by LPS or exposed to an inflammatory environment by the cytomix, the production of IL-6 was significantly upregulated (Figure 4F). Nevertheless, we found no dose-dependent effect of the LPS stimulation, and the release of LPS- and cytokine-stimulated IL-6 protein was nearly comparable (LPS 10: 29.3 ± 3.3; LPS 100: 30.5 ± 7.2; LPS 1000: 32.5 ± 4.9; cytomix 33.5 ± 9.3 ng/mL, mean $\pm$ SD, $n = 4$). The LTA also induced an increase in IL-6 release, but the effect was not significant (17.0 ± 7.1 ng/mL; mean $\pm$ SD, $n = 4$) (Figure 4F).

These results suggest that, under these culture conditions, prASCs are capable of initiating an inflammation-like response upon stimulation with LPS or cytokines. Interestingly, only LPS (from gram negative bacteria) induced a significant stimulation of prASCs, but no significant stimulation was found by after incubation with the pathogen of gram-positive bacteria.

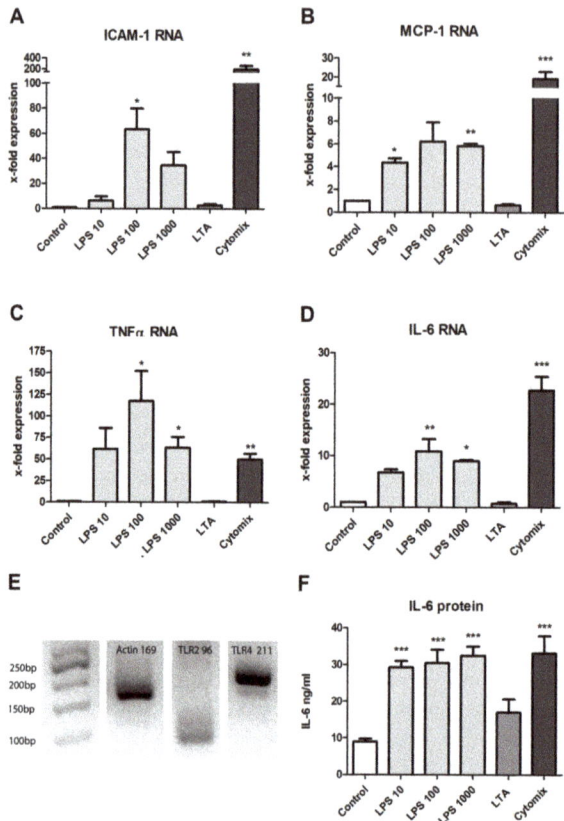

Figure 4. Effect of lipopolysaccharide (LPS) (10, 100, 1000 ng/mL), LTA (1000 ng/mL) or a cytokine mix (cytomix). (**A–D**) Assessment at the mRNA level by qPCR for ICAM-1, MCP-1, IL-6, and TNFα after 4 h stimulation. The expression levels in each experiment were normalized to a housekeeping gene (β-actin) and are expressed relative to the control using the ΔΔCT method. (mean ± SD; * $p < 0.05$, ** $p < 0.01$, *** $p < 0.001$ versus control), $n = 4$.; (**E**) Constitutive expression of TLR-2- and TLR-4-mRNA of prASCs in vitro. The PCR products were separated by agarose electrophoresis and observed under UV illumination (TLR-2: 96 kb, TLR-4: 211 kb, and β-actin: 169 kb (housekeeper)); (**F**) Quantification of IL-6 protein in the supernatant after 48 h stimulation. Data from four independent immunoassays (ELISA) are represented as mean ± SD (*** $p < 0.0001$).

To investigate the effects of LPS, LTA and the cytomix on prASCs viability, we used two viability assays using XTT or calcein-AM. The XTT assay is a colorimetric assay used to determine viability based on the metabolic activity of the cultured cells. Calcein-AM is a cell permeant non-fluorescent dye, which is in live cells intracellularly converted into calcein, a dye with intense green fluorescence. Whereas a slightly reduced metabolic activity after each stimulation regimen could be detected with the XTT assay (XTT calculated in percent: control, 100%; LPS 10, 80.02%; LPS 100, 76.86%; LPS 1000, 74.86%; LTA, 83.91%; cytomix, 84.24%), the differences in live cell detection were very low. No statistically significant difference could be found, either with the XTT assay (Figure 5A) or with the calcein assay (Figure 5B).

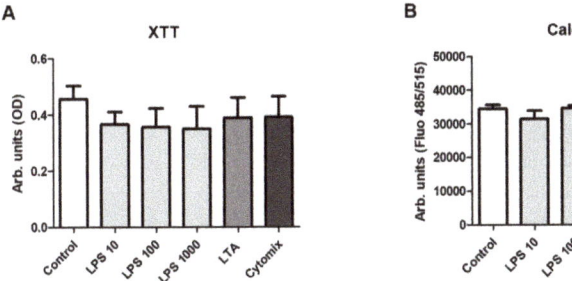

Figure 5. Cell viability after stimulation with LPS, LTA or cytomix for 96 h. A total of 5000 cells were cultured in 96 well plates ($n = 3$, each in quintuplicate) and stimulated for 96 h. (**A**) The XTT assay was performed and optical density (OD) was measured in a microplate reader at 492 vs. 650 nm (arbitrary units). (**B**) The calcein assay was performed and fluorescence was measured in a reader at 485 nm (excitation) and 515 nm (emission). No significant effects of the different stimulations could be detected with both assays (mean ± SD, $n = 3$, each in quintuplicate).

3.4. Infection with HCMV

Experiments with prASCs infection were done by HCMV strain Hi91, using a MOI of 0.05, 0.5, 1 and 4. Our results showed prASCs to be susceptible to HCMV even at MOI 0.05. The increase of viral load resulted in an augmented number of infected prASCs and progressive CPE (Figure 6B). Only very few cells were still adherent at 96 h post infection (MOI of 4), all being highly positive for HCMV gB/late antigen (Figure 6B). The HCMV specific mRNA of UL83-coded phosphoprotein HCMV virion protein was absent in controls and strongly expressed in prASCs 96 h after infection (Figure 6C), thus showing permissiveness of the cells.

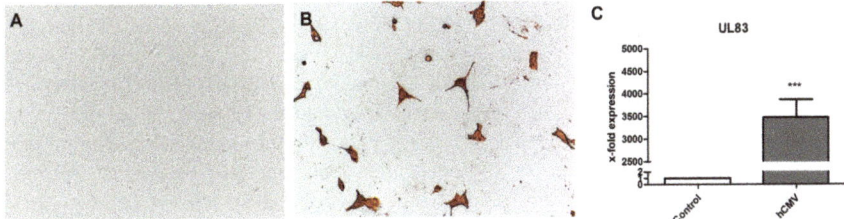

Figure 6. Infection of prASCs with HCMV Hi 91 for 96h. (**A**, **B**) Bright field microscopy of mock-infected prASCs (**A**) and HCMV-infected cells (**B**). Compared to the mock-infected controls (**A**) a strong CPE with very few adherent cells is seen 96 h after infection with HCMV at a MOI of 4 (**B**). All remaining cells are positive for HCMV late antigen, as shown by immunostaining. (**C**) Levels of UL83 mRNA were assessed after 96h. The expression levels in each experiment were normalized to β-actin and are calculated relative to the control using the ΔΔCT method (mean ± SD; * $p < 0.05$ versus control, $n = 3$).

4. Discussion

The abundance of MSCs, their multipotency and ability to secrete various cytokines, and their immunomodulatory effects account for their key role in current tissue regeneration approaches (i.e., Regenerative Medicine) [6]. The MSCs are present in all organs and tissues in vivo [2], and it has also been demonstrated that adipose tissue is a rich source of MSCs. Recent studies have explored the isolation, culture and characterization of MSCs from different adipose tissue depots [32]. The differences in gene expression between subcutaneous and visceral adipose tissue depots—when looking at total fat—have been described [32]. Regarding the tissue source, attention has also been paid to differences between cells derived from subcutaneous and visceral adipose tissue, and emerging evidence shows that there is also a significant variation between different visceral depots [32,33]. There is clear evidence that distinct differences in the expression profiles of developmental genes exist between all adipose tissue depots [32]. Nevertheless, we have not compared the ASCs isolated from different adipose origin in our current study. Adipose tissues have generally been classified as loose connective tissues [14]. Perirenal fat shares the same developmental origin as typical visceral fat. However, the perirenal adipose tissue is an atypical visceral fat pad with a complete system of blood supply, lymph fluid drainage and innervation [14] with near proximity to the kidneys. Perirenal adipose tissue is rarely described as the source of MSCs (or ASCs in particular). One possible reason for this is that the perirenal tissue cannot be easily recovered and an intervention in the perirenal space must be indicated for the removal. Our current study was conducted to characterize cultured MSCs from this cell source and to prove the potential of prASCs. The possible clinical use of prASCs for regenerative therapies is clearly restricted due to the limited tissue source. Thus, liposuction aspirate is easier to access as a cell source and, thus, better explored. In this study, we described the isolation and culture of human prASCs in detail, characterized cultured cells, investigated their multipotential differentiation, including epithelial differentiation, and their immunomodulatory capabilities in response to inflammatory stimuli. The isolation of prASCs could be done according to a protocol from liposuction aspirate established already [25,26]. Perirenal fat is another suitable source of ASC isolation, as also shown by others [21,22]. However, not all of our isolations could be successfully cultured. The cells were from morbid donors who had to be nephrectomized due to a malignant disease. Variability in the tumor dignity could be an explanation, in addition to genetic factors, for the inadequate growth of some isolations. A comparison of MSCs from different tissues, however, showed that MSCs from perirenal fat tissue have the same morphology and phenotypic characteristics as MSCs from other sources.

Since the first description of ASCs and their trilineage differentiation potential by Zuk and co-workers in 2001, many other lineages have been explored where ASCs can differentiate and how this differentiation can be induced. Several studies have shown that ASCs are able to differentiate into epithelial cells when cultured in media containing a retinoid (ATRA) [26], conditioned medium from epithelial cells [34] or a breast cancer cell line [35]. ATRA is an active metabolite of vitamin A and belongs to the retinoids. Retinoids have important functions in the growth and differentiation of tissues in vertebrates. An earlier study from our group showed the de novo expression of CK-18 and a reduction expression of the mesenchymal intermediate filament vimentin [26]. The type I intermediate filament CK-18 is characteristic of cells of single-layered epithelia and essential for normal tissue structure and function. Thus, CK-18 forms an important marker for the identification of epithelial cells. This result is considered to be the first step towards epithelial differentiation, because the intermediate filament vimentin is expressed exclusively in cells of mesenchymal origin. In the present work, medium containing ATRA was also used to stimulate the epithelial differentiation of prASCs. After two weeks of culture in induction media, we verified the epithelial differentiation by the induced expression of the characteristic marker CK-18.

The ASCs were also shown to play a role in the control of tissue inflammation and immunomodulation. The MSCs adopt an immunoregulatory phenotype in response to incubation (or pre-conditioning) with inflammatory factors (e.g., γ-Interferon (IFNγ), Interleukin 1β (IL-1β) or Tumor Necrosis Factor-α (TNFα)), in vivo secreted by activated immune cells [36]. In this context, administration of (pre-conditioned) ASCs could be used to decrease the severity of inflammation. Exemplarily, pre-conditioning of ASCs with inflammatory cytokines prior to cell transplantation is considered as a way to boost their immune regulatory function [37]. IFNγ, a pro-inflammatory cytokine acting against viral and bacterial infections, is one representative source for a pre-conditioning regimen for functional enhancement and upregulation of (pro- and anti-) inflammatory mediators [38,39]. The ASCs incubated with TNFα increased the secretion of IL-6 and IL-8, resulting in promoting endothelial progenitor cell homing and stimulating angiogenesis in an ischemic hindlimb model [40]. The ASCs pre-conditioned with IFNγ, TNFα and IL-6 showed enhanced immunosuppressive properties in vitro [41]. MSCs have also been shown to execute an immunosuppressive effect on lymphocyte proliferation in vitro [42]. In this context,, the inhibitory effect of histocompatibility locus antigen

(HLA)—G, expressed and released by MSCs, has been shown [43]. Nevertheless, we did not evaluate the effects of stimulated prASCs on lymphocyte populations and also have not determined the HLA-G expression of prASCs. In the current study, we used a mixture of three cytokines to investigate the stimulatory response of prASCs and measured the induction of pro-inflammatory cytokines (IL-6 and TNFα), a chemokine (MCP-1) and a cell adhesion molecule (ICAM-1). Taken together, pre-conditioning with inflammatory cytokines is a potential way to improve the therapeutic effectiveness for tissue injury and inflammatory disease [37,38].

In addition, ASCs also get in contact with bacterial components during invasive infections. Not much is known about how these pathogens (i.e., LPS and LTA) interact with ASCs and how contact to bacteria influences the secretome in ASCs. The TLRs mediate the activation process of cells by recognizing pathogen-associated molecular patterns, such as LPS or LTA. Activation of TLRs promotes the expression of various inflammatory cytokines, such as TNFα and other costimulatory molecules, and, therefore, initiates adaptive immune responses. Nevertheless, we were not able to show a significant stimulation via TLR-2 induced by LTA. Whereas most reports describe the anti-inflammatory properties (or immune suppressive) of MSCs, other reports target the pro-inflammatory characteristics of pre-conditioned MSCs. Studies reported that the activation of TLR-4 via LPS turned MSCs into a pro-inflammatory phenotype, whereas TLR-3 activation modified MSCs into an anti-inflammatory phenotype [38,44]. Incubation with low-dose LPS limited the immunosuppressive effects of ASCs by increasing IL-6 and TNFα expression, and also some growth factors [45]. Furthermore, it has been demonstrated that proliferation and osteogenic differentiation of adipose-derived MSCs is influenced by LPS [46,47]. Another study showed no significant influence of LPS or LTA on the migration rate and chemotaxis of MSCs [48]. More in vivo studies are needed to understand the immunomodulatory mechanisms of MSCs and the enhancement of this potential by in vitro pre-conditioning regimens.

The susceptibility and permissibility of prASCs to HCMV was not known before our experiments, but is consistent with reported productive infection of MSC derived from bone marrow [20], umbilical cord Wharton's jelly [49], placenta [50] and MSC from subcutaneous adipose tissue [51] The perivascular niche was described as a relevant MSC origin across the human organs [1]. In addition perivascular stromal cells host HCMV and are a likely long term reservoir [52]. Cell susceptibility to HCMV depends on entry receptor expression, like e.g., b3-Integrin (CD61), which is expressed on ASC [53] and the expression pattern of b1-integrin ((CD29) [54] which is also present on prASCs (see Figure 1C). Pathophysiologically, HCMV can induce an impairment of bone marrow-derived MSCs effector functions [55] and MSCs' differentiation potential [51]. Because of the perivascular cells' impact on vascular health further studies elucidating the in vitro and in vivo effects of HCMV infection in prASCs are warranted.

In summary, this study is the first comprehensive description of MSCs from perirenal adipose tissue in vitro. Our current study describes the isolation and culture of human prASCs, characterized cultured cells and the differentiation potential of prASCs into adipocytes, chondrocytes, osteoblasts and, for the first time, into epithelial cells. Furthermore, we showed the immunomodulatory potential of prASCs after stimulation with LPS or cytomix, and—also for the first time—high susceptibility as well as permissivity to HCMV. Interestingly, only LPS (from gram negative bacteria) induced a significant stimulation of prASCs, but no significant stimulation was found by after incubation with the pathogen of gram-positive bacteria.

Author Contributions: Investigation, P.C.B., B.K., E.H., J.C.J.; conceptualization, P.C.B., B.K., E.H., R.S., I.A.H., H.G.; formal analysis, P.C.B., E.H., J.C.J., I.A.H.; writing, review, and editing, P.C.B., B.K., R.S., H.G.

Funding: This research received no external funding.

Conflicts of Interest: The authors declare no conflict of interest.

Abbreviations

ASCs	Adipose-derived MSCs
ATRA	All-trans retinoic acid
CK	Cytokeratin
CPE	Viral load dependent cytopathological effect
FBS	Fetal bovine serum
HCMV	Human cytomegalovirus
ICAM-1	Intercellular adhesion molecule 1
IFNγ	γ−Interferon
IL	Interleukin
MCP-1	Monocyte chemotactic protein
MSCs	Mesenchymal stromal/stem cells
MOI	Multiplicity of infection
PCR	Polymerase chain reaction
prASCs	ASCs from perirenal adipose tissue
qPCR	Quantitative real-time polymerase chain reaction
RT	Room temperature
TLR	Toll-like receptor
TNFα	Tumor necrosis factor-α
UL83	HCMV-specific mRNA of UL83-coded phosphoprotein 65

References

1. Crisan, M.; Yap, S.; Casteilla, L.; Chen, C.-W.; Corselli, M.; Park, T.S.; Andriolo, G.; Sun, B.; Zheng, B.; Zhang, L.; et al. A perivascular origin for mesenchymal stem cells in multiple human organs. *Cell Stem Cell* **2008**, *3*, 301–313. [CrossRef] [PubMed]
2. Da Silva Meirelles, L.; Chagastelles, P.C.; Nardi, N.B. Mesenchymal stem cells reside in virtually all post-natal organs and tissues. *J. Cell Sci.* **2006**, *119*, 2204–2213. [CrossRef] [PubMed]
3. Baer, P.C.; Geiger, H. Adipose-derived mesenchymal stromal/stem cells: Tissue localization, characterization, and heterogeneity. *Stem Cells Int.* **2012**, *2012*, 812693. [CrossRef] [PubMed]
4. Durand, N.; Russell, A.; Zubair, A.C. Effect of Comedications and Endotoxins on Mesenchymal Stem Cell Secretomes, Migratory and Immunomodulatory Capacity. *J. Clin. Med.* **2019**, *8*, 497. [CrossRef] [PubMed]
5. Ponte, A.L.; Marais, E.; Gallay, N.; Langonné, A.; Delorme, B.; Hérault, O.; Charbord, P.; Domenech, J. The in vitro migration capacity of human bone marrow mesenchymal stem cells: Comparison of chemokine and growth factor chemotactic activities. *Stem Cells* **2007**, *25*, 1737–1745. [CrossRef] [PubMed]
6. Han, Y.; Li, X.; Zhang, Y.; Han, Y.; Chang, F.; Ding, J. Mesenchymal Stem Cells for Regenerative Medicine. *Cells* **2019**, *8*, 886. [CrossRef]
7. Gao, F.; Chiu, S.M.; Motan, D.A.L.; Zhang, Z.; Chen, L.; Ji, H.-L.; Tse, H.-F.; Fu, Q.-L.; Lian, Q. Mesenchymal stem cells and immunomodulation: Current status and future prospects. *Cell Death Dis.* **2016**, *7*, e2062. [CrossRef]
8. Raicevic, G.; Rouas, R.; Najar, M.; Stordeur, P.; Boufker, H.I.; Bron, D.; Martiat, P.; Goldman, M.; Nevessignsky, M.T.; Lagneaux, L. Inflammation modifies the pattern and the function of Toll-like receptors expressed by human mesenchymal stromal cells. *Hum. Immunol.* **2010**, *71*, 235–244. [CrossRef]
9. Liotta, F.; Angeli, R.; Cosmi, L.; Filì, L.; Manuelli, C.; Frosali, F.; Mazzinghi, B.; Maggi, L.; Pasini, A.; Lisi, V.; et al. Toll-like receptors 3 and 4 are expressed by human bone marrow-derived mesenchymal stem cells and can inhibit their T-cell modulatory activity by impairing Notch signaling. *Stem Cells* **2008**, *26*, 279–289. [CrossRef]
10. Cook, D.N.; Pisetsky, D.S.; Schwartz, D.A. Toll-like receptors in the pathogenesis of human disease. *Nat. Immunol.* **2004**, *5*, 975–979. [CrossRef]
11. Lynes, M.D.; Tseng, Y.-H. Deciphering adipose tissue heterogeneity. *Ann. N.Y. Acad. Sci.* **2018**, *1411*, 5–20. [CrossRef] [PubMed]
12. Pellegrinelli, V.; Carobbio, S.; Vidal-Puig, A. Adipose tissue plasticity: How fat depots respond differently to pathophysiological cues. *Diabetologia* **2016**, *59*, 1075–1088. [CrossRef] [PubMed]

13. Kwok, K.H.M.; Lam, K.S.L.; Xu, A. Heterogeneity of white adipose tissue: Molecular basis and clinical implications. *Exp. Mol. Med.* **2016**, *48*, e215. [CrossRef] [PubMed]
14. Liu, B.-X.; Sun, W.; Kong, X.-Q. Perirenal Fat: A Unique Fat Pad and Potential Target for Cardiovascular Disease. *Angiology* **2019**, *70*, 584–593. [CrossRef] [PubMed]
15. Chau, Y.-Y.; Bandiera, R.; Serrels, A.; Martínez-Estrada, O.M.; Qing, W.; Lee, M.; Slight, J.; Thornburn, A.; Berry, R.; McHaffie, S.; et al. Visceral and subcutaneous fat have different origins and evidence supports a mesothelial source. *Nat. Cell Biol.* **2014**, *16*, 367–375. [CrossRef] [PubMed]
16. Favre, G.; Grangeon-Chapon, C.; Raffaelli, C.; François-Chalmin, F.; Iannelli, A.; Esnault, V. Perirenal fat thickness measured with computed tomography is a reliable estimate of perirenal fat mass. *PLoS ONE* **2017**, *12*, e0175561. [CrossRef]
17. Foster, M.C.; Hwang, S.-J.; Porter, S.A.; Massaro, J.M.; Hoffmann, U.; Fox, C.S. Fatty kidney, hypertension, and chronic kidney disease: The Framingham Heart Study. *Hypertension* **2011**, *58*, 784–790. [CrossRef]
18. Czaja, K.; Kraeling, R.R.; Barb, C.R. Are hypothalamic neurons transsynaptically connected to porcine adipose tissue? *Biochem. Biophys. Res. Commun.* **2003**, *311*, 482–485. [CrossRef]
19. Sundin, M.; Orvell, C.; Rasmusson, I.; Sundberg, B.; Ringdén, O.; Le Blanc, K. Mesenchymal stem cells are susceptible to human herpesviruses, but viral DNA cannot be detected in the healthy seropositive individual. *Bone Marrow Transplant.* **2006**, *37*, 1051–1059. [CrossRef]
20. Smirnov, S.V.; Harbacheuski, R.; Lewis-Antes, A.; Zhu, H.; Rameshwar, P.; Kotenko, S.V. Bone-marrow-derived mesenchymal stem cells as a target for cytomegalovirus infection: Implications for hematopoiesis, self-renewal and differentiation potential. *Virology* **2007**, *360*, 6–16. [CrossRef]
21. Hoogduijn, M.J.; Crop, M.J.; Peeters, A.M.A.; van Osch, G.J.V.M.; Balk, A.H.M.M.; Ijzermans, J.N.M.; Weimar, W.; Baan, C.C. Human heart, spleen, and perirenal fat-derived mesenchymal stem cells have immunomodulatory capacities. *Stem Cells Dev.* **2007**, *16*, 597–604. [CrossRef] [PubMed]
22. Crop, M.J.; Baan, C.C.; Korevaar, S.S.; Ijzermans, J.N.M.; Alwayn, I.P.J.; Weimar, W.; Hoogduijn, M.J. Donor-derived mesenchymal stem cells suppress alloreactivity of kidney transplant patients. *Transplantation* **2009**, *87*, 896–906. [CrossRef] [PubMed]
23. Crop, M.J.; Baan, C.C.; Korevaar, S.S.; Ijzermans, J.N.M.; Weimar, W.; Hoogduijn, M.J. Human adipose tissue-derived mesenchymal stem cells induce explosive T-cell proliferation. *Stem Cells Dev.* **2010**, *19*, 1843–1853. [CrossRef] [PubMed]
24. Griesche, N.; Luttmann, W.; Luttmann, A.; Stammermann, T.; Geiger, H.; Baer, P.C. A simple modification of the separation method reduces heterogeneity of adipose-derived stem cells. *Cells Tissues Organs (Print)* **2010**, *192*, 106–115. [CrossRef]
25. Baer, P.C.; Brzoska, M.; Geiger, H. Epithelial differentiation of human adipose-derived stem cells. *Methods Mol. Biol.* **2011**, *702*, 289–298. [CrossRef]
26. Brzoska, M.; Geiger, H.; Gauer, S.; Baer, P. Epithelial differentiation of human adipose tissue-derived adult stem cells. *Biochem. Biophys. Res. Commun.* **2005**, *330*, 142–150. [CrossRef]
27. Michaelis, M.; Paulus, C.; Löschmann, N.; Dauth, S.; Stange, E.; Doerr, H.W.; Nevels, M.; Cinatl, J. The multi-targeted kinase inhibitor sorafenib inhibits human cytomegalovirus replication. *Cell. Mol. Life Sci.* **2011**, *68*, 1079–1090. [CrossRef]
28. Cinatl, J.; Weber, B.; Rabenau, H.; Gümbel, H.O.; Chenot, J.F.; Scholz, M.; Encke, A.; Doerr, H.W. In vitro inhibition of human cytomegalovirus replication in human foreskin fibroblasts and endothelial cells by ascorbic acid 2-phosphate. *Antivir. Res.* **1995**, *27*, 405–418. [CrossRef]
29. Overath, J.M.; Gauer, S.; Obermüller, N.; Schubert, R.; Schäfer, R.; Geiger, H.; Baer, P.C. Short-term preconditioning enhances the therapeutic potential of adipose-derived stromal/stem cell-conditioned medium in cisplatin-induced acute kidney injury. *Exp. Cell Res.* **2016**, *342*, 175–183. [CrossRef]
30. Pfaffl, M.W. A new mathematical model for relative quantification in real-time RT–PCR. *Nucleic Acids Res.* **2001**, *29*, e45. [CrossRef]
31. Baer, P.C.; Bereiter-Hahn, J.; Schubert, R.; Geiger, H. Differentiation status of human renal proximal and distal tubular epithelial cells in vitro: Differential expression of characteristic markers. *Cells Tissues Organs (Print)* **2006**, *184*, 16–22. [CrossRef] [PubMed]
32. Cleal, L.; Aldea, T.; Chau, Y.-Y. Fifty shades of white: Understanding heterogeneity in white adipose stem cells. *Adipocyte* **2017**, *6*, 205–216. [CrossRef]

33. Ritter, A.; Friemel, A.; Fornoff, F.; Adjan, M.; Solbach, C.; Yuan, J.; Louwen, F. Characterization of adipose-derived stem cells from subcutaneous and visceral adipose tissues and their function in breast cancer cells. *Oncotarget* **2015**, *6*, 34475–34493. [CrossRef] [PubMed]

34. Baer, P.C.; Bereiter-Hahn, J.; Missler, C.; Brzoska, M.; Schubert, R.; Gauer, S.; Geiger, H. Conditioned medium from renal tubular epithelial cells initiates differentiation of human mesenchymal stem cells. *Cell Prolif.* **2009**, *42*, 29–37. [CrossRef] [PubMed]

35. Yang, J.; Xiong, L.; Wang, R.; Yuan, Q.; Xia, Y.; Sun, J.; Horch, R.E. In vitro expression of cytokeratin 18, 19 and tube formation of adipose-derived stem cells induced by the breast epithelial cell line HBL-100. *J. Cell. Mol. Med.* **2015**, *19*, 2827–2831. [CrossRef] [PubMed]

36. Hoogduijn, M.J.; Lombardo, E. Concise Review: Mesenchymal Stromal Cells Anno 2019: Dawn of the Therapeutic Era? *Stem Cells Transl. Med.* **2019**. [CrossRef] [PubMed]

37. Schäfer, R.; Spohn, G.; Baer, P.C. Mesenchymal Stem/Stromal Cells in Regenerative Medicine: Can Preconditioning Strategies Improve Therapeutic Efficacy? *Transfus. Med. Hemother.* **2016**, *43*, 256–267. [CrossRef]

38. Seo, Y.; Shin, T.-H.; Kim, H.-S. Current Strategies to Enhance Adipose Stem Cell Function: An Update. *Int. J. Mol. Sci.* **2019**, *20*, 3827. [CrossRef]

39. Krampera, M.; Cosmi, L.; Angeli, R.; Pasini, A.; Liotta, F.; Andreini, A.; Santarlasci, V.; Mazzinghi, B.; Pizzolo, G.; Vinante, F.; et al. Role for interferon-gamma in the immunomodulatory activity of human bone marrow mesenchymal stem cells. *Stem Cells* **2006**, *24*, 386–398. [CrossRef]

40. Kwon, Y.W.; Heo, S.C.; Jeong, G.O.; Yoon, J.W.; Mo, W.M.; Lee, M.J.; Jang, I.-H.; Kwon, S.M.; Lee, J.S.; Kim, J.H. Tumor necrosis factor-α-activated mesenchymal stem cells promote endothelial progenitor cell homing and angiogenesis. *Biochim. Biophys. Acta* **2013**, *1832*, 2136–2144. [CrossRef]

41. Crop, M.J.; Baan, C.C.; Korevaar, S.S.; Ijzermans, J.N.M.; Pescatori, M.; Stubbs, A.P.; van Ijcken, W.F.J.; Dahlke, M.H.; Eggenhofer, E.; Weimar, W.; et al. Inflammatory conditions affect gene expression and function of human adipose tissue-derived mesenchymal stem cells. *Clin. Exp. Immunol.* **2010**, *162*, 474–486. [CrossRef] [PubMed]

42. Nasef, A.; Zhang, Y.Z.; Mazurier, C.; Bouchet, S.; Bensidhoum, M.; Francois, S.; Gorin, N.C.; Lopez, M.; Thierry, D.; Fouillard, L.; et al. Selected Stro-1-enriched bone marrow stromal cells display a major suppressive effect on lymphocyte proliferation. *Int. J. Lab. Hematol.* **2009**, *31*, 9–19. [CrossRef] [PubMed]

43. Nasef, A.; Mathieu, N.; Chapel, A.; Frick, J.; François, S.; Mazurier, C.; Boutarfa, A.; Bouchet, S.; Gorin, N.-C.; Thierry, D.; et al. Immunosuppressive effects of mesenchymal stem cells: Involvement of HLA-G. *Transplantation* **2007**, *84*, 231–237. [CrossRef] [PubMed]

44. Waterman, R.S.; Tomchuck, S.L.; Henkle, S.L.; Betancourt, A.M. A new mesenchymal stem cell (MSC) paradigm: Polarization into a pro-inflammatory MSC1 or an Immunosuppressive MSC2 phenotype. *PLoS ONE* **2010**, *5*, e10088. [CrossRef] [PubMed]

45. Lee, S.C.; Jeong, H.J.; Lee, S.K.; Kim, S.-J. Lipopolysaccharide preconditioning of adipose-derived stem cells improves liver-regenerating activity of the secretome. *Stem Cell Res. Ther.* **2015**, *6*, 75. [CrossRef] [PubMed]

46. Fiedler, T.; Salamon, A.; Adam, S.; Herzmann, N.; Taubenheim, J.; Peters, K. Impact of bacteria and bacterial components on osteogenic and adipogenic differentiation of adipose-derived mesenchymal stem cells. *Exp. Cell Res.* **2013**, *319*, 2883–2892. [CrossRef]

47. Herzmann, N.; Salamon, A.; Fiedler, T.; Peters, K. Lipopolysaccharide induces proliferation and osteogenic differentiation of adipose-derived mesenchymal stromal cells in vitro via TLR4 activation. *Exp. Cell Res.* **2017**, *350*, 115–122. [CrossRef]

48. Herzmann, N.; Salamon, A.; Fiedler, T.; Peters, K. Analysis of migration rate and chemotaxis of human adipose-derived mesenchymal stem cells in response to LPS and LTA in vitro. *Exp. Cell Res.* **2016**, *342*, 95–103. [CrossRef]

49. Qiao, G.-H.; Zhao, F.; Cheng, S.; Luo, M.-H. Multipotent mesenchymal stromal cells are fully permissive for human cytomegalovirus infection. *Virol. Sin.* **2016**, *31*, 219–228. [CrossRef]

50. Avanzi, S.; Leoni, V.; Rotola, A.; Alviano, F.; Solimando, L.; Lanzoni, G.; Bonsi, L.; Di Luca, D.; Marchionni, C.; Alvisi, G.; et al. Susceptibility of human placenta derived mesenchymal stromal/stem cells to human herpesviruses infection. *PLoS ONE* **2013**, *8*, e71412. [CrossRef]

51. Zwezdaryk, K.J.; Ferris, M.B.; Strong, A.L.; Morris, C.A.; Bunnell, B.A.; Dhurandhar, N.V.; Gimble, J.M.; Sullivan, D.E. Human cytomegalovirus infection of human adipose-derived stromal/stem cells restricts differentiation along the adipogenic lineage. *Adipocyte* **2016**, *5*, 53–64. [CrossRef] [PubMed]
52. Soland, M.A.; Keyes, L.R.; Bayne, R.; Moon, J.; Porada, C.D.; St Jeor, S.; Almeida-Porada, G. Perivascular stromal cells as a potential reservoir of human cytomegalovirus. *Am. J. Transplant.* **2014**, *14*, 820–830. [CrossRef] [PubMed]
53. Baer, P.C.; Kuçi, S.; Krause, M.; Kuçi, Z.; Zielen, S.; Geiger, H.; Bader, P.; Schubert, R. Comprehensive phenotypic characterization of human adipose-derived stromal/stem cells and their subsets by a high throughput technology. *Stem Cells Dev.* **2013**, *22*, 330–339. [CrossRef] [PubMed]
54. Kawasaki, H.; Kosugi, I.; Meguro, S.; Iwashita, T. Pathogenesis of developmental anomalies of the central nervous system induced by congenital cytomegalovirus infection. *Pathol. Int.* **2017**, *67*, 72–82. [CrossRef] [PubMed]
55. Meisel, R.; Heseler, K.; Nau, J.; Schmidt, S.K.; Leineweber, M.; Pudelko, S.; Wenning, J.; Zimmermann, A.; Hengel, H.; Sinzger, C.; et al. Cytomegalovirus infection impairs immunosuppressive and antimicrobial effector functions of human multipotent mesenchymal stromal cells. *Mediat. Inflamm.* **2014**, *2014*, 898630. [CrossRef] [PubMed]

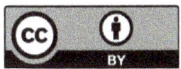

© 2019 by the authors. Licensee MDPI, Basel, Switzerland. This article is an open access article distributed under the terms and conditions of the Creative Commons Attribution (CC BY) license (http://creativecommons.org/licenses/by/4.0/).

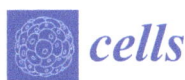

Article

Murine Mesenchymal Stromal Cells Retain Biased Differentiation Plasticity Towards Their Tissue of Origin

Ting Ting Ng [1], Kylie Hin-Man Mak [1], Christian Popp [1] and Ray Kit Ng [1,2,*]

[1] School of Biomedical Sciences, Li Ka Shing Faculty of Medicine, The University of Hong Kong, Hong Kong SAR, China; karinetingting.ng@gmail.com (T.T.N.); kyliehm@connect.hku.hk (K.H.-M.M.); christianpopp123@gmail.com (C.P.)
[2] Shenzhen Institute of Research and Innovation, The University of Hong Kong, Hong Kong SAR, China
* Correspondence: raykitng@hku.hk

Received: 29 February 2020; Accepted: 18 March 2020; Published: 19 March 2020

Abstract: Mesenchymal stromal/stem cells (MSCs) reside in many human tissues and comprise a heterogeneous population of cells with self-renewal and multi-lineage differentiation potential, making them useful in regenerative medicine. It remains inconclusive whether MSCs isolated from different tissue sources exhibit variations in biological features. In this study, we derived MSCs from adipose tissue (AT-MSC) and compact bone (CB-MSC). We found that early passage of MSCs was readily expandable ex vivo, whereas the prolonged culture of MSCs showed alteration of cell morphology to fibroblastoid and reduced proliferation. CB-MSCs and AT-MSCs at passage 3 were $CD29^+$, $CD44^+$, $CD105^+$, $CD106^+$, and $Sca-1^+$; however, passage 7 MSCs showed a reduction of MSC markers, indicating loss of stem cell population after prolonged culturing. Strikingly, CB-MSC was found more efficient at undergoing osteogenic differentiation, while AT-MSC was more efficient to differentiate into adipocytes. The biased differentiation pattern of MSCs from adipogenic or osteogenic tissue source was accompanied by preferential expression of the corresponding lineage marker genes. Interestingly, CB-MSCs treated with DNA demethylation agent 5-azacytidine showed enhanced osteogenic and adipogenic differentiation, whereas the treated AT-MSCs are less competent to differentiate. Our results suggest that the epigenetic state of MSCs is associated with the biased differentiation plasticity towards its tissue of origin, proposing a mechanism related to the retention of epigenetic memory. These findings facilitate the selection of optimal tissue sources of MSCs and the ex vivo expansion period for therapeutic applications.

Keywords: mesenchymal stromal cell; differentiation; tissue of origin; prolonged culture; epigenetic memory

1. Introduction

Mesenchymal stromal cells (MSCs), also referred to mesenchymal stem cells [1], represent a heterogeneous population of cells that can be isolated from a wide range of tissues, including bone marrow, compact bone, placenta and adipose tissue [2–6]. MSC was first isolated from mouse bone marrow as fibroblast colony-forming units, which were distinguished by their ability to adhere to plastic culture dishes [2]. They display fibroblastic morphology and are capable of differentiation to chondrocytes, adipocytes, and osteoblasts in vitro [1,7]. Differentiation to other non-mesodermal cell types, such as neurons, muscles, endothelial cells, and hepatocytes, has also been reported [8–11]. MSCs are intensely studied in clinical research because of their multi-lineage potential and ease of isolation and culture [1,12]. In addition, their ability to evade the host immune system by suppressing T cells, B cells, and natural killer cells [13], and releasing anti-inflammatory proteins [14,15] have made them an important tool for disease treatment. Clinical trials using MSCs for the treatment of osteoarthritis, degenerative disc disease, ischemic heart disease, and stroke are currently undergoing to explore their therapeutic applications [12].

Harvesting MSCs from the non-bone marrow tissue sources can be done by less invasive methods and the primary isolated MSCs can be expanded ex vivo to yield a larger number. Therefore, these non-bone marrow-derived MSCs are considered as an attractive repertoire for stem cell and regenerative medicine. In light of the broad potentials for therapeutic applications and the variety of sources for MSCs, it has been reported that MSCs, regardless of their tissue of origins, displayed similar characteristics in the differentiation to adipocytes, chondrocytes and osteocytes [16–18]. However, other studies comparing MSCs from human bone marrow, skin and adipose tissues showed considerable differences in their growth rate and differentiation potentials [19,20], supporting the hypothesis of preferential differentiation hierarchies [21,22]. It, therefore, remains inconclusive on the characteristics and the differentiation potentials of MSCs obtained from various tissue sources.

With such variability in mind, a better understanding of the differences between MSCs from different tissue origins can help identify the most suitable cell source for specific clinical purposes. Here we compared and characterized murine MSCs obtained from the adipose tissues (AT-MSC) and compact bone (CB-MSC) using standard isolation methods and expanded ex vivo at early and late cell passages. Both MSCs cultured for an extended period of time showed morphological changes and a decline in cell proliferation. We also demonstrated the tissue origin of MSC is associated with the alterations of cell surface marker patterns and differentiation potential towards osteogenic and adipogenic lineages. Removal of DNA methylation by pharmacological agent can alter the biased differentiation potential of MSCs dependent on the tissue source.

2. Materials and Methods

2.1. MSC Isolation and Culture

MSCs were harvested from 8-week old C57BL/6 mice (Laboratory Animal Unit, The University of Hong Kong). Written informed consent to use the animals was approved by the Committee on the Use of Live Animals in Teaching and Research of the University of Hong Kong (Reference no.: 2416-11). Three mice were used for the MSC isolation experiment and a total of five experiments were performed. The male to female ratio was 2:1. Mice were sacrificed by over-dosage of isoflurane inhalation. The MSC isolation procedures were described previously [5,23]. For CB-MSC isolation, muscles from femur, humerus, and tibia were removed. The epiphyseal ends of the bone were cut and discarded. Bone marrow was released by gently crushing the bones in cold PBS with 2% FBS (Gibco, Invitrogen, Grand Island, NY, USA) and 1 mM EDTA (Sigma-Aldrich, St. Louis, MO, USA). The cleaned bone fragments were digested in 0.25% collagenase I (Gibco) with 20% FBS for 5 min at 37 °C. The bone fragments were further chopped into 1–2 mm bits and digested for another 45 min at 37 °C. CB-MSCs were separated from the bone fragments by filtering the cell suspension through a 70 μm cell strainer (BD Biosciences, Franklin Lakes, NJ, USA). For AT-MSC isolation, adipose tissue dissected from inguinal and subcutaneous sites was digested in 5% collagenase I (Gibco) for 1 h at 37 °C. Cells were released from the adipose tissue by centrifuging for 5 min at 500× g. The released cells were treated with ammonium-chloride-potassium (ACK) lysing buffer (Sigma-Aldrich) for 3 min at room temperature to lyse red blood cells. The cell suspension was washed twice with α-MEM and tissue debris was removed by filtering through a 70 μm cell strainer. The isolated cell suspension (5×10^6) were cultured in α-MEM with 10% fetal bovine serum (FBS) (HyClone, Logan, UT, USA) and 1× penicillin-streptomycin-glutamine (Gibco) on a 100 mm culture dish at 37 °C with 5% CO_2. MSCs were adhered within 48 h. The culture medium was changed every 2 days. MSCs were passaged in a 1:4 ratio when reaching 80% confluence by Accutase (Gibco) for 5 min at 37 °C.

2.2. Cell Proliferation and Immunophenotypic Analysis

AT-MSCs and CB-MSCs (2×10^4 cells) were seeded into 6-well plates on day 0. The total number of expanded cells were counted at day 1, 3 and 5. Cell doubling time (DT) was calculated by the following formula: $DT = T \times \ln2/\ln \times (Xe/Xb)$, where T is the incubation time in any units; Xb is the cell number at the beginning of the incubation time; Xe is the cell number at the end of the incubation time.

Cultured cells were stained with FITC-conjugated anti-CD29 or anti-c-kit, PE-conjugated anti-CD44, anti-CD45, anti-CD106 or anti-Sca-1, APC-conjugated anti-CD105, and APC-Cy7-conjugated anti-CD11b (all from Biolegend, San Diego, CA, USA) at a concentration of 0.5 µg/mL for 30 min at 4 °C. The corresponding fluorophore-conjugated isotype controls were used for the gating of the positive-stained cells. Immunophenotypic analysis of 5000–10,000 cells of each sample was performed using FACSCanto II flow cytometer (BD Biosciences). The flow cytometry data were analyzed using Flowjo software (Tree Star, Ashland, OR, USA, ver. 10.0.7). Both assays were performed three times with duplicated samples.

2.3. MSC Differentiation Assays

MSCs at passage 3 or 7 (6×10^4 cells) were seeded into 24-well plates. One group of MSCs was treated with 0.5 µM 5-azacytidine (5-aza, Sigma-Aldrich) for 48 h prior to differentiation. For osteogenic differentiation, MSCs were differentiated in α-MEM with 10% FBS and StemXVivo Mouse/Rat Osteogenic Supplement (R&D Systems, Minneapolis, MN, USA) for 18 days. Differentiated cells were fixed in 4% formaldehyde (Sigma-Aldrich) for 10 min at room temperature and stained with 2% Alizarin Red solution (Chemicon, Merck Millipore, Billerica, MA, USA) for 15 min at room temperature. For adipogenic differentiation, MSCs were differentiated in α-MEM with 10% FBS and StemXVivo Adipogenic Supplement (R&D Systems) for 14 days. Differentiated cells were fixed in 4% formaldehyde (Sigma-Aldrich) for 10 min at room temperature and stained with 0.5% Oil Red O solution (Sigma-Aldrich) for 15 min at room temperature. For chondrogenic differentiation, MSCs were centrifuged for 5 min at 200× *g* in a 1.5 mL tube and differentiated in DMEM /F-12 with 1× Insulin-Transferrin-Selenium (Gibco) and StemXVivo Human/Mouse Chondrogenic Supplement (R&D Systems) for 21 days. Chondrocyte spheroids were fixed in 4% formaldehyde (Sigma-Aldrich) for 1 h at room temperature and stained with Alcian Blue 8GX solution (Sigma-Aldrich) for 30 min at room temperature. MSCs cultured in the differentiation medium without supplements were served as controls. The differentiation assay was performed three times with duplicated samples.

2.4. RNA Extraction and Quantitative RT-PCR (qRT-PCR)

Total RNA was extracted from the differentiated MSCs using MiniBEST Universal RNA Extraction Kit (Takara, Kusatsu, Japan). Genomic DNA eraser column and DNaseI treatment were used to remove genomic DNA. cDNA was synthesized using PrimeScriptTM RT reagent kit with gDNA Eraser (Takara) according to the manufacturer's protocol. qRT-PCR was performed with the 7900HT Fast Real-Time PCR System (Applied Biosystems, Waltham, MA, USA) using SYBR Premix Ex TaqTM (Takara) with the oligo primers listed in Supplementary Table S1. *Gapdh* and *β-Actin* served as house-keeping genes for normalization of gene expression. All samples were analyzed in triplicate. Three independent experiments were performed and relative gene expression was calculated using $2^{-\Delta\Delta CT}$ method.

2.5. Statistical Analysis

A statistically significant difference was calculated by two-tailed unpaired Student's *t*-test.

3. Results

3.1. Ex Vivo Expansion of MSC Isolated from Compact Bone and Adipose Tissue

Murine MSCs isolated from the adipose tissue (AT) and compact bone (CB) were expanded ex vivo. Both AT-MSCs and CB-MSCs displayed spindle-like to fibroblastoid cell morphology [4,5,23]. It was observed that cells at passage one (P1) contain a small number of cells with spherical shape, which were presumably dividing cells or non-MSCs (Figure 1a,e). However, continuous passaging of cells to the third passage (P3), which is one week of culture, gradually eliminated the non-MSC populations and enriched for MSCs (Figure 1b,f). From passage three (P3) onwards, cell morphology changed from elongated to fibroblastoid in both cultures (Figure 1b–d,f–h).

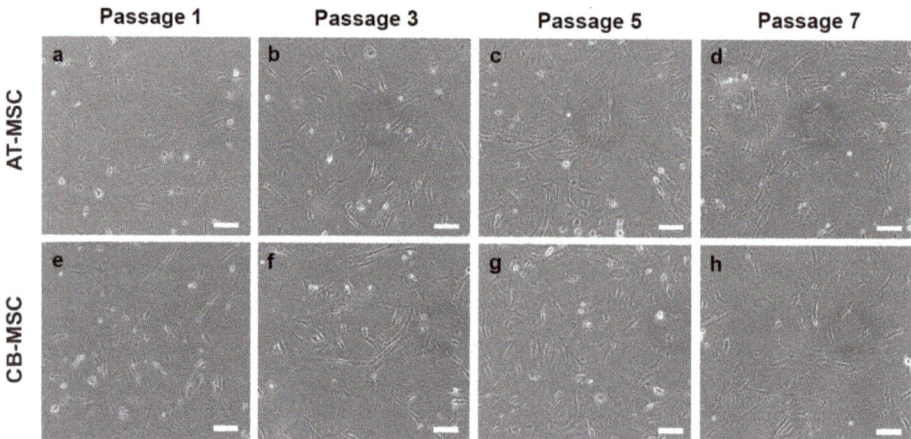

Figure 1. Cell morphology of AT-MSC and CB-MSC. Morphologies of MSCs at (**a,e**) passage 1, (**b,f**) passage 3, (**c,g**) passage 5, and (**d,h**) passage 7 were shown. Cell morphology changed gradually from spindle-like to flat and fibroblastoid with increasing passage number. Representative images were taken at 20× magnification. Scale bars: 100 μm.

Ex vivo culture of AT-MSC and CB-MSC at P3 or P7 for 5 days demonstrated cell number expansion. P3 and P7 AT-MSC showed limited expansion by 2.2- and 1.5-fold, respectively; whereas P3 and P7 CB-MSC were expanded 4.3- and 3.3-fold, respectively (Figure 2a,b). Besides, it was found that the doubling time of CB-MSC was comparable between both passages (2.4 days and 2.8 days for P4 and P7, respectively); however, AT-MSC demonstrated a significant increase in doubling time from P4 (4.3 days) to P7 (8.9 days) (Figure 2c). These results demonstrated different cell proliferation patterns between MSCs isolated from different tissue origins. Nevertheless, prolonged culture of both types of MSCs gradually reduced proliferation rate beyond passage 7.

3.2. Alterations of MSC Immunophenotypes by Prolonged Culture

Previous studies have shown that prolonged culture of MSC altered their immunophenotypes [24]. This prompt us to examine the expression of a panel of mesenchymal stromal cell surface markers, including CD29, CD44, CD105, CD106, and stem cell antigen-1 (Sca-1) [25–28], in the ex vivo expanded cells. Hematopoietic markers c-kit, CD11b, and CD45 were served as negative markers for the detection of contamination of hematopoietic cells from the MSC isolation procedures [27,29]. c-kit$^+$ and CD11b$^+$ populations were generally low in both types of MSCs, particularly for the late passage culture (Figure S1). It was observed that 38.4% of CD45$^+$ populations were present in P3 CB-MSC, suggesting a low degree of hematopoietic cell contamination from compact bone during MSC isolation.

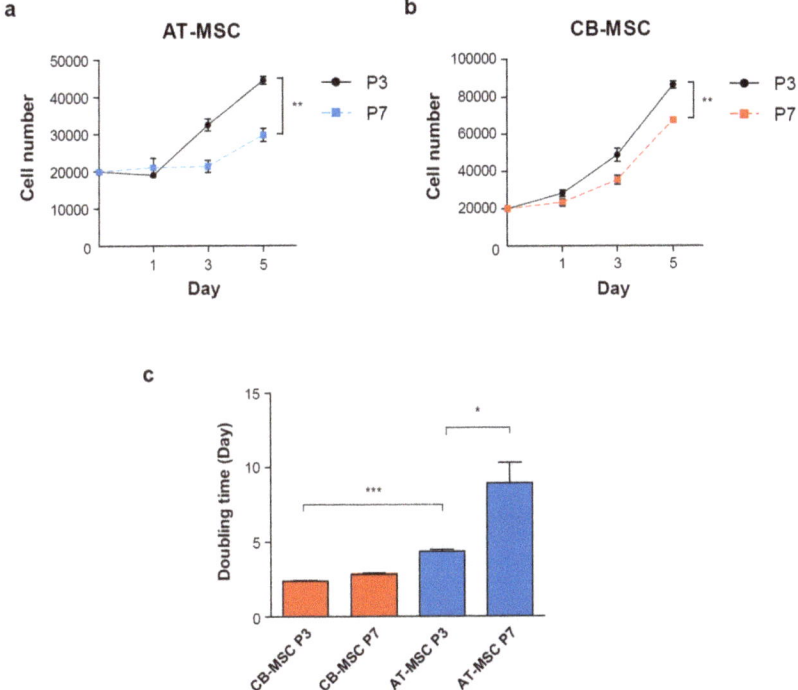

Figure 2. Ex vivo expansion of MSCs at different passage numbers. Cell proliferation assay was performed to determine the growth rate of early (Passage 3) and late passage (Passage 7) of (**a**) AT-MSC and (**b**) CB-MSC. Cells were counted on day 1, 3 and 5 (n = 3). (**c**) Doubling times of MSCs were calculated over 5 days of culture. CB-MSCs demonstrated a higher cell proliferation rate than AT-MSCs. The doubling time of AT-MSC was significantly increased at late passage. Experiments were performed with three replicates. Data represent mean ± SD; *p < 0.05, ** p < 0.01 and *** p < 0.001.

Nevertheless, the $CD45^+$ hematopoietic cells were gradually lost when cells passaging to P7. Both AT-MSCs and CB-MSCs demonstrated high expression of most of the MSC markers at passage 3. It was noted that $CD29^+$, $CD44^+$, and $CD106^+$ populations showed further increased in passage 7 (Table 1, Figure 3). However, $CD105^+$ population was reduced significantly at late passage MSCs. While a significant portion of the AT-MSC population retained as $CD105^+$ (33.6 ± 4.3%) at P7, the $CD105^+$ population in CB-MSC reduced drastically from 34.2% at P3 to 7.5% at P7. In contrast, CB-MSC consisted of over 83% Sca-1^+ cells at P3 and P7, whereas the Sca-1^+ population dropped from 98.5% to 26.3% in AT-MSC from P3 to P7. These immunophenotypic results demonstrated the alteration of MSC surface marker pattern during ex vivo culture, suggesting that prolonged culture of MSC is accompanied by the loss of MSC identity.

Table 1. Percentage of cell populations in AT-MSC and CB-MSC.

Sample	Passage	CD29	CD44	CD105	CD106	Sca-1	c-kit	CD11b	CD45
AT-MSC	P3	99.8 ± 0.1	18.3 ± 1.3	50.1 ± 2.4	38.1 ± 3.2	98.5 ± 0.7	2.1 ± 0.6	0.99 ± 0.2	0.71 ± 0.2
	P7	99.9 ± 0.0	41.8 ± 3.4 *	33.6 ± 4.3 *	54.3 ± 3.6 *	26.3 ± 4.4 **	1.8 ± 1.0	0.11 ± 0.1 *	0.1 ± 0.0 *
CB-MSC	P3	89.6 ± 4.2	87.9 ± 2.6	34.2 ± 3.3	60.2 ± 4.1	83.9 ± 5.4	6.7 ± 1.3	0.84 ± 0.4	38.4 ± 3.6
	P7	99.9 ± 0.1	94.5 ± 2.7	7.5 ± 1.7 *	99.1 ± 0.5 **	97.0 ± 1.8 *	0.3 ± 0.2 *	0.51 ± 0.3	1.1 ± 0.3 *

* p < 0.05 and ** p < 0.01 in the comparison between P3 and P7.

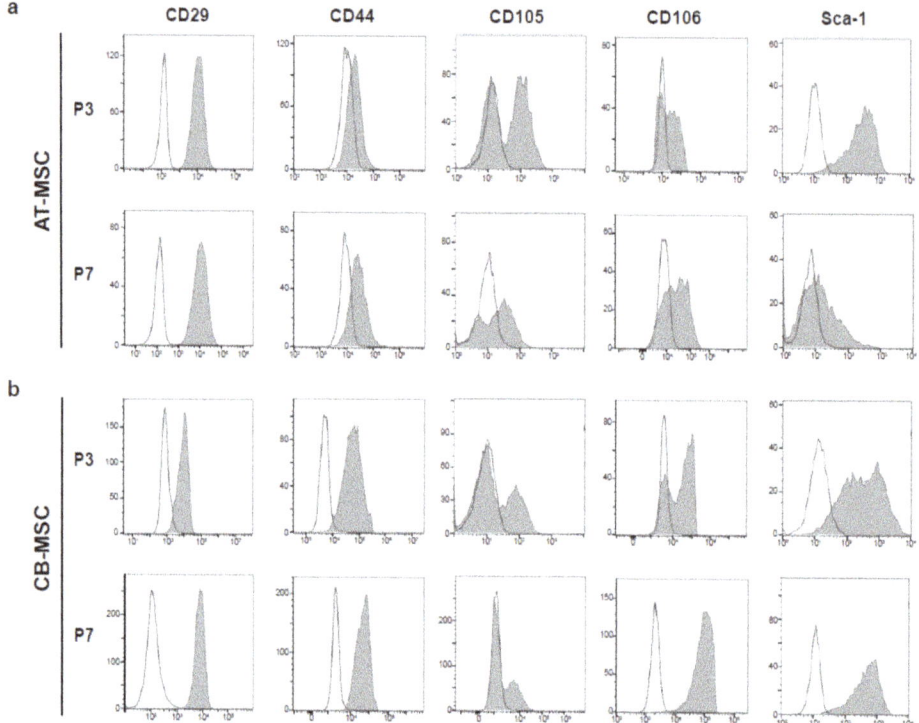

Figure 3. Immunophenotypes of MSCs. Cell surface markers for MSCs, CD29, CD44, CD105, CD106, and Sca-1 were used to characterize (**a**) AT-MSC and (**b**) CB-MSC at passage 3 (P3) and 7 (P7), respectively. Representative flow cytometry patterns were shown. Shaded peaks represent antibody-labeled population; blank peaks represented isotype controls.

3.3. Biased Differentiation Towards the Tissue Origin

A defining feature of MSC is their ability to differentiate into multiple mesodermal lineages. To examine the multi-lineage differentiation potentials of MSCs derived from different tissue origins, we induced in vitro differentiation of early and late passage (P3 and P7) AT-MSC and CB-MSC into the osteogenic, adipogenic, and chondrogenic lineages. We observed that both AT-MSCs and CB-MSCs were able to differentiate into the three lineages (Figure 4), indicating that MSCs from adipose tissue or compact bone are multipotent in nature. However, although both types of MSCs were able to form the positive Alcian Blue stained chondrocyte spheroids efficiently (Figure 4i–l), we observed that fewer cells stained positive with Alizarin Red in the AT-MSC sample (Figure 4a–d) and lower number of Oil Red O stained cells from CB-MSC sample (Figure 4e–h). Besides, the P7 MSCs of both types appeared to have weaker positive staining patterns when compared to the early P3 samples. These results suggest that MSCs derived from different tissue origins exhibit differentiation bias and their differentiation capacities reduce after prolonged culture.

To further elucidate the differentiation bias associated with the tissue origin of MSCs, we examined the expression of osteogenic (*Ocn* and *Opn*), adipogenic (*Adipoq* and *Pparg*) and chondrogenic (*Sox9* and *Col2a1*) markers in the differentiated MSC samples. Induction of *Ocn* and *Opn* were high in the osteogenic differentiation of P3 CB-MSC when compared to the P7 CB-MSC (over 4-fold for both genes). Importantly, osteogenic differentiated AT-MSC demonstrated significantly lower expression of these two osteogenic markers, regardless of the length of culture (Figure 5a, Figure S2a).

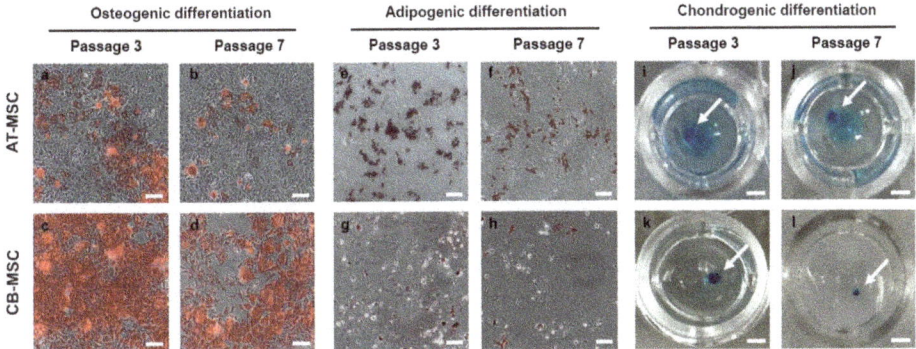

Figure 4. Osteogenic and adipogenic differentiation of MSCs. AT-MSCs and CB-MSCs underwent 18-day of osteogenic, 14-day of adipogenic, or 21-days of chondrogenic differentiation conditions. (**a–d**) Alizarin red staining, (**e–h**) Oil Red O staining, and (**i–l**) Alcian blue staining were used to assess osteogenic, adipogenic and chondrogenic differentiation, respectively. Passage 3 of CB-MSCs displayed stronger staining for Alizarin red; whereas passage 3 of AT-MSCs displayed stronger Oil-Red-O staining. Late passage MSCs showed weaker staining in both lineage differentiations. Chondrogenic differentiation is comparable in both types of MSCs. The white arrows indicate the stained chondrocyte spheroids. Representative images were taken at 20× (**a–h**) or 5× (**i–l**) magnification. Scale bars: (**a–h**) 100 µm; (**i–l**) 1 mm.

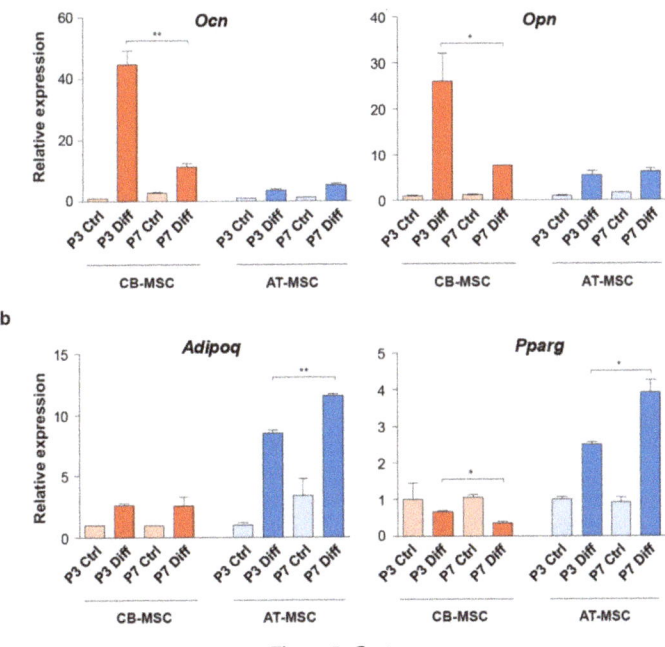

Figure 5. *Cont.*

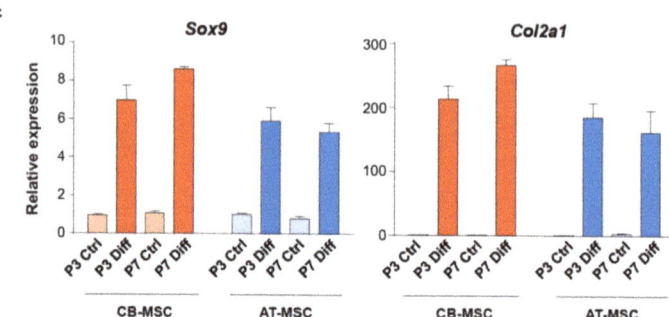

Figure 5. Expression of lineage marker genes in the differentiated MSCs. (**a**) Osteogenic markers, *Ocn* and *Opn*, (**b**) adipogenic markers, *Adipoq* and *Pparg*, and (**c**) chondrogenic markers, *Sox9* and *Col2a1*, were used to determine the multi-lineage differentiation of AT-MSCs and CB-MSCs. MSCs cultured in basic medium without differentiation agents for the same period of time were served as controls. Gene expressions were normalized with housekeeping gene *Gapdh*. Experiments were performed with three replicates. Data represent mean ± SD; *$p < 0.05$ and **$p < 0.01$.

In contrast, AT-MSCs were able to express a high level of *Adipoq* and *Pparg* when compared to the CB-MSCs in adipogenic differentiation (over 4-fold for both genes) (Figure 5b and Figure S2b). The expression of adipogenic markers was less pronounced between different passages of MSCs. We also noticed that the expression of *Sox9* and *Col2a1* was high in both types of differentiated MSCs (Figure 5c and Figure S2c), which implies comparable chondrogenic differentiation efficiency. Taken together, the differential expressions of osteogenic and adipogenic markers are in agreement with the Alizarin red and Oil Red O staining patterns (Figure 4), suggesting that MSCs, although harboring multi-lineage differentiation potential, have a preference to differentiate towards their tissues of origin.

3.4. Inhibition of DNA Methylation Alters MSC Multipotency

MSCs derived from different tissues could be modulated by the microenvironment which confers a differential epigenetic state associated with stem cell multipotency. To determine whether DNA methylation, a well-known epigenetic modification, is involved in the differentiation bias of CB-MSC and AT-MSC, we treated MSCs with the DNA methylation inhibitor, 5-azacytidine (5-aza), for 48 h prior in vitro differentiation. The 48-h treatment period was chosen based on the rationale that the epigenetic function of 5-aza as a DNA methylation inhibitor is dependent on cell division [30], which takes roughly 2 days (determined by the doubling time in Figure 2c) for both types of MSCs. Both types of MSCs under 5-aza treatment were able to differentiate into osteogenic and adipogenic lineages (Figure 6a). Interestingly, we observed that there were more osteogenic differentiated cells stained with Alizarin red from the 5-aza-treated CB-MSCs when comparing to the untreated sample. However, the number of osteogenic differentiated AT-MSCs remains low by the 5-aza treatment. This observation is in agreement with the qRT-PCR results of the osteogenic marker expression, which showed a significant increase in *Ocn* and *Opn* expression in the 5-aza-treated CB-MSCs (Figure 6b and Figure S3a). Unexpectedly, although the AT-MSCs are more competent to undergo adipogenic differentiation, the 5-aza treatment resulted in a lower number of Oil Red O stained cells (Figure 6a), with a significant decrease in the expression of adipogenic markers *Adipoq* and *Pparg* (Figure 6b and Figure S3b). By contrast, the treated CB-MSCs showed enhanced adipogenic differentiation with a comparable level of adipogenic marker gene expression to the untreated AT-MSCs. These results suggest that inhibition of DNA methylation can restore the biased differentiation capacity of CB-MSC to the adipogenic lineage, whereas AT-MSC loses its multipotency under the same epigenetic condition. It thus implies a differential epigenetic effect of 5-aza on the MSCs derived from different tissue sources.

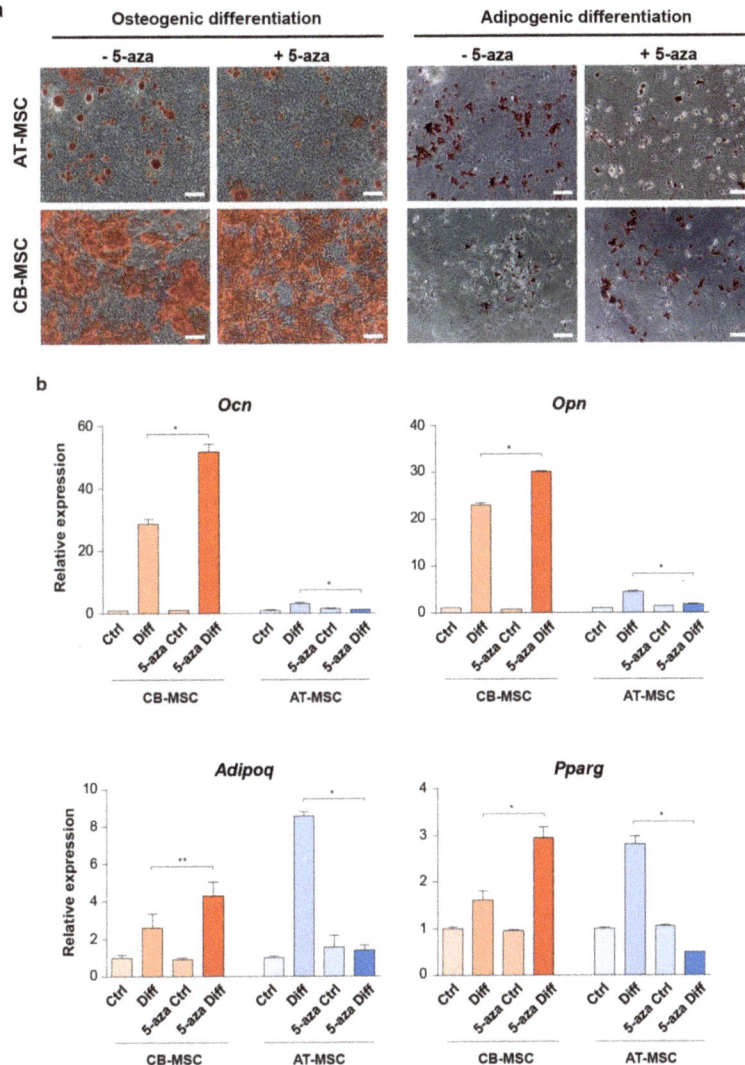

Figure 6. Osteogenic and adipogenic differentiation of the 5-aza-treated MSCs. (**a**) AT-MSCs and CB-MSCs were pre-treated with 5-aza for 48 h prior to osteogenic (Alizarin red staining) or adipogenic differentiation (Oil Red O staining). Representative images were taken at 20×. Scale bars: 100 μm. (**b**) The expression of osteocyte markers (*Ocn* and *Opn*) and adipocyte markers (*Adipoq* and *Pparg*) were determined by qRT-PCR. MSCs cultured in basic medium without differentiation agents for the same period of time were served as controls. Gene expressions were normalized with housekeeping gene *Gapdh*. Experiments were performed with three replicates. Data represent mean ± SD; * $p < 0.05$ and ** $p < 0.01$.

4. Discussion

In this study, murine MSCs were isolated from compact bone and adipose tissue. Our results showed that prolonged culture of MSC leads to changes in cell morphology and cell surface marker patterns, and cell proliferation rate. Importantly, the tissue origins of MSC have impact on their differentiation capacity towards the corresponding cell lineages, indicating the presence of epigenetic memory in the MSCs. The multipotency of CB-MSC, but not AT-MSC, can be enhanced through inhibition of DNA methylation prior differentiation, which suggests a possible strategy to erase the epigenetic memory in certain tissue-derived MSCs. Although we were using murine MSCs in our study, cross-species comparisons of MSC corroborated that the surface markers [31] and biological functions [32] of MSC are similar, even though not identical, between different species. There are numerous studies of the therapeutic applications of MSCs using mouse models for the investigation of the molecular mechanisms and the safety concerns prior to human clinical trials [33]. With the findings of preferential differentiation of murine MSCs derived from different tissues and the possible manipulation of the epigenetic memory in MSCs, we propose that our findings can be applied to human MSCs for the selection of optimal tissue source and the strategy to enhance the multipotency of human MSCs for therapeutic applications.

The immunophenotype of MSCs is dynamic over the culture period. MSCs isolated from various tissues were reported to express a common set of cell surface markers, such as CD105, CD90, CD73, CD29, and CD44, with a lack of CD34, CD45, CD11b, and major histocompatibility complex (MHC) class II expression [25]. The MSC isolation protocols retained the plastic adherent cells from the tissue, which invariably consist of a heterogeneous cell population including hematopoietic cells and other tissue cells. Nevertheless, the non-MSC populations presumably undergo depletion gradually in the MSC culture condition, resulting in a more homogeneous MSC population. In our study, we observed that nearly all the early passage MSCs from both compact bone and adipose tissue expressed CD29 and Sca-1, but only 34–50% are CD105$^+$ and 38–60% are CD106$^+$, suggesting the heterogeneity of MSC immunophenotypes. Prolonged culture of MSCs leads to loss of Sca-1 and CD105 expression, which is particularly obvious in the AT-MSCs and CB-MSCs, respectively. Similar observation for the loss of CD15, CD90, and CD309 was also reported in the neoplastic transformation of bone marrow-derived MSCs after numerous passages [34]. The loss of MSC immunophenotype is correlated with the findings of fibroblastoid morphology change, reduced cell proliferation and differentiation potentials of the late passage MSCs, suggesting that the "stemness" of MSCs cannot be maintained by prolonged culture. This is in agreement with the previous study of the prolonged culture of human bone marrow-derived MSCs with a loss of osteogenic potential [35]. However, the loss of stemness could be less prominent in other tissue-derived MSCs, for example, umbilical cord MSCs, which retained comparable growth rate and osteogenic capacity after 16 passages when compared to the freshly isolated one [36]. Although the MSC culture condition used in this study follows a common protocol in the field, the alterations of MSC phenotypes and cell functions owing to the prolonged culture might reflect a suboptimal condition that needs to be further optimized for better maintenance of the stemness of MSCs. In addition, it has been reported that a subpopulation of MSC is CD105 negative [37,38], which varies in the differentiation potentials and modulation of CD4$^+$ T cell proliferation when comparing to the CD105$^+$ counterpart. Interestingly, the CD105 expression in the CD105$^+$ MSCs can be altered by the culture condition, such as passage number, cell density, and medium composition [37,39]. Being a component of the TGF-β receptor, CD105 also serves as a proliferation marker of endothelial cells [40]. As we observed a reduction of MSC proliferation upon prolonged culturing, we speculate that this could be associated with the loss of CD105 expression in the P7 MSCs.

The biased differentiation capacity of MSCs derived from different tissues remains controversial. While several studies have reported that bone marrow-derived MSCs were more prone to osteogenic differentiation [17,41,42] and adipose tissue-derived MSCs showed decreased chondrogenic differentiation capacity [43,44], others demonstrated no significant differences in differentiation potentials of MSCs derived from various tissues [16–18]. In our study, we observed that both types of MSCs showed comparable chondrogenic differentiation, but preferential differentiation of AT-MSCs to adipo-lineage and CB-MSCs to osteo-lineage. It is proposed that the isolation procedures, culture condition, such as with serum or serum-free, and the heterogeneity of MSC populations may account for the preferential differentiation to certain lineages through enrichment of distinct MSC subpopulations. In addition, MSCs resided in different tissues are subjected to the distinct cellular microenvironments, e.g., signaling molecules, extracellular matrix components, metabolites, etc. These extrinsic factors can induce alterations of the MSC epigenome, leading to potential variations in transcriptomes and biological responses related to stemness [45]. This is indeed supported by the global transcriptomic and proteomic studies which demonstrated substantial differences in the expression of genes or proteins between MSCs derived from bone marrow and adipose tissue [17,20,46,47]. The biased differentiation of CB-MSC and AT-MSC also suggests that the altered epigenome is retained as the "epigenetic memory" of tissue origin. It is reported that the reprogrammed stem cells showed preferential differentiation towards their somatic lineage origins. The epigenetic memory of donor cell origin was found in *Xenopus* nuclear transplanted embryos [48] and early passage of induced pluripotent stem cells (iPSCs) [49,50]. It has been shown that blood-derived iPSCs were preferentially differentiated towards blood lineages and were defective to osteogenic differentiation, whereas bone marrow-derived iPSC demonstrated the opposite [50]. Although the derivation of MSCs does not involve cellular reprogramming, MSCs located at different tissues might be epigenetically reprogrammed by the tissue niche environment. Previous studies reported that the memory status in iPSC can be erased by extensive cell culture passages [49] or by epigenetic modifying agents, such as DNA methylation inhibitor [50]. It remains a challenge to test if the memory status of MSCs can be erased by prolonged culture because late passage MSCs undergo senescence and reduced overall differentiation capacity. Interestingly, our data showed that inhibition of DNA methylation can partially restore the adipogenic differentiation capacity of CB-MSCs, suggesting a possible way to erase the epigenetic memory in MSCs. However, we noticed that AT-MSCs failed to restore osteogenic differentiation after 5-aza treatment, suggesting the involvement of other types of epigenetic modifications, e.g., histone protein methylation or acetylation. Therefore, it is worth evaluating the effects of other epigenetic inhibitors, such as histone deacetylase inhibitors, on the multipotency of MSCs derived from other tissues.

5. Conclusions

We have demonstrated that early passage MSCs derived from compact bone or adipose tissue are highly proliferative and retain multipotent nature. The tissue origin of the MSCs results in epigenetic memory which implicates a preference for lineage differentiation. A better understanding of the molecular nature of such tissue origin memory can facilitate the choice of optimal sources of MSCs for tissue engineering and regenerative medicine.

Supplementary Materials: The following are available online at http://www.mdpi.com/2073-4409/9/3/756/s1, Figure S1: Immunophenotypes of hematopoietic markers on MSCs, Figure S2: Expression of lineage marker genes in the differentiated MSCs with reference to β-Actin gene, Figure S3: Expression of lineage marker genes in the differentiated 5-aza-treated MSCs with reference to β-Actin gene, Table S1: Primer sequences for qRT-PCR.

Author Contributions: Conceptualization, T.T.N. and R.K.N.; methodology, T.T.N.; validation, T.T.N., K.H.-M.M. and C.P.; formal analysis, T.T.N., R.K.N.; investigation, T.T.N.; data curation, K.H.-M.M., C.P.; writing—original draft preparation, T.T.N.; writing—review and editing, R.K.N.; supervision, R.K.N.; project administration, R.K.N.; funding acquisition, R.K.N. All authors have read and agreed to the published version of the manuscript

Funding: This research was funded by Research Grants Council General Research Fund, grant number HKU774712M, and Theme-based Research Scheme, grant number T12-708/12-N. The APC was funded by National Natural Science Foundation of China (NSFC) - Science Fund for Young Scholars, grant number 026-NG KIT_81200341, and NSFC-Shenzhen Matching Fund 2013, grant number 121-NG KIT_SIRI/04/04/2014/22.

Acknowledgments: The authors thank the Faculty Core Facility of the University of Hong Kong Li Ka Shing Faculty of Medicine for assistance with the flow cytometry analyses.

Conflicts of Interest: The authors declare no conflict of interest. The funders had no role in the design of the study; in the collection, analyses, or interpretation of data; in the writing of the manuscript, or in the decision to publish the results.

References

1. Nombela-Arrieta, C.; Ritz, J.; Silberstein, L.E. The elusive nature and function of mesenchymal stem cells. *Nat. Rev. Mol. Cell Biol.* **2011**, *12*, 126–131. [CrossRef] [PubMed]
2. Friedenstein, A.J.; Chailakhyan, R.K.; Latsinik, N.V.; Panasyuk, A.F.; Keiliss-Borok, I.V. Stromal cells responsible for transferring the microenvironment of the hemopoietic tissues. Cloning in vitro and retransplantation in vivo. *Transplantation* **1974**, *17*, 331–340. [CrossRef] [PubMed]
3. Fukuchi, Y.; Nakajima, H.; Sugiyama, D.; Hirose, I.; Kitamura, T.; Tsuji, K. Human placenta-derived cells have mesenchymal stem/progenitor cell potential. *Stem Cells* **2004**, *22*, 649–658. [CrossRef]
4. Short, B.; Wagey, R. Isolation and culture of mesenchymal stem cells from mouse compact bone. *Methods Mol. Biol.* **2013**, *946*, 335–347. [PubMed]
5. Zhu, H.; Guo, Z.K.; Jiang, X.X.; Li, H.; Wang, X.Y.; Yao, H.Y.; Zhang, Y.; Mao, N. A protocol for isolation and culture of mesenchymal stem cells from mouse compact bone. *Nat. Protoc.* **2010**, *5*, 550–560. [CrossRef] [PubMed]
6. Zhu, Y.; Liu, T.; Song, K.; Fan, X.; Ma, X.; Cui, Z. Adipose-derived stem cell: A better stem cell than BMSC. *Cell Biochem. Funct.* **2008**, *26*, 664–675. [CrossRef]
7. Pittenger, M.F.; Mackay, A.M.; Beck, S.C.; Jaiswal, R.K.; Douglas, R.; Mosca, J.D.; Moorman, M.A.; Simonetti, D.W.; Craig, S.; Marshak, D.R. Multilineage potential of adult human mesenchymal stem cells. *Science* **1999**, *284*, 143–147. [CrossRef]
8. Anghileri, E.; Marconi, S.; Pignatelli, A.; Cifelli, P.; Galie, M.; Sbarbati, A.; Krampera, M.; Belluzzi, O.; Bonetti, B. Neuronal differentiation potential of human adipose-derived mesenchymal stem cells. *Stem Cells Dev.* **2008**, *17*, 909–916. [CrossRef]
9. Mizuno, H.; Zuk, P.A.; Zhu, M.; Lorenz, H.P.; Benhaim, P.; Hedrick, M.H. Myogenic differentiation by human processed lipoaspirate cells. *Plast. Reconstr. Surg.* **2002**, *109*, 199–209, discussion 210–211. [CrossRef]
10. Oswald, J.; Boxberger, S.; Jorgensen, B.; Feldmann, S.; Ehninger, G.; Bornhauser, M.; Werner, C. Mesenchymal stem cells can be differentiated into endothelial cells in vitro. *Stem Cells* **2004**, *22*, 377–384. [CrossRef]
11. Snykers, S.; De Kock, J.; Rogiers, V.; Vanhaecke, T. In vitro differentiation of embryonic and adult stem cells into hepatocytes: State of the art. *Stem Cells* **2009**, *27*, 577–605. [CrossRef] [PubMed]
12. Trounson, A.; McDonald, C. Stem Cell Therapies in Clinical Trials: Progress and Challenges. *Cell Stem Cell* **2015**, *17*, 11–22. [CrossRef] [PubMed]
13. Spaggiari, G.M.; Capobianco, A.; Becchetti, S.; Mingari, M.C.; Moretta, L. Mesenchymal stem cell-natural killer cell interactions: Evidence that activated NK cells are capable of killing MSCs, whereas MSCs can inhibit IL-2-induced NK-cell proliferation. *Blood* **2006**, *107*, 1484–1490. [CrossRef] [PubMed]
14. Aggarwal, S.; Pittenger, M.F. Human mesenchymal stem cells modulate allogeneic immune cell responses. *Blood* **2005**, *105*, 1815–1822. [CrossRef] [PubMed]
15. Beyth, S.; Borovsky, Z.; Mevorach, D.; Liebergall, M.; Gazit, Z.; Aslan, H.; Galun, E.; Rachmilewitz, J. Human mesenchymal stem cells alter antigen-presenting cell maturation and induce T-cell unresponsiveness. *Blood* **2005**, *105*, 2214–2219. [CrossRef]
16. Kern, S.; Eichler, H.; Stoeve, J.; Kluter, H.; Bieback, K. Comparative analysis of mesenchymal stem cells from bone marrow, umbilical cord blood, or adipose tissue. *Stem Cells* **2006**, *24*, 1294–1301. [CrossRef]
17. Noel, D.; Caton, D.; Roche, S.; Bony, C.; Lehmann, S.; Casteilla, L.; Jorgensen, C.; Cousin, B. Cell specific differences between human adipose-derived and mesenchymal-stromal cells despite similar differentiation potentials. *Exp. Cell Res.* **2008**, *314*, 1575–1584. [CrossRef]
18. De Ugarte, D.A.; Morizono, K.; Elbarbary, A.; Alfonso, Z.; Zuk, P.A.; Zhu, M.; Dragoo, J.L.; Ashjian, P.; Thomas, B.; Benhaim, P.; et al. Comparison of multi-lineage cells from human adipose tissue and bone marrow. *Cells Tissues Organs* **2003**, *174*, 101–109. [CrossRef]
19. Al-Nbaheen, M.; Vishnubalaji, R.; Ali, D.; Bouslimi, A.; Al-Jassir, F.; Megges, M.; Prigione, A.; Adjaye, J.; Kassem, M.; Aldahmash, A. Human stromal (mesenchymal) stem cells from bone marrow, adipose tissue and skin exhibit differences in molecular phenotype and differentiation potential. *Stem Cell Rev.* **2013**, *9*, 32–43. [CrossRef]
20. Izadpanah, R.; Trygg, C.; Patel, B.; Kriedt, C.; Dufour, J.; Gimble, J.M.; Bunnell, B.A. Biologic properties of mesenchymal stem cells derived from bone marrow and adipose tissue. *J. Cell. Biochem.* **2006**, *99*, 1285–1297. [CrossRef]

21. Muraglia, A.; Cancedda, R.; Quarto, R. Clonal mesenchymal progenitors from human bone marrow differentiate in vitro according to a hierarchical model. *J. Cell Sci.* **2000**, *113*, 1161–1166. [PubMed]
22. Satomura, K.; Krebsbach, P.; Bianco, P.; Gehron Robey, P. Osteogenic imprinting upstream of marrow stromal cell differentiation. *J. Cell. Biochem.* **2000**, *78*, 391–403. [CrossRef]
23. Bunnell, B.A.; Flaat, M.; Gagliardi, C.; Patel, B.; Ripoll, C. Adipose-derived stem cells: Isolation, expansion and differentiation. *Methods* **2008**, *45*, 115–120. [CrossRef] [PubMed]
24. Mosna, F.; Sensebe, L.; Krampera, M. Human bone marrow and adipose tissue mesenchymal stem cells: A user's guide. *Stem Cells Dev.* **2010**, *19*, 1449–1470. [CrossRef]
25. Dominici, M.; Le Blanc, K.; Mueller, I.; Slaper-Cortenbach, I.; Marini, F.; Krause, D.; Deans, R.; Keating, A.; Prockop, D.; Horwitz, E. Minimal criteria for defining multipotent mesenchymal stromal cells. The International Society for Cellular Therapy position statement. *Cytotherapy* **2006**, *8*, 315–317. [CrossRef]
26. Houlihan, D.D.; Mabuchi, Y.; Morikawa, S.; Niibe, K.; Araki, D.; Suzuki, S.; Okano, H.; Matsuzaki, Y. Isolation of mouse mesenchymal stem cells on the basis of expression of Sca-1 and PDGFR-alpha. *Nat. Protoc.* **2012**, *7*, 2103–2111. [CrossRef]
27. Lee, R.H.; Kim, B.; Choi, I.; Kim, H.; Choi, H.S.; Suh, K.; Bae, Y.C.; Jung, J.S. Characterization and expression analysis of mesenchymal stem cells from human bone marrow and adipose tissue. *Cell. Physiol. Biochem.* **2004**, *14*, 311–324. [CrossRef]
28. Yamamoto, N.; Akamatsu, H.; Hasegawa, S.; Yamada, T.; Nakata, S.; Ohkuma, M.; Miyachi, E.; Marunouchi, T.; Matsunaga, K. Isolation of multipotent stem cells from mouse adipose tissue. *J. Dermatol. Sci.* **2007**, *48*, 43–52. [CrossRef]
29. Sung, J.H.; Yang, H.M.; Park, J.B.; Choi, G.S.; Joh, J.W.; Kwon, C.H.; Chun, J.M.; Lee, S.K.; Kim, S.J. Isolation and characterization of mouse mesenchymal stem cells. *Transpl. Proc.* **2008**, *40*, 2649–2654. [CrossRef]
30. Taylor, S.M.; Jones, P.A. Mechanism of action of eukaryotic DNA methyltransferase. Use of 5-azacytosine-containing DNA. *J. Mol. Biol.* **1982**, *162*, 679–692. [CrossRef]
31. Ghaneialvar, H.; Soltani, L.; Rahmani, H.R.; Lotfi, A.S.; Soleimani, M. Characterization and Classification of Mesenchymal Stem Cells in Several Species Using Surface Markers for Cell Therapy Purposes. *Indian J. Clin. Biochem.* **2018**, *33*, 46–52. [CrossRef] [PubMed]
32. Laing, A.G.; Fanelli, G.; Ramirez-Valdez, A.; Lechler, R.I.; Lombardi, G.; Sharpe, P.T. Mesenchymal stem cells inhibit T-cell function through conserved induction of cellular stress. *PLoS ONE* **2019**, *14*, e0213170. [CrossRef] [PubMed]
33. Uder, C.; Bruckner, S.; Winkler, S.; Tautenhahn, H.M.; Christ, B. Mammalian MSC from selected species: Features and applications. *Cytom. Part A* **2018**, *93*, 32–49. [CrossRef]
34. Miura, M.; Miura, Y.; Padilla-Nash, H.M.; Molinolo, A.A.; Fu, B.; Patel, V.; Seo, B.M.; Sonoyama, W.; Zheng, J.J.; Baker, C.C.; et al. Accumulated chromosomal instability in murine bone marrow mesenchymal stem cells leads to malignant transformation. *Stem Cells* **2006**, *24*, 1095–1103. [CrossRef] [PubMed]
35. Derubeis, A.R.; Cancedda, R. Bone marrow stromal cells (BMSCs) in bone engineering: Limitations and recent advances. *Ann. Biomed. Eng.* **2004**, *32*, 160–165. [CrossRef] [PubMed]
36. Shi, Z.; Zhao, L.; Qiu, G.; He, R.; Detamore, M.S. The effect of extended passaging on the phenotype and osteogenic potential of human umbilical cord mesenchymal stem cells. *Mol. Cell. Biochem.* **2015**, *401*, 155–164. [CrossRef] [PubMed]
37. Anderson, P.; Carrillo-Galvez, A.B.; Garcia-Perez, A.; Cobo, M.; Martin, F. CD105 (endoglin)-negative murine mesenchymal stromal cells define a new multipotent subpopulation with distinct differentiation and immunomodulatory capacities. *PLoS ONE* **2013**, *8*, e76979. [CrossRef]
38. Leyva-Leyva, M.; Barrera, L.; Lopez-Camarillo, C.; Arriaga-Pizano, L.; Orozco-Hoyuela, G.; Carrillo-Casas, E.M.; Calderon-Perez, J.; Lopez-Diaz, A.; Hernandez-Aguilar, F.; Gonzalez-Ramirez, R.; et al. Characterization of mesenchymal stem cell subpopulations from human amniotic membrane with dissimilar osteoblastic potential. *Stem Cells Dev.* **2013**, *22*, 1275–1287. [CrossRef]
39. Mark, P.; Kleinsorge, M.; Gaebel, R.; Lux, C.A.; Toelk, A.; Pittermann, E.; David, R.; Steinhoff, G.; Ma, N. Human Mesenchymal Stem Cells Display Reduced Expression of CD105 after Culture in Serum-Free Medium. *Stem Cells Int.* **2013**, *2013*, 698076. [CrossRef]

40. Li, C.; Guo, B.; Ding, S.; Rius, C.; Langa, C.; Kumar, P.; Bernabeu, C.; Kumar, S. TNF alpha down-regulates CD105 expression in vascular endothelial cells: A comparative study with TGF beta 1. *Anticancer Res.* **2003**, *23*, 1189–1196.
41. Sakaguchi, Y.; Sekiya, I.; Yagishita, K.; Muneta, T. Comparison of human stem cells derived from various mesenchymal tissues: Superiority of synovium as a cell source. *Arthritis Rheum.* **2005**, *52*, 2521–2529. [CrossRef] [PubMed]
42. Bochev, I.; Elmadjian, G.; Kyurkchiev, D.; Tzvetanov, L.; Altankova, I.; Tivchev, P.; Kyurkchiev, S. Mesenchymal stem cells from human bone marrow or adipose tissue differently modulate mitogen-stimulated B-cell immunoglobulin production in vitro. *Cell Biol. Int.* **2008**, *32*, 384–393. [CrossRef] [PubMed]
43. Winter, A.; Breit, S.; Parsch, D.; Benz, K.; Steck, E.; Hauner, H.; Weber, R.M.; Ewerbeck, V.; Richter, W. Cartilage-like gene expression in differentiated human stem cell spheroids: A comparison of bone marrow-derived and adipose tissue-derived stromal cells. *Arthritis Rheum.* **2003**, *48*, 418–429. [CrossRef] [PubMed]
44. Huang, J.I.; Kazmi, N.; Durbhakula, M.M.; Hering, T.M.; Yoo, J.U.; Johnstone, B. Chondrogenic potential of progenitor cells derived from human bone marrow and adipose tissue: A patient-matched comparison. *J. Orthop. Res.* **2005**, *23*, 1383–1389. [CrossRef]
45. Ho, Y.T.; Shimbo, T.; Wijaya, E.; Ouchi, Y.; Takaki, E.; Yamamoto, R.; Kikuchi, Y.; Kaneda, Y.; Tamai, K. Chromatin accessibility identifies diversity in mesenchymal stem cells from different tissue origins. *Sci. Rep.* **2018**, *8*, 17765. [CrossRef]
46. Park, H.W.; Shin, J.S.; Kim, C.W. Proteome of mesenchymal stem cells. *Proteomics* **2007**, *7*, 2881–2894. [CrossRef]
47. Wagner, W.; Wein, F.; Seckinger, A.; Frankhauser, M.; Wirkner, U.; Krause, U.; Blake, J.; Schwager, C.; Eckstein, V.; Ansorge, W.; et al. Comparative characteristics of mesenchymal stem cells from human bone marrow, adipose tissue, and umbilical cord blood. *Exp. Hematol.* **2005**, *33*, 1402–1416. [CrossRef]
48. Ng, R.K.; Gurdon, J.B. Epigenetic memory of active gene transcription is inherited through somatic cell nuclear transfer. *Proc. Natl. Acad. Sci. USA* **2005**, *102*, 1957–1962. [CrossRef]
49. Polo, J.M.; Liu, S.; Figueroa, M.E.; Kulalert, W.; Eminli, S.; Tan, K.Y.; Apostolou, E.; Stadtfeld, M.; Li, Y.; Shioda, T.; et al. Cell type of origin influences the molecular and functional properties of mouse induced pluripotent stem cells. *Nat. Biotechnol.* **2010**, *28*, 848–855. [CrossRef]
50. Kim, K.; Doi, A.; Wen, B.; Ng, K.; Zhao, R.; Cahan, P.; Kim, J.; Aryee, M.J.; Ji, H.; Ehrlich, L.I.; et al. Epigenetic memory in induced pluripotent stem cells. *Nature* **2010**, *467*, 285–290. [CrossRef]

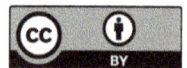

© 2020 by the authors. Licensee MDPI, Basel, Switzerland. This article is an open access article distributed under the terms and conditions of the Creative Commons Attribution (CC BY) license (http://creativecommons.org/licenses/by/4.0/).

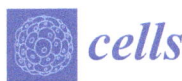

Review

Spheroid Culture System Methods and Applications for Mesenchymal Stem Cells

Na-Eun Ryu [1], Soo-Hong Lee [2,*] and Hansoo Park [1,*]

[1] Department of Integrative Engineering, Chung-Ang University, Seoul 06974, Korea; ryuskdms234@gmail.com
[2] Department of Medical Biotechnology, Dongguk University, Seoul 06974, Korea
* Correspondence: soohong@dongguk.edu (S.-H.L.); heyshoo@gmail.com (H.P.); Tel.: +82-31-961-5153 (S.-H.L.); +82-2-820-5940 (H.P.)

Received: 26 November 2019; Accepted: 9 December 2019; Published: 12 December 2019

Abstract: Owing to the importance of stem cell culture systems in clinical applications, researchers have extensively studied them to optimize the culture conditions and increase efficiency of cell culture. A spheroid culture system provides a similar physicochemical environment in vivo by facilitating cell–cell and cell–matrix interaction to overcome the limitations of traditional monolayer cell culture. In suspension culture, aggregates of adjacent cells form a spheroid shape having wide utility in tumor and cancer research, therapeutic transplantation, drug screening, and clinical study, as well as organic culture. There are various spheroid culture methods such as hanging drop, gel embedding, magnetic levitation, and spinner culture. Lately, efforts are being made to apply the spheroid culture system to the study of drug delivery platforms and co-cultures, and to regulate differentiation and pluripotency. To study spheroid cell culture, various kinds of biomaterials are used as building forms of hydrogel, film, particle, and bead, depending upon the requirement. However, spheroid cell culture system has limitations such as hypoxia and necrosis in the spheroid core. In addition, studies should focus on methods to dissociate cells from spheroid into single cells.

Keywords: 3D cell culture; spheroid culture; biomaterials

1. Introduction

Stem cells are valuable resources in regenerative medicine with clinical and research applications (Table 1). Particularly, human mesenchymal stem cells have secretory properties constituted by anti-inflammation, angiogenesis, and immune reaction regulation factors [1,2]. The primary characteristic of stem cells is stemness, represented by their ability of self-renewal, which generate new same cells from the original stem cells, and multipotency, which allows production of new differentiated cells having relatively limited potential [3]. Another characteristic of stem cells is clonality, which is related to lineage of stem cells [4]. Stemness enables the stem cells to have potential for application in numerous biological therapeutic tools such as cell-based therapy, high-throughput pharmacology, drug screening, and tissue engineering. However, stemness is actually maintained in the in vivo microenvironment, which provides growth factors in addition to the cell–cell or cell– extracellular matrix interactions. Therefore, conditions of the cell culture are very essential to facilitate the properties of stemness, maintenance, and proliferation. To fully exploit the properties of stem cells, development of cell culture methods that can increase the proliferation of cells in terms of cell count and superior quality are important. Previously, studies have attempted to develop methods for enhancing stemness and proliferation during in vitro cell culture process [5,6].

Cells constantly require biological signals from the substrates in cellular niches. These signals encourage proliferation and enhance cellular viability. However, the signals can also inhibit proliferation and biological activation of cells, thereby checking the growth [7]. In general, traditional two-dimension cell culture systems, wherein the cells grow as a monolayer, face some limitations in the realization of in vivo multi-cellular conditions [8]. These limitations restrict the cellular studies involving multi-cellular features and cancer cells [9]. When stem cells grow in two-dimensional cultures, maintenance of the differentiation potential and stemness is relatively more difficult than in stem cells growing in actual multi-cellular conditions [6]. However, three-dimensional cell culture systems can reconstitute conditions similar to that in an in vivo microenvironment (Table 2). Three dimensional systems construct cell–cell and cell–extracellular matrix (ECM) interaction networks (Table 2), which play a significant role in various cellular mechanisms, subsequently maintaining the cellular properties [10]. Researchers can attempt to decrease the limitations of conventional monolayer culturing and develop progressive cellular study methods (Table 2).

Spheroid culture system is a promising three-dimensional cell culture method. Morphology of stem cells cultured in spheroid culture system is different from that of cells in the monolayer culture system. In addition, mesenchymal stem cells of spheroids maintain their intrinsic phenotypic properties by cell–extracellular matrix interactions (Table 2) [11].

Spheroid stem cell cultures promote the expression of transcriptional factors of stemness markers such as Oct-4 and Nanog (Table 2). Spheroid stem cells secrete higher levels of cytokines and chemokines that affect the proliferation, viability, and migration of cells and also secrete higher angiogenesis than those secreted in the monolayer stem cells (Table 2). Spheroid stem cells regulated by hypoxia-induced upregulation of gene expression have properties of apoptosis resistance, improved viability, and secretion of angiogenic factors and chemokines (Table 2) [12,13].

Table 1. Applications of spheroid of Mesenchymal stem cells.

Applications of Spheroid	Examples
Tumor model	MSCs have resistance to chemotherapies and produce biochemical responses similar to parental tumors. Therefore MSCs-based modeling is usable to predict in vivo therapeutic efficacy [9].
Biology research	Co-culture of MSCs with other cells has been used to analyze cell–cell interaction. The cell–cell interactions are crucial to function of tissues [9].
Tissue Engineering	MSCs have been used for organ reconstruction. Spheroid of MSCs provide advantageous conditions for organ reconstruction. The MSCs can be transplanted to patient [9].
Transplantation therapy	Differentiation of MSCs is enhanced by spheroid culture system. In vivo tissue (cartilage [14,15], bone [16], spinal cord [17], nerve [18]) formation may be enhanced after MSCs spheroid transplantation.

Table 2. Advantages and disadvantages of spheroid culture.

Advantages	Disadvantages
• facilitate cell–cell and cell–matrix interaction • provide a similar physicochemical environment to the in vivo • maintain intrinsic phenotypic properties • promote the stemness marker expression • secrete cytokines, chemokines and angiogenic factors • improve viability and proliferation	• have diffusion gradient with increased spheroid size and lack of nutrients in the core of spheroid

2. Mechanism of Spheroid Formation

In a cell culture suspension, cells tend to aggregate and go through the process of self-assembly. Self-assembly means single cells constitute multi-cellular spheroids by themselves. Self-assembly is a natural phenomenon that happens during embryogenesis, morphogenesis, and organogenesis. It is affected by various factors, including gradients of nutrients, oxygen, and growth factors in cell culture medium, as well as cellular paracrine factors. Cell culture medium permeates inside the spheroids by diffusion. The gradient of diffusion is induced by increasing the spheroid size during spheroid culture. The bigger the size attained by the spheroids, the harder it becomes for the medium to reach the core of the spheroids. In addition, the rate of production and consumption of factors can affect self-assembly [19].

Adhesion and differentiation of cells affect the formation of multi-cellular spheroids. In particular, cadherin and integrin are directly related to the mechanism of spheroid formation. The process of spheroid formation is divided into several steps. Firstly, single cells present within the suspension agglomerate to form loosely adhesive cell spheroids. In this step, extracellular matrix fibers including complementary binding of peripheral cell surface to integrin encourages preliminary aggregation. Next, E-cadherin promotes strong adhesion of initial cell aggregate by creating homophilic binding between cadherins of peripheral cells. In addition, β-catenin complex facilitates cellular signal transduction. Actin can also affect agglomeration and stemness by promoting contacts between adjacent cells [20]. As a result, strong adhesive multi-cellular spheroids are formed [21].

E-cadherin (CDH1), a Ca^{2+}-dependent homophilic transmembrane adhesion molecule, could be a central component of spheroid formation [22,23]. The effects of E-cadherin have been demonstrated in cellular experiments involving human breast cancer cell lines and mouse embryonic stem cells [24]. For example, in a mouse embryonic stem cell study, E-cadherin-mediated cell attachment initiates embryonic body agglomeration. In addition, if the reaction of E-cadherin on the embryonic body with α-mouse E-cadherin antibodies is blocked, there is considerable inhibition of embryonic body agglomeration [25]. Integrins are transmembrane adhesion proteins composed of α-subunits and β-subunits of heterodimers that facilitate the cell-ECM connection during cell invasion and migration. Apart from E-cadherin, $β_1$-integrin also plays a role in the attachment of the early spheroid formation. Interaction of integrin-ECM affects multi-cellular spheroid formation rates [21].

3. Spheroid Formation Methods

3.1. Technical Methods

3.1.1. Pellet Culture

In this system, cells are concentrated to the bottom of the tube by centrifugal force. Cell–cell adhesions are maximized by proximity of the single cells at the bottom of the tube (Figure 1a), (Table 3). To harvest the cell pellet, supernatants are removed, and cell pellets are resuspended in spheroid formation cell culture medium. After estimating the cell count, cells in medium are dispensed into each well of a 96-well U bottom plate with cell repellent surface [19,26].

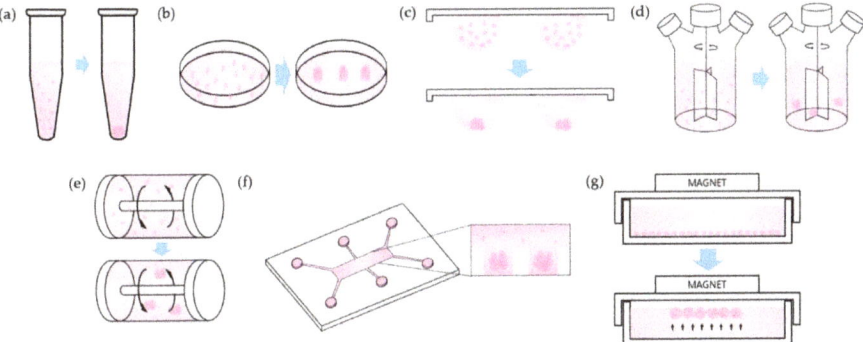

Figure 1. Schemes of technical methods. (**a**) Pellet Culture, (**b**) Liquid Overlay, (**c**) Hanging Drop, (**d**) Spinner Culture, (**e**) Rotating Wall Vessel, (**f**) Microfluidics, (**g**) Magnetic Levitation.

Table 3. Properties of technical methods.

Technical Method	Properties
Pellet Culture	use centrifugal force to concentrate cells
Liquid Overlay	use non-adhesive materials to inhibit cell attachment
Hanging Drop	use surface tension and gravitational force
Spinner Culture	use convectional force by stirring bar
Rotating Wall Vessel	use constant circular rotation of vessel
Microfluidics	use microfluid flow and materials permeable to soluble factors
Magnetic Levitation	use magnetic force to levitate cells

Pellet culture can be used to induce differentiation of mesenchymal stem cells. In particular, a pellet culture system is suitable for stem cell differentiation by chondrogenesis since the interaction between adjacent cells in a pellet culture microenvironment is similar to the interaction in pre-cartilage condensation occurring during embryonic development. In pellet culture, mesenchymal stem cells can change their morphological shape from fibroblastic to polygonal in a manner similar to that in chondrocytes. Therefore, pellet culture system can be used for the study of signal pathways of chondrogenesis and for assessing the chondrogenic potentiality of stem cells [27,28].

3.1.2. Liquid Overlay

Liquid overlay culture technique, also called the static suspension culture, forms spheroids by interrupting the adhesion of cells on non-adherent culture plates (Figure 1b), (Table 3). A non-adherent culture layer is typically composed of agar or agarose gel. Agarose is a very efficient material for the inhibition of cell attachment and is superior to agar with respect to its non-adherent properties. Since the cell attachments are inhibited, cells spontaneously form spheroids above the non-adherent surface by promoting cell–cell adhesive molecules [19,29,30].

Despite excellent non-adherent properties of agarose, this biomaterial has drawbacks in terms of culturing cancer cells. Agarose has trouble in interacting with tumor cells and is unable to activate the specific signaling pathways related to reaction of tumor cells to therapy process. Recently, hyaluronic acid can be a suitable alternative biomaterial that can replace agarose. It has the capability to interact with surface receptors of cancer cells during cancer progression. This interaction enhances transduction of cellular signals related to proliferation, angiogenesis, survival, and differentiation, as well as resistance to therapeutics [31,32].

3.1.3. Hanging Drop

Hanging drop culture technique allows single cells to aggregate and fabricate spheroids in the form of droplets (Figure 1c), (Table 3). By controlling the volume of the drop or density of cell suspension, it is possible to control the spheroid size [33]. The novel hanging drop array platform is capable of efficiently forming definite size spheroids [34]. This technique can form circular spheroids having a narrow distribution of size with 10% to 15% variation coefficient, while the spheroid growth in non-adherent surface culture methods has 40% to 60% variation coefficient [35]. A general method involves starting from a monolayer cell culture, after which the cells are prepared as suspension and diluted with culture medium to attain the desired cell density. Subsequently, the cell suspension is dispensed into wells of a mini-tray with the help of a compatible multistep or multichannel pipette. A lid is placed on the mini-tray and the entire mini-tray is reversed upside down. The cell suspension drops attached on the mini-tray would stay on the reversed surface by surface tension. In this method, spheroids are formed as droplets owing to simultaneous action of surface tension and gravitational force [19,36].

Besides the adjustable size of a spheroid, hanging drop system has other advantages. There is no requirement of expensive or professional equipment to form spheroids for small scale experiments. A huge quantity of spheroids can be produced readily by multichannel pipetting and can be harvested by scraping lids of culture dishes [33]. In addition, mesenchymal stem cells cultured via hanging drop system can secrete considerable quantities of potent anti-inflammatory as well as anti-tumorigenic factors [37].

3.1.4. Spinner Culture

Spinner culture technique refers to the technique wherein the cell suspension in spinner flask bioreactor containers is continuously mixed by stirring (Figure 1d), (Table 3). The resultant spheroid is dependent on size of the bioreactor container [9,38]. Conditions of the fluid and mass in the containers are affected by the convectional force of the stirring bar, which is crucial to form the spheroid. A high stirring rate induces damage to the spheroid cells. However, an extremely slow rate of stirring allows spheroid cells to sink to the bottom of the container, resulting in inhibition of spheroid formation in the container [19].

In addition to adipogenesis, osteogenic differentiation of mesenchymal stem cells is also boosted by improved expression of osteogenic markers such as osteopontin and osteocalcin in the spinner system [39].

3.1.5. Rotating Wall Vessel

Rotating wall vessel reconstructs microgravity by constant circular rotation [40]. Due to constant rotation, cells are continuously in a suspended state in the vessel (Figure 1e), (Table 3) [41]. This microgravity can affect gene expression of mesenchymal stem cells. In microgravity conditions, chondrogenic and osteogenic gene expression of stem cells reduces, whereas adipogenic gene expression is elevated [42]. This is because microgravity inhibits expression of *Collagen I* of the osteoblastic marker gene and integrin/Collagen I signaling pathway during the osteoblastic differentiation [43]. In addition, microgravity suppresses stress fiber development and improves intracellular lipid accumulation. However, reduction of osteogenic gene expression by microgravity can be regulated. Expression of RhoA protein switches these microgravitational effects and improves expression of the markers of osteoblastic differentiation of mesenchymal stem cells [44]. Expression of chondrogenic genes is increased by regulation of the p38 MAPK activation pathways [45].

3.1.6. Microfluidics

This microfluidic culture technique, also called lab-on-a-chip technique, is used for applications such as single cell analysis, genetic assays, and drug toxicity studies. This culture method has microscale dimensions corresponding to the scale of in vivo microstructures (Figure 1f), (Table 3). In addition, microfluidic devices easily enable microscale control of the environment, mimicking the in vivo three-dimensional environment. One of the features of the microfluidic method is that it integrates multiple processes including cell capture, mixing, detection, and cell culturing. Another feature is a considerably high cell throughput for cell analysis. Microfluidic devices employ materials permeable to oxygen and growth factors affecting proliferation. This characteristic feature of microfluidics technology can decrease hypoxia, which is an unavoidable disadvantage of spheroid culture [46].

Recently developed fluidic systems overcome the limitations posed by the conventional fluidic system and offer advantages such as diversity of design and cost reduction through smaller requirements for specimens and reagents for cell transport assays [47]. Presently, the fluidic system can produce a distinct concentration of analyte mixtures and facilitates real-time monitoring of living cells. In addition, this system can optimize cell culture conditions for the proliferation and differentiation of stem cells, and be used for tissue engineering processes such as organ replacement and tissue regeneration, and in future clinical trials [48–50]. The currently used microfluidics system can be used to develop a co-culturing system related to the generation of microvascular network using mesenchymal stem cells. The co-culture system can also induce formation of a human microvascular network [51].

3.1.7. Magnetic Levitation

Magnetic levitation-based culturing makes use of magnetic particles and integration with hydrogels according to the given conditions. In the magnetic levitation system, cells are mixed with magnetic particles and subjected to magnetic force during cell culture (Figure 1g), (Table 3). This system utilizes negative magnetophoresis, which can imitate a weightlessness condition, because positive magnetophoresis can hinder the attainment of weightlessness [52]. Due to magnetic force, the cells incorporated with magnetic particles stay levitated against gravity. This condition induces the geometry change of cell mass and promotes contact between cells, leading to cell aggregation. In addition, this system can facilitate multi-cellular co-culturing with agglomeration of different cell types [53,54].

When mesenchymal stem cells and magnetic particles are cultured with collagen gel, particle internalization takes place. Spheroid formation can be reproducible and reduces necrosis in the spheroid core, thus maintaining its stemness as a spheroid [54]. However, some groups have demonstrated that artificially manipulated gravity can lead to changes in cellular structures and can result in apoptosis [55,56].

3.2. Using Biomaterials Methods

3.2.1. Hydrogels

Hydrogels are widely used for cell culture studies. Hydrogels have been fabricated using biocompatible materials such as alginate [57,58], fibrin [59,60], collagen [54] and hyaluronic acid [61,62]. The primary properties of hydrogels is that mesenchymal stem cells can be entrapped in them (Figure 2a), (Table 4). This method effectively improves the viability of cells while reducing cellular apoptosis. Furthermore, osteogenic differentiation potential is stably maintained and secretion of proangiogenic factors is activated in the hydrogel-entrapped cells compared to that in the non-entrapped cells of the monolayer culture [11,57,59]. Activated secretion of proangiogenic factors implies increased angiogenic potential and highly correlates to improved osteogenesis [63,64].

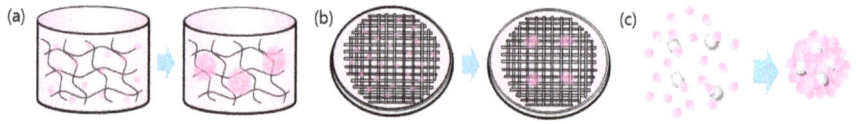

Figure 2. Schemes of using biomaterials methods. (a) Hydrogels, (b) biofilms, (c) particles.

Table 4. Properties of biomaterials.

Biomaterial	Properties
Hydrogel	• entrap cells during culture and can deliver cells as injectable form. • provide an environment similar to extracellular matrix and improve viability, stemness and angiogenetic capacity of stem cells.
Biofilms	• increase stemness, differentiation potential, adhesion and proliferation of stem cells.
Particles	• control mechanotransductional mechanisms inside the spheroid and improve viability and proliferation.

Physicochemical biomimetic properties of hydrogels similar to those of the extracellular matrix are capable of offering functional niches promoting the self-renewal potential and wound healing. These properties of hydrogels improve angiogenetic capacity and stemness of the cells (Table 4) [65]. By adjusting the physical properties of hydrogel materials, the size of a spheroid can be optimized. To control the size of spheroids, weak adhesive materials can be used and physically embossed patterns on the surface of the hydrogel should be fabricated [66]. In addition, another main property of a hydrogel is the capability to deliver cells directly. Hydrogels can also be prepared in an injectable form that can directly deliver stem cells to in vivo models and compensate for the necrotic or defective tissues [65,67].

Hydrogels have been developed to study the microenvironment of cancer cells. The stiffness of hydrogels can affect the phenotype and growth of cancer cells. The number and size of cancer cells tend to reduce when cultured in stiff hydrogels. However, tumorigenicity of cancer cells increases after in vivo transfer in softer hydrogels. This stiffness of hydrogels can be optimized by modifying the concentrations of the composing materials [68].

3.2.2. Biofilms

Films made of biomaterials can be constructed by various methods such as photolithography and stamping (Figure 2b). Tumor cell spheroids can be cultured on films for their role in cancer drug discovery [69,70]. Apart from tumor cells, stem cells can be cultured on films. Stemness marker expression and differentiation potential are increased during culturing on film (Table 4) [71,72]. Adhesion and proliferation of stem cells can be enhanced by changing the composition and concentration of the film materials (Table 4) [73]. The component ratios used in the films are critical to the size of spheroids and rate of spheroid fabrication, as well as cellular adhesion and proliferation. In a previous study, hyaluronic acid(HA) modified chitosan film was found to form larger spheroids and induce cell aggregation in lesser time than the unmodified chitosan film [74]. The size of spheroids is also affected by the thickness of the film. Reducing thickness of the film leads to decreased spheroid size [75].

One of the biomaterials used in such films is chitosan. Culturing on chitosan films can improve angiogenesis, chemotaxis, and self-renewal [13,76]. Recently, graphene has been investigated as a cell culturing material [77,78]. Graphene films can provide distinctive environments beneficial to neurogenesis. Moreover, the neurons differentiated on graphene films have a remarkably keen sense of external stimulations. Graphene is believed to be capable of adjusting neural differentiation and growth of mesenchymal stem cells [79].

3.2.3. Particles

Particulate factors have been used in spheroid cultures to control the cell culture microenvironment (Figure 2c). A drawback of spheroid cultures is the inadequate supply of nutrients and oxygen to the core of the spheroid. This is accounted by a rise in the diffusion gradient with increased spheroid size. However, particles within spheroids are capable of controlling conditions inside the spheroids during culturing. Consequently, the viability and proliferation of cells improve (Table 4) [80,81].

Particles are capable of regulating stem cell differentiation by controlling the extracellular environment [82]. Differentiation is also regulated by encapsulating stem cells in these particles. A previous study demonstrated that mesenchymal stem cell encapsulating particles, including a nanofibrous meshwork, could induce osteogenic differentiation [83]. However, particles can inhibit specific stem cell differentiation while inducing differentiation of other stem cells. This is achieved by controlling mechanotransductional mechanisms. Particles act as obstacles of internal adhesion between adjacent cells of spheroids. Alteration of mechanical force, including internal adhesion, surface tension, and interfacial tension in a spheroid, leads to biased differentiation of the stem cells [84].

The desired delivery of growth factors using particles can modulate the spheroid microenvironment. By transferring suitable growth factors into spheroids, differentiation can be spatially controlled [85,86].

4. Applications of Spheroid

4.1. Study of Tumors

Tumor cells are affected by cellular structures and extracellular matrix. The conventional 2D culture system has limitations pertaining to tumor cell culture. Spheroid culture system is a promising method for the study of tissue structure, signaling pathways, and immune activation of cancer cells.

Single tumor cells may form multi-cellular tumor spheroids mixed with other types of cells in a non-adherent 3D culture system, which is more effective in creating cellular heterogeneity [87]. Morphologies of these tumor spheroids are affected by spheroid culture microenvironment. In accordance with the conditions of culture microenvironment, morphologies may form aggregated circles, entangled bundles, elongated ovals, or star-shaped spheroids.

Spheroid form is the most suitable model for cancer study because it has a limited oxygen concentration at its core. This hypoxic nature of spheroids is the primary advantage of spheroid culture. However, in the case of tumors, spheroids larger than 500 μm in diameter undergo necrosis at their core [87] and have a concentration gradient of biological factors similar to tumor cells due to restricted diffusion of nutrients, oxygen, and growth factors [88].

4.2. Drug Screening

A study using an animal model has a limitation in disease modelling [89]. Presently, parameters of drug screening studies using a mouse model can possibly be overcome by adopting spheroid cell culture [90]. However, lack of uniformity in diameter or morphology of spheroids appears as new parameters for reproducible drug screening. By increasing the uniformity during the spheroid culture period, tumor spheroids can provide precise information on the diseases and suppress undesired side effects of the drugs under development [90,91].

In the context of tumor cell culture for drug screening, co-culture of normal cell and tumor cells can be a potential technique for reconstruction of the heterogenous multi-cellular environment for solid tumors as well as for promoting migration in tumors. The co-culture enables the investigation of interactions between tumor cells and peripheral multi-cellular environments. In addition, because normal host cells proximal to tumor cells can influence drug sensitivity of tumor cells, spheroid co-cultures can be used for drug screening study.

4.3. Regenerative Medicine

Transplantation is one of the most promising strategies for regenerative therapy. The currently used transplantation therapy has some drawbacks. In case of autografts, the amount of cellular supply is limited and the process of cell collection is cumbersome for the donor. However, allograft transplantation results in problems such as infection, inflammation, and host rejection [16]. Besides, injection in the form of single cells results in the limited immobility of injected cells at the site of the defect [92]. Injectable spheroids of stem cells are considered to improve the engraftment efficiency after transplantation [93]. After the implantation of spheroids, stem cells may be induced to differentiate into suitable cells for reconstructing the defective site [16,94]. Differentiation potential of spheroids has been demonstrated in vitro. Spheroid culture method improves differentiation potential compared to monolayer culturing [95].

Genetically modified spheroids have been developed for cell transplantation therapy [17,96]. These spheroids are prepared in the form of injectable suspensions. After transplanting these spheroids, the altered gene expression is maintained for a longer period of time in host tissues, whereas expression of cells cultured from monolayer plates decreases soon after transplantation. Thus, desired properties of cells transplanted in the host tissues are preserved by the process of spheroid culture [97].

5. Conclusions

Stem cells have shown applicability in various fields such as regenerative medicine as well as tumor and cancer research. Three-dimensional cultures enhance the applicability of stem cells by increasing the efficiency of culture. Spheroid culture system is an attractive method to overcome limitations of traditional monolayer culture. This system can resolve problems of monolayer culture such as the limited realization of in vivo multi-cellular microenvironments and it can reconstruct biological signal pathways of cell–cell and cell–ECM interactions, which encourage proliferation and viability of cells. Therefore, maintenance of the differentiation potential, stemness and intrinsic phenotypic properties is improved. To conclude, development of spheroid culture is essential to further optimize formation of spheroids and utilize them as resource in the medical field.

Author Contributions: All authors have contributed to the conceptualization, writing and approved the final version of this manuscript.

Funding: This work was supported by Research of Korea Centers for Disease Control and Prevention (2018ER610300) and by the Chung-Ang University Research Scholarship Grants in 2018.

Conflicts of Interest: The authors declare no conflict of interest.

References

1. Prockop, D.J.; Kota, D.J.; Bazhanov, N.; Reger, R.L. Evolving paradigms for repair of tissues by adult stem/progenitor cells (MSCs). *J. Cell. Mol. Med.* **2010**, *14*, 2190–2199. [CrossRef] [PubMed]
2. Stroncek, D.F.; Sabatino, M.; Ren, J.; England, L.; Kuznetsov, S.A.; Klein, H.G.; Robey, P.G. Establishing a bone marrow stromal cell transplant program at the National Institutes of Health Clinical Center. *Tissue Eng. Part B Rev.* **2014**, *20*, 200–205. [CrossRef] [PubMed]
3. Ramalho-Santos, M.; Yoon, S.; Matsuzaki, Y.; Mulligan, R.C.; Melton, D.A. "Stemness": Transcriptional profiling of embryonic and adult stem cells. *Science* **2002**, *298*, 597–600. [CrossRef] [PubMed]
4. Melton, D. Chapter 2—'Stemness': Definitions, criteria, and standards. In *Essentials of Stem Cell Biology*, 3rd ed.; Lanza, R., Atala, A., Eds.; Academic Press: Boston, MA, USA, 2014; pp. 7–17. [CrossRef]
5. Zhang, S.; Liu, P.; Chen, L.; Wang, Y.; Wang, Z.; Zhang, B. The effects of spheroid formation of adipose-derived stem cells in a microgravity bioreactor on stemness properties and therapeutic potential. *Biomaterials* **2015**, *41*, 15–25. [CrossRef] [PubMed]
6. Lei, Y.; Schaffer, D.V. A fully defined and scalable 3D culture system for human pluripotent stem cell expansion and differentiation. *Proc. Natl. Acad. Sci. USA* **2013**, *110*, E5039–E5048. [CrossRef] [PubMed]
7. Li, L.; Neaves, W.B. Normal stem cells and cancer stem cells: The niche matters. *Cancer Res.* **2006**, *66*, 4553–4557. [CrossRef] [PubMed]
8. Pampaloni, F.; Reynaud, E.G.; Stelzer, E.H.K. The third dimension bridges the gap between cell culture and live tissue. *Nat. Rev. Mol. Cell Biol.* **2007**, *8*, 839. [CrossRef] [PubMed]
9. Lin, R.Z.; Chang, H.Y. Recent advances in three-dimensional multicellular spheroid culture for biomedical research. *Biotechnol. J.* **2008**, *3*, 1172–1184. [CrossRef]
10. Rosso, F.; Giordano, A.; Barbarisi, M.; Barbarisi, A. From cell-ECM interactions to tissue engineering. *J. Cell Physiol.* **2004**, *199*, 174–180. [CrossRef]
11. Murphy, K.C.; Hoch, A.I.; Harvestine, J.N.; Zhou, D.; Leach, J.K. Mesenchymal stem cell spheroids retain osteogenic phenotype through alpha2beta1 signaling. *Stem Cells Transl. Med.* **2016**, *5*, 1229–1237. [CrossRef]
12. Zhang, Q.; Nguyen, A.L.; Shi, S.; Hill, C.; Wilder-Smith, P.; Krasieva, T.B.; Le, A.D. Three-dimensional spheroid culture of human gingiva-derived mesenchymal stem cells enhances mitigation of chemotherapy-induced oral mucositis. *Stem Cells Dev.* **2012**, *21*, 937–947. [CrossRef] [PubMed]
13. Cheng, N.C.; Chen, S.Y.; Li, J.R.; Young, T.H. Short-term spheroid formation enhances the regenerative capacity of adipose-derived stem cells by promoting stemness, angiogenesis, and chemotaxis. *Stem Cells Transl. Med.* **2013**, *2*, 584–594. [CrossRef] [PubMed]
14. Yoon, H.H.; Bhang, S.H.; Shin, J.Y.; Shin, J.; Kim, B.S. Enhanced cartilage formation via three-dimensional cell engineering of human adipose-derived stem cells. *Tissue Eng. Part A* **2012**, *18*, 1949–1956. [CrossRef] [PubMed]
15. Lee, J.; Sato, M.; Kim, H.; Mochida, J. Transplantation of scaffold-free spheroids composed of synovium-derived cells and chondrocytes for the treatment of cartilage defects of the knee. *Eur. Cell Mater.* **2011**, *22*, 90. [CrossRef] [PubMed]
16. Suenaga, H.; Furukawa, K.S.; Suzuki, Y.; Takato, T.; Ushida, T. Bone regeneration in calvarial defects in a rat model by implantation of human bone marrow-derived mesenchymal stromal cell spheroids. *J. Mater. Sci. Mater. Med.* **2015**, *26*, 254. [CrossRef] [PubMed]
17. Uchida, S.; Hayakawa, K.; Ogata, T.; Tanaka, S.; Kataoka, K.; Itaka, K. Treatment of spinal cord injury by an advanced cell transplantation technology using brain-derived neurotrophic factor-transfected mesenchymal stem cell spheroids. *Biomaterials* **2016**, *109*, 1–11. [CrossRef] [PubMed]

18. Zhang, Q.; Nguyen, P.D.; Shi, S.; Burrell, J.C.; Cullen, D.K.; Le, A.D. 3D bio-printed scaffold-free nerve constructs with human gingiva-derived mesenchymal stem cells promote rat facial nerve regeneration. *Sci. Rep.* **2018**, *8*, 6634. [CrossRef] [PubMed]
19. Achilli, T.M.; Meyer, J.; Morgan, J.R. Advances in the formation, use and understanding of multi-cellular spheroids. *Expert Opin. Biol. Ther.* **2012**, *12*, 1347–1360. [CrossRef] [PubMed]
20. Tsai, A.C.; Liu, Y.; Yuan, X.; Ma, T. Compaction, fusion, and functional activation of three-dimensional human mesenchymal stem cell aggregate. *Tissue Eng. Part A* **2015**, *21*, 1705–1719. [CrossRef] [PubMed]
21. Lin, R.Z.; Chou, L.F.; Chien, C.C.; Chang, H.Y. Dynamic analysis of hepatoma spheroid formation: Roles of E-cadherin and beta1-integrin. *Cell Tissue Res.* **2006**, *324*, 411–422. [CrossRef]
22. Batlle, E.; Sancho, E.; Francí, C.; Domínguez, D.; Monfar, M.; Baulida, J.; García de Herreros, A. The transcription factor Snail is a repressor of E-cadherin gene expression in epithelial tumour cells. *Nat. Cell Biol.* **2000**, *2*, 84–89. [CrossRef] [PubMed]
23. Comijn, J.; Berx, G.; Vermassen, P.; Verschueren, K.; van Grunsven, L.; Bruyneel, E.; Mareel, M.; Huylebroeck, D.; van Roy, F. The two-handed E box binding zinc finger protein SIP1 downregulates E-cadherin and induces invasion. *Mol. Cell* **2001**, *7*, 1267–1278. [CrossRef]
24. Konze, S.A.; van Diepen, L.; Schroder, A.; Olmer, R.; Moller, H.; Pich, A.; Weissmann, R.; Kuss, A.W.; Zweigerdt, R.; Buettner, F.F. Cleavage of E-cadherin and beta-catenin by calpain affects Wnt signaling and spheroid formation in suspension cultures of human pluripotent stem cells. *Mol. Cell Proteomics* **2014**, *13*, 990–1007. [CrossRef] [PubMed]
25. Dang, S.M.; Gerecht-Nir, S.; Chen, J.; Itskovitz-Eldor, J.; Zandstra, P.W. Controlled, scalable embryonic stem cell differentiation culture. *Stem Cells* **2004**, *22*, 275–282. [CrossRef] [PubMed]
26. Maritan, S.M.; Lian, E.Y.; Mulligan, L.M. An efficient and flexible cell aggregation method for 3D spheroid production. *J. Vis. Exp.* **2017**. [CrossRef] [PubMed]
27. Zhang, L.; Su, P.; Xu, C.; Yang, J.; Yu, W.; Huang, D. Chondrogenic differentiation of human mesenchymal stem cells: A comparison between micromass and pellet culture systems. *Biotechnol. Lett.* **2010**, *32*, 1339–1346. [CrossRef]
28. Bosnakovski, D.; Mizuno, M.; Kim, G.; Ishiguro, T.; Okumura, M.; Iwanaga, T.; Kadosawa, T.; Fujinaga, T. Chondrogenic differentiation of bovine bone marrow mesenchymal stem cells in pellet cultural system. *Exp. Hematol.* **2004**, *32*, 502–509. [CrossRef]
29. Carlsson, J.; Yuhas, J.M. Liquid-overlay culture of cellular spheroids. *Recent Results Cancer Res.* **1984**, *95*, 1–23.
30. Costa, E.C.; de Melo-Diogo, D.; Moreira, A.F.; Carvalho, M.P.; Correia, I.J. Spheroids formation on non-adhesive surfaces by liquid overlay technique: Considerations and practical approaches. *Biotechnol. J.* **2018**, *13*. [CrossRef]
31. Carvalho, M.P.; Costa, E.C.; Miguel, S.P.; Correia, I.J. Tumor spheroid assembly on hyaluronic acid-based structures: A review. *Carbohydr. Polym.* **2016**, *150*, 139–148. [CrossRef]
32. Carvalho, M.P.; Costa, E.C.; Correia, I.J. Assembly of breast cancer heterotypic spheroids on hyaluronic acid coated surfaces. *Biotechnol. Prog.* **2017**, *33*, 1346–1357. [CrossRef] [PubMed]
33. Bartosh, T.J.; Ylostalo, J.H. Preparation of anti-inflammatory mesenchymal stem/precursor cells (MSCs) through sphere formation using hanging-drop culture technique. *Curr. Protoc. Stem Cell Biol.* **2014**, *28*. [CrossRef] [PubMed]
34. Tung, Y.C.; Hsiao, A.Y.; Allen, S.G.; Torisawa, Y.S.; Ho, M.; Takayama, S. High-throughput 3D spheroid culture and drug testing using a 384 hanging drop array. *Analyst* **2011**, *136*, 473–478. [CrossRef] [PubMed]
35. Kelm, J.M.; Timmins, N.E.; Brown, C.J.; Fussenegger, M.; Nielsen, L.K. Method for generation of homogeneous multicellular tumor spheroids applicable to a wide variety of cell types. *Biotechnol. Bioeng.* **2003**, *83*, 173–180. [CrossRef] [PubMed]
36. Timmins, N.E.; Nielsen, L.K. Generation of multicellular tumor spheroids by the hanging-drop method. *Methods Mol. Med.* **2007**, *140*, 141–151. [PubMed]
37. Bartosh, T.J.; Ylostalo, J.H.; Mohammadipoor, A.; Bazhanov, N.; Coble, K.; Claypool, K.; Lee, R.H.; Choi, H.; Prockop, D.J. Aggregation of human mesenchymal stromal cells (MSCs) into 3D spheroids enhances their antiinflammatory properties. *Proc. Natl. Acad. Sci. USA* **2010**, *107*, 13724–13729. [CrossRef]
38. Kim, J.B. Three-dimensional tissue culture models in cancer biology. *Semin. Cancer Biol.* **2005**, *15*, 365–377. [CrossRef]

39. Frith, J.E.; Thomson, B.; Genever, P.G. Dynamic three-dimensional culture methods enhance mesenchymal stem cell properties and increase therapeutic potential. *Tissue Eng. Part C Methods* 2010, *16*, 735–749. [CrossRef]
40. Carpenedo, R.L.; Sargent, C.Y.; McDevitt, T.C. Rotary suspension culture enhances the efficiency, yield, and homogeneity of embryoid body differentiation. *Stem Cells* 2007, *25*, 2224–2234. [CrossRef]
41. Manley, P.; Lelkes, P.I. A novel real-time system to monitor cell aggregation and trajectories in rotating wall vessel bioreactors. *J. Biotechnol.* 2006, *125*, 416–424. [CrossRef]
42. Sheyn, D.; Pelled, G.; Netanely, D.; Domany, E.; Gazit, D. The effect of simulated microgravity on human mesenchymal stem cells cultured in an osteogenic differentiation system: A bioinformatics study. *Tissue Eng. Part A* 2010, *16*, 3403–3412. [CrossRef]
43. Meyers, V.E.; Zayzafoon, M.; Gonda, S.R.; Gathings, W.E.; McDonald, J.M. Modeled microgravity disrupts collagen I/integrin signaling during osteoblastic differentiation of human mesenchymal stem cells. *J. Cell Biochem.* 2004, *93*, 697–707. [CrossRef] [PubMed]
44. Meyers, V.E.; Zayzafoon, M.; Douglas, J.T.; McDonald, J.M. RhoA and cytoskeletal disruption mediate reduced osteoblastogenesis and enhanced adipogenesis of human mesenchymal stem cells in modeled microgravity. *J. Bone Miner. Res.* 2005, *20*, 1858–1866. [CrossRef] [PubMed]
45. Yu, B.; Yu, D.; Cao, L.; Zhao, X.; Long, T.; Liu, G.; Tang, T.; Zhu, Z. Simulated microgravity using a rotary cell culture system promotes chondrogenesis of human adipose-derived mesenchymal stem cells via the p38 MAPK pathway. *Biochem. Biophys. Res. Commun.* 2011, *414*, 412–418. [CrossRef] [PubMed]
46. Ziolkowska, K.; Jedrych, E.; Kwapiszewski, R.; Lopacinska, J.; Skolimowski, M.; Chudy, M. PDMS/glass microfluidic cell culture system for cytotoxicity tests and cells passage. *Sens. Actuators B Chem.* 2010, *145*, 533–542. [CrossRef]
47. Nie, F.Q.; Yamada, M.; Kobayashi, J.; Yamato, M.; Kikuchi, A.; Okano, T. On-chip cell migration assay using microfluidic channels. *Biomaterials* 2007, *28*, 4017–4022. [CrossRef]
48. Chung, B.G.; Flanagan, L.A.; Rhee, S.W.; Schwartz, P.H.; Lee, A.P.; Monuki, E.S.; Jeon, N.L. Human neural stem cell growth and differentiation in a gradient-generating microfluidic device. *Lab Chip* 2005, *5*, 401–406. [CrossRef]
49. Ju, X.; Li, D.; Gao, N.; Shi, Q.; Hou, H. Hepatogenic differentiation of mesenchymal stem cells using microfluidic chips. *Biotechnol. J.* 2008, *3*, 383–391. [CrossRef]
50. Li, F.; Truong, V.X.; Thissen, H.; Frith, J.E.; Forsythe, J.S. Microfluidic encapsulation of human mesenchymal stem cells for articular cartilage tissue regeneration. *ACS Appl. Mater. Interfaces* 2017, *9*, 8589–8601. [CrossRef]
51. Jeon, J.S.; Bersini, S.; Whisler, J.A.; Chen, M.B.; Dubini, G.; Charest, J.L.; Moretti, M.; Kamm, R.D. Generation of 3D functional microvascular networks with human mesenchymal stem cells in microfluidic systems. *Integr. Biol.* 2014, *6*, 555–563. [CrossRef]
52. Anil-Inevi, M.; Yaman, S.; Yildiz, A.A.; Mese, G.; Yalcin-Ozuysal, O.; Tekin, H.C.; Ozcivici, E. Biofabrication of in situ self assembled 3D cell cultures in a weightlessness environment generated using magnetic levitation. *Sci. Rep.* 2018, *8*, 7239. [CrossRef] [PubMed]
53. Kim, J.A.; Choi, J.H.; Kim, M.; Rhee, W.J.; Son, B.; Jung, H.K.; Park, T.H. High-throughput generation of spheroids using magnetic nanoparticles for three-dimensional cell culture. *Biomaterials* 2013, *34*, 8555–8563. [CrossRef] [PubMed]
54. Lewis, N.S.; Lewis, E.E.; Mullin, M.; Wheadon, H.; Dalby, M.J.; Berry, C.C. Magnetically levitated mesenchymal stem cell spheroids cultured with a collagen gel maintain phenotype and quiescence. *J. Tissue Eng.* 2017, *8*, 2041731417704428. [CrossRef] [PubMed]
55. Meng, R.; Xu, H.Y.; Di, S.M.; Shi, D.Y.; Qian, A.R.; Wang, J.F.; Shang, P. Human mesenchymal stem cells are sensitive to abnormal gravity and exhibit classic apoptotic features. *Acta Biochim. Biophys. Sin.* 2011, *43*, 133–142. [CrossRef] [PubMed]
56. Sytkowski, A.J.; Davis, K.L. Erythroid cell growth and differentiation in vitro in the simulated microgravity environment of the NASA rotating wall vessel bioreactor. *In Vitro Cell Dev. Biol. Anim.* 2001, *37*, 79–83. [CrossRef]
57. Ho, S.S.; Murphy, K.C.; Binder, B.Y.; Vissers, C.B.; Leach, J.K. Increased survival and function of mesenchymal stem cell spheroids entrapped in instructive alginate hydrogels. *Stem Cells Transl. Med.* 2016, *5*, 773–781. [CrossRef]

58. Ho, S.S.; Keown, A.T.; Addison, B.; Leach, J.K. Cell Migration and Bone Formation from Mesenchymal Stem Cell Spheroids in Alginate Hydrogels Are Regulated by Adhesive Ligand Density. *Biomacromolecules* **2017**, *18*, 4331–4340. [CrossRef]
59. Murphy, K.C.; Fang, S.Y.; Leach, J.K. Human mesenchymal stem cell spheroids in fibrin hydrogels exhibit improved cell survival and potential for bone healing. *Cell Tissue Res.* **2014**, *357*, 91–99. [CrossRef]
60. Murphy, K.C.; Whitehead, J.; Zhou, D.; Ho, S.S.; Leach, J.K. Engineering fibrin hydrogels to promote the wound healing potential of mesenchymal stem cell spheroids. *Acta Biomater.* **2017**, *64*, 176–186. [CrossRef]
61. Mineda, K.; Feng, J.; Ishimine, H.; Takada, H.; Doi, K.; Kuno, S.; Kinoshita, K.; Kanayama, K.; Kato, H.; Mashiko, T.; et al. Therapeutic Potential of Human Adipose-Derived Stem/Stromal Cell Microspheroids Prepared by Three-Dimensional Culture in Non-Cross-Linked Hyaluronic Acid Gel. *Stem Cells Transl. Med.* **2015**, *4*, 1511–1522. [CrossRef]
62. Gwon, K.; Kim, E.; Tae, G. Heparin-hyaluronic acid hydrogel in support of cellular activities of 3D encapsulated adipose derived stem cells. *Acta Biomater.* **2017**, *49*, 284–295. [CrossRef] [PubMed]
63. He, J.; Genetos, D.C.; Leach, J.K. Osteogenesis and trophic factor secretion are influenced by the composition of hydroxyapatite/poly(lactide-co-glycolide) composite scaffolds. *Tissue Eng. Part A* **2010**, *16*, 127–137. [CrossRef] [PubMed]
64. Cheung, W.K.; Working, D.M.; Galuppo, L.D.; Leach, J.K. Osteogenic comparison of expanded and uncultured adipose stromal cells. *Cytotherapy* **2010**, *12*, 554–562. [CrossRef] [PubMed]
65. Rustad, K.C.; Wong, V.W.; Sorkin, M.; Glotzbach, J.P.; Major, M.R.; Rajadas, J.; Longaker, M.T.; Gurtner, G.C. Enhancement of mesenchymal stem cell angiogenic capacity and stemness by a biomimetic hydrogel scaffold. *Biomaterials* **2012**, *33*, 80–90. [CrossRef] [PubMed]
66. Kim, S.J.; Park, J.; Byun, H.; Park, Y.W.; Major, L.G.; Lee, D.Y.; Choi, Y.S.; Shin, H. Hydrogels with an embossed surface: An all-in-one platform for mass production and culture of human adipose-derived stem cell spheroids. *Biomaterials* **2019**, *188*, 198–212. [CrossRef] [PubMed]
67. Wang, L.S.; Chung, J.E.; Chan, P.P.; Kurisawa, M. Injectable biodegradable hydrogels with tunable mechanical properties for the stimulation of neurogenesic differentiation of human mesenchymal stem cells in 3D culture. *Biomaterials* **2010**, *31*, 1148–1157. [CrossRef] [PubMed]
68. Li, Y.; Kumacheva, E. Hydrogel microenvironments for cancer spheroid growth and drug screening. *Sci. Adv.* **2018**, *4*, eaas8998. [CrossRef]
69. LaBarbera, D.V.; Reid, B.G.; Yoo, B.H. The multicellular tumor spheroid model for high-throughput cancer drug discovery. *Expert Opin. Drug Discov.* **2012**, *7*, 819–830. [CrossRef]
70. Frimat, J.P.; Sisnaiske, J.; Subbiah, S.; Menne, H.; Godoy, P.; Lampen, P.; Leist, M.; Franzke, J.; Hengstler, J.G.; van Thriel, C.; et al. The network formation assay: A spatially standardized neurite outgrowth analytical display for neurotoxicity screening. *Lab Chip* **2010**, *10*, 701–709. [CrossRef]
71. Cheng, N.C.; Wang, S.; Young, T.H. The influence of spheroid formation of human adipose-derived stem cells on chitosan films on stemness and differentiation capabilities. *Biomaterials* **2012**, *33*, 1748–1758. [CrossRef]
72. Lu, T.J.; Chiu, F.Y.; Chiu, H.Y.; Chang, M.C.; Hung, S.C. Chondrogenic Differentiation of Mesenchymal Stem Cells in Three-Dimensional Chitosan Film Culture. *Cell Transplant.* **2017**, *26*, 417–427. [CrossRef] [PubMed]
73. Cheng, N.C.; Chang, H.H.; Tu, Y.K.; Young, T.H. Efficient transfer of human adipose-derived stem cells by chitosan/gelatin blend films. *J. Biomed. Mater. Res. B Appl. Biomater.* **2012**, *100*, 1369–1377. [CrossRef] [PubMed]
74. Huang, G.S.; Dai, L.G.; Yen, B.L.; Hsu, S.H. Spheroid formation of mesenchymal stem cells on chitosan and chitosan-hyaluronan membranes. *Biomaterials* **2011**, *32*, 6929–6945. [CrossRef] [PubMed]
75. Yeh, H.Y.; Liu, B.H.; Hsu, S.H. The calcium-dependent regulation of spheroid formation and cardiomyogenic differentiation for MSCs on chitosan membranes. *Biomaterials* **2012**, *33*, 8943–8954. [CrossRef]
76. Hsu, S.-H.; Lin, Y.; Lin, T.-C.; Tseng, T.-C.; Lee, H.-T.; Liao, Y.-C.; Chiu, I.-M. Spheroid formation from neural stem cells on chitosan membranes. *J. Med. Biol. Eng.* **2012**, *32*, 85–90. [CrossRef]
77. Ryu, S.; Kim, B.-S. Culture of neural cells and stem cells on graphene. *Tissue Eng. Regen. Med.* **2013**, *10*, 39–46. [CrossRef]
78. Li, N.; Zhang, Q.; Gao, S.; Song, Q.; Huang, R.; Wang, L.; Liu, L.; Dai, J.; Tang, M.; Cheng, G. Three-dimensional graphene foam as a biocompatible and conductive scaffold for neural stem cells. *Sci. Rep.* **2013**, *3*, 1604. [CrossRef]

79. Kim, J.; Park, S.; Kim, Y.J.; Jeon, C.S.; Lim, K.T.; Seonwoo, H.; Cho, S.P.; Chung, T.D.; Choung, P.H.; Choung, Y.H.; et al. Monolayer graphene-directed growth and neuronal differentiation of mesenchymal stem cells. *J. Biomed. Nanotechnol.* **2015**, *11*, 2024–2033. [CrossRef] [PubMed]
80. Kim, Y.; Baipaywad, P.; Jeong, Y.; Park, H. Incorporation of gelatin microparticles on the formation of adipose-derived stem cell spheroids. *Int. J. Biol. Macromol.* **2018**, *110*, 472–478. [CrossRef] [PubMed]
81. Hayashi, K.; Tabata, Y. Preparation of stem cell aggregates with gelatin microspheres to enhance biological functions. *Acta Biomater.* **2011**, *7*, 2797–2803. [CrossRef] [PubMed]
82. Bratt-Leal, A.M.; Carpenedo, R.L.; Ungrin, M.D.; Zandstra, P.W.; McDevitt, T.C. Incorporation of biomaterials in multicellular aggregates modulates pluripotent stem cell differentiation. *Biomaterials* **2011**, *32*, 48–56. [CrossRef] [PubMed]
83. Chan, B.P.; Hui, T.Y.; Wong, M.Y.; Yip, K.H.; Chan, G.C. Mesenchymal stem cell-encapsulated collagen microspheres for bone tissue engineering. *Tissue Eng. Part C Methods* **2010**, *16*, 225–235. [CrossRef] [PubMed]
84. Abbasi, F.; Ghanian, M.H.; Baharvand, H.; Vahidi, B.; Eslaminejad, M.B. Engineering mesenchymal stem cell spheroids by incorporation of mechanoregulator microparticles. *J. Mech. Behav. Biomed. Mater.* **2018**, *84*, 74–87. [CrossRef] [PubMed]
85. Baraniak, P.R.; Cooke, M.T.; Saeed, R.; Kinney, M.A.; Fridley, K.M.; McDevitt, T.C. Stiffening of human mesenchymal stem cell spheroid microenvironments induced by incorporation of gelatin microparticles. *J. Mech. Behav. Biomed. Mater.* **2012**, *11*, 63–71. [CrossRef] [PubMed]
86. Bratt-Leal, A.M.; Nguyen, A.H.; Hammersmith, K.A.; Singh, A.; McDevitt, T.C. A microparticle approach to morphogen delivery within pluripotent stem cell aggregates. *Biomaterials* **2013**, *34*, 7227–7235. [CrossRef]
87. Vinci, M.; Gowan, S.; Boxall, F.; Patterson, L.; Zimmermann, M.; Court, W.; Lomas, C.; Mendiola, M.; Hardisson, D.; Eccles, S.A. Advances in establishment and analysis of three-dimensional tumor spheroid-based functional assays for target validation and drug evaluation. *BMC Biol.* **2012**, *10*, 29. [CrossRef]
88. Nath, S.; Devi, G.R. Three-dimensional culture systems in cancer research: Focus on tumor spheroid model. *Pharmacol. Ther.* **2016**, *163*, 94–108. [CrossRef]
89. Frese, K.K.; Tuveson, D.A. Maximizing mouse cancer models. *Nat. Rev. Cancer* **2007**, *7*, 645–658. [CrossRef]
90. Langhans, S.A. Three-dimensional in vitro cell culture models in drug discovery and drug repositioning. *Front. Pharmacol.* **2018**, *9*, 6. [CrossRef]
91. Sant, S.; Johnston, P.A. The production of 3D tumor spheroids for cancer drug discovery. *Drug Discov. Today Technol.* **2017**, *23*, 27–36. [CrossRef]
92. Teng, C.J.; Luo, J.; Chiu, R.C.; Shum-Tim, D. Massive mechanical loss of microspheres with direct intramyocardial injection in the beating heart: Implications for cellular cardiomyoplasty. *J. Thorac. Cardiovasc. Surg.* **2006**, *132*, 628–632. [CrossRef] [PubMed]
93. Lee, W.-Y.; Chang, Y.-H.; Yeh, Y.-C.; Chen, C.-H.; Lin, K.M.; Huang, C.-C.; Chang, Y.; Sung, H.-W. The use of injectable spherically symmetric cell aggregates self-assembled in a thermo-responsive hydrogel for enhanced cell transplantation. *Biomaterials* **2009**, *30*, 5505–5513. [CrossRef] [PubMed]
94. Tseng, T.C.; Hsu, S.H. Substrate-mediated nanoparticle/gene delivery to MSC spheroids and their applications in peripheral nerve regeneration. *Biomaterials* **2014**, *35*, 2630–2641. [CrossRef] [PubMed]
95. Yamaguchi, Y.; Ohno, J.; Sato, A.; Kido, H.; Fukushima, T. Mesenchymal stem cell spheroids exhibit enhanced in-vitro and in-vivo osteoregenerative potential. *BMC Biotechnol.* **2014**, *14*, 105. [CrossRef] [PubMed]
96. Yanagihara, K.; Uchida, S.; Ohba, S.; Kataoka, K.; Itaka, K. Treatment of bone defects by transplantation of genetically modified mesenchymal stem cell spheroids. *Mol. Ther. Methods Clin. Dev.* **2018**, *9*, 358–366. [CrossRef]
97. Uchida, S.; Itaka, K.; Nomoto, T.; Endo, T.; Matsumoto, Y.; Ishii, T.; Kataoka, K. An injectable spheroid system with genetic modification for cell transplantation therapy. *Biomaterials* **2014**, *35*, 2499–2506. [CrossRef]

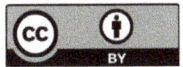

© 2019 by the authors. Licensee MDPI, Basel, Switzerland. This article is an open access article distributed under the terms and conditions of the Creative Commons Attribution (CC BY) license (http://creativecommons.org/licenses/by/4.0/).

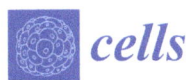

Brief Report

Human Platelet Lysate as a Functional Substitute for Fetal Bovine Serum in the Culture of Human Adipose Derived Stromal/Stem Cells

Mathew Cowper [1,†], Trivia Frazier [1,2,3], Xiying Wu [2,3], J. Lowry Curley [2,4], Michelle H. Ma [3], Omair A. Mohiuddin [1], Marilyn Dietrich [5], Michelle McCarthy [1], Joanna Bukowska [1,6] and Jeffrey M. Gimble [1,2,3,*]

1. School of Medicine, Tulane University, New Orleans, LA 70112, USA
2. LaCell LLC, New Orleans, LA 70148, USA
3. Obatala Sciences Inc., New Orleans, LA 70148, USA
4. Axosim Inc., New Orleans, LA 70112, USA
5. Louisiana State University School of Veterinary Medicine, Baton Rouge, LA 70803, USA
6. Institute for Animal Reproduction and Food Research, Polish Academy of Science, 10-748 Olsztyn, Poland
* Correspondence: jeffrey.gimble@lacell-usa.com; Tel.: +1-(504)-300-0266
† Current Affiliations: Department of Urology, Bowman Gray School of Medicine, Wake Forest University, Winston Salem, NC 27101, USA.

Received: 15 May 2019; Accepted: 9 July 2019; Published: 15 July 2019

Abstract: Introduction: Adipose derived stromal/stem cells (ASCs) hold potential as cell therapeutics for a wide range of disease states; however, many expansion protocols rely on the use of fetal bovine serum (FBS) as a cell culture nutrient supplement. The current study explores the substitution of lysates from expired human platelets (HPLs) as an FBS substitute. Methods: Expired human platelets from an authorized blood center were lysed by freeze/thawing and used to examine human ASCs with respect to proliferation using hematocytometer cell counts, colony forming unit-fibroblast (CFU-F) frequency, surface immunophenotype by flow cytometry, and tri-lineage (adipocyte, chondrocyte, osteoblast) differentiation potential by histochemical staining. Results: The proliferation assays demonstrated that HPLs supported ASC proliferation in a concentration dependent manner, reaching levels that exceeded that observed in the presence of 10% FBS. The concentration of 0.75% HPLs was equivalent to 10% FBS when utilized in cell culture media with respect to proliferation, immunophenotype, and CFU-F frequency. When added to osteogenic, adipogenic, and chondrogenic differentiation media, both supplements showed appropriate differentiation by staining. Conclusion: HPLs is an effective substitute for FBS in the culture, expansion and differentiation of human ASCs suitable for pre-clinical studies; however, additional assays and analyses will be necessary to validate HPLs for clinical applications and regulatory approval.

Keywords: adipogenesis; adipose-derived stromal/stem cells; chondrogenesis; colony forming unit-fibroblast; fetal bovine serum; human platelet lysate; mesenchymal stem cell; osteogenesis; regenerative medicine

1. Introduction

Human adipose-derived stromal/stem cells (ASCs) are derived from culture expanded stromal vascular fraction (SVF) cells isolated by collagenase digestion from adipose tissue harvested by tumescent liposuction or abdominoplasty [1]. The ASCs are multipotent progenitors that can be distinguished based on their surface antigen immunophenotypic profile and their differentiation potential along the adipocyte, chondrocyte, and osteoblast lineage pathways [1,2]. In addition, there is considerable interest in the ability of ASCs to modulate inflammation in vivo via their secretion of cytokines and exosome vesicles containing microRNAs and proteins [3–9]. Due to the ease of collection, multipotent differentiation, and paracrine function, ASCs are now being applied in clinical settings to regenerate and repair human tissues impacted by biological aging and disease processes [10,11].

In order to use human ASCs to treat disease, it has been necessary to standardize the methodology for ex vivo expansion in accordance with Current Good Manufacturing Practice (cGMP). Due to the presence of bovine spongiform encephalopathy (BSE) in many herds worldwide, their remains considerable regulatory concern for potential use of FBS as a cell culture nutrient to introduce xenogeneic material [12,13]. Historically, proliferation of ASCs has largely been performed using growth media supplemented fetal bovine serum. While FBS has been an effective medium for cell culture, it does have several additional disadvantages beyond those relating to the risk of BSE contamination. First, FBS products introduce considerable cost to the manufacturing process relative to human platelet lysate due in part to reduced proliferation rates and the need for extended culture expansion periods [14]. Second, FBS use introduces xenoproteins that bind to isolated ASCs, thereby increasing the risk of immune rejection due to antibody development against surface protein complexes on the transplanted ASCs. Indeed, consistent with this concern, the examination of allogeneic transplantation of ASCs in rat models has detected subsequent FBS-related antibody production [15].

To address the potential shortcomings of FBS as a nutrient for clinical expansion of ASCs, investigators have turned to human blood-derived products as alternatives. For example, Finnish investigators have used human serum successfully to expand autologous ASCs for tissue regeneration of craniofacial defects [16]. Likewise, human platelet lysates have long been used as a potential nutrient for the growth of human cells in vitro [17,18]. Independent investigators have begun to explore the use of human platelet lysates as an FBS substitute in culture medium for human ASC expansion [19–30]. To extend this line of research, the current study evaluated a human platelet lysate-derived substitute for FBS based on human ASC proliferation, colony forming unit-fibroblast (CFU-F), and differentiation assays.

2. Methods

2.1. Materials

All reagents were obtained from Thermo Fisher Scientific (Rochester, NY, USA) or LaCell LLC (New Orleans LA) unless stated otherwise.

2.2. Human Platelet Lysate Preparation

Platelet lysate was generated from expired bags of concentrated platelets donated by anonymous consenting donors (n = 3 to 4 donors per lot) obtained from a local blood bank (LifeShare Blood Center, Shreveport & Baton Rouge, LA). The platelets were stored on dry ice during transport. Platelets underwent three rounds of freezing (−80 °C overnight) and thawing (18–24 h at 4–8 °C) and were subsequently transferred to sterile centrifugation tubes (Thermo Scientific, Rochester, NY, USA) within a BSL2 cabinet (Class II A/B3 Biological Safety Cabinet, Thermo Forma, USA). In order to remove particulates, the samples were centrifuged at 4000 rpm for 15 min (Sorval Legend T, Kendro, Germany) and the supernatant was aspirated above the pelleted material. The aspirated platelet lysate solution from n = 3 individual donors was pooled, 0.22 µM sterile filtered, and stored at −20 °C prior to use.

2.3. Adipose Derived Stromal/Stem Cells

Primary human ASCs were isolated from the lipoaspirate of multiple anonymous healthy female donors (n = 7) with a mean body mass index (BMI) of 25.77 ± 2.82 (± standard deviation) and a mean age of 46.14 ± 14.34 years as previously described (Table 1) [31,32]. All subjects provided informed written consent under a LaCell sponsored protocol reviewed and approved by the Western Institutional Review Board (Pulyallup, WA, USA) as Study Number 1,138,160 and IRB (Institutional Review Board) Tracking Number 20,130,449 with a most recent approval date of March 9, 2019. The donors were either

Caucasian (n = 5) or African-American (n = 2). Lipoaspirate was transferred to a sterile 250 mL bottle. The tissue was washed with an equal volume of prewarmed (37 °C) sterile phosphate buffered saline (PBS), and then centrifuged at 1200 rpm for 5 min. The infranatant was aspirated before the tissue was washed and centrifuged again. An equal volume of prewarmed (37 °C) sterile PBS supplemented with type I collagenase (1 mg/mL of tissue) (Worthington Biochemical Corporation, Lakewood, NJ, USA), Fraction V bovine serum albumin (BSA) (10 mg/mL) (Sigma-Aldrich, Saint Louis, MO, USA), and 2 mM $CaCl_2$ was added to the tissue. The resulting suspension was then put on a shaker (Innova 4200 Incubator Shaker, New Brunswick Scientific, Edison, NJ, USA) between 180 and 200 rpm at 37 °C for between 50 and 70 min. The digested tissue was then centrifuged at 1200 rpm for five minutes. After gently resuspending the separated tissue, this step was repeated. The supernatant was aspirated and the cell pellet, the stromal vascular fraction (SVF), was transferred to a sterile centrifugation tube and resuspended in prewarmed (37 °C) sterile PBS. The resulting solution was centrifuged at 1200 rpm for five minutes. The PBS was aspirated before the cell pellet was resuspended in LaCell StromaQual™ media (LaCell, New Orleans, LA, USA) containing 10% FBS and plated in T150 or T175 flasks at a density of 0.19 to 0.22 mL of digested lipoaspirate per cm^2 and incubated in a humidified 5% CO_2 incubator (Heratherm® microbiological incubators, Thermo Scientific, Logan, UT, USA) for 24 to 48 h. The media was vacuum aspirated, and the flask was washed with prewarmed (37 °C) sterile PBS, fed with 35 mL of fresh stromal media, and the flask returned to the incubator. Upon reaching 80% to 90% confluence, the adherent cell layer, composed of ASCs, was detached using 0.05% trypsin/EDTA (ethylenediamine tetraacetic acid). ASCs were resuspended and stored at a density of 1.0×10^6/mL in cryopreservation media (LaCell, LA, USA) in 2.0 mL cryogenic vials in a liquid nitrogen tank (LS 3000 Lab Systems Taylor Warton, Minnetonka, MN, USA) until use. All subsequent studies were performed with cryopreserved and thawed ASCs used between passages 1 to 3.

Table 1. Adipose derived stromal/stem cell donor demographic information.

Donor	Race	Age	BMI
L111110W	AA	55	24.56
L110411W	C	66	25.28
L110822W	C	56	26.62
L100401T	C	41	23.73
L100723W	C	22	23.59
L100910W	C	44	24.89
L145	AA	39	31.75
Average		46.14 ± 14.35	25.77 ± 2.82

2.4. Proliferation Assay

ASCs (n = 7) were seeded in stromal media containing 10% FBS, 1.0% PL (Platelet Lysate), 0.75% PL (n = 4), 0.33% PL, or 0.1% PL in 12 well plates (Olympus Plastic, Genesee Scientific, San Diego, CA, USA) at a density of 10,000 cells/cm^2. Every 24 h for four days, one well of ASCs from each media condition was detached using 0.05% trypsin/EDTA, stained using trypan blue, and counted using a hemocytometer counting chamber with a phase contrast microscope (Motic Microscope, Hong Kong, China).

2.5. Colony Forming Unit Assay

ASCs (n = 7) were seeded in six well plates (Olympus Plastic, Genesee Scientific, San Diego, CA, USA) containing LaCell StromaQual™ media supplemented with 10% FBS or 0.75% PL at densities of 100, 200, and 400 cells per well. ASCs were proliferated for two weeks, with the media being changed each week. Colonies were stained with toluidine blue and counted using a phase-contrast microscope.

Colonies containing 32 or more cells were counted. Linear regression was performed on the counted colonies, and data are reported as colonies per 100 cells seeded.

2.6. Flow Cytometry Assay

Cryopreserved ASCs isolated from n = 4 donors with mean ± S.D. ages of 46.5 ± 7.8 years and BMI of 27.50 ± 3.89 were thawed, cultured in StromaQual supplemented with either 10% FBS or 0.75% PL until confluent, harvested by trypsin digestion, stained with fluorochrome conjugated antibodies (anti-CD29, anti-CD105, anti-CD45, anti-CD34, anti-CD31, anti-CD73, anti-CD90, and isotype control IgG1 (Immunoglobulin G1)), and evaluated by flow cytometry (FACSAria instrument, BD Biosciences, San Jose, CA, USA) as previously described [31].

2.7. Differentiation Capacity of ASCs

Confluent ASCs were cultured with adipogenic, osteogenic, as well as stromal media as a control. Passage 1 ASCs (n = 4) were cultured with LaCell StromaQual media containing 10% FBS in T-25 flasks until fully confluent. ASCs were washed with PBS, resuspended in stromal media containing either 10% FBS or 0.75% PL, and seeded on a 12 well plate at a density of 40,000 cells/cm^2. Once fully confluent, the stromal media was aspirated, and adipogenic and osteogenic differentiation media was introduced.

Pellet ASCs were cultured with chondrogenic containing 10% FBS or 0.75% PL, as well as stromal media with the same concentrations of nutrient supplements as a control. Passage 1 ASCs were (n = 3) cultured with LaCell StromaQual media containing 10% FBS in T-175 flasks until fully confluent. ASCs were washed with PBS, and resuspended in 0.5 mL of chondrogenic differentiation media at a density of 500,000 cells/cm^2 in 15 mL conical tubes. The ASCs were centrifuged at 300 G at 22 °C for 5 min to form a pellet at the bottom of the tube. The tops of the conical tubes were loosened to facilitate gas exchange and the pellets were incubated at 37 °C and 5% CO_2 overnight. Five pellets were then aggregated into 50 mL conical tubes.

2.8. Adipogenic Induction

Confluent ASCs were exposed to adipogenic differentiation media (AdipoQual™ LaCell, LA, USA) containing either 3% FBS or 0.75% PL for three days as previously described [32,33]. Adipogenic maintenance media containing the same concentrations of FBS or PL was then introduced, and the cells were maintained for an additional five to six more days, with the media being changed every two to three days. Differentiated cells were fixed by aspirating the differentiation media, washing three times with PBS, adding PBS containing 10% formalin (Thermo Scientific, Boston, UT, USA), and then placed at 4 °C for one hour. The PBS containing 10% formalin was aspirated and 0.22 µm sterile filtered 5% Oil Red O (Sigma-Aldrich, Saint Louis, MO, USA) in isopropanol was added for 15 min at room temperature. The stain was removed, and the sample rinsed three times or more with distilled water until completely clear. Images were captured using Motic Images Plus 2.0 software (Motic, Hong Kong, China) and a phase contrast microscope.

2.9. Osteogenic Induction

Confluent ASCs were exposed to osteogenic differentiation media (OsteoQual™, LaCell, LA, USA) containing either 10% FBS or 0.75% PL for eight to nine days, with the media being changed every two to three days according to a modification of previously described methods [31–34]. Differentiated cells were fixed by aspirating the differentiation media, washing three times with 150 mM NaCl, adding ice cold 70% ethanol (Sigma-Aldrich, Saint Louis, MO, USA), and then placed at 4 °C for one hour. The 70% ethanol was aspirated, and the sample washed three times with distilled water. Then, 0.22 µm sterile filtered 2% Alizarin Red (Sigma-Aldrich, Saint Louis, MO, USA) stain was added for 10 min at room temperature. The stain was removed, and the sample rinsed five times or more with distilled water until completely clear. Images were captured using Motic Images Plus 2.0 software and a phase contrast microscope.

2.10. Chondrogenic Induction

ASC pellets were exposed to complete chondrogenic differentiation media (ChondroQual™, LaCell, LA, USA) containing either 10% FBS or 0.75% PL for 14 days in pellet cultures prepared with 0.25×10^6 ASCs, with media being changed every other day according to a modification of previously described methods [35]. As controls, equivalent pellets were maintained in StromaQual medium over the same time period. Differentiated and undifferentiated cell pellets were fixed by aspirating the media, and washing once with PBS. The pellets were fixed in 4% paraformaldehyde solution, paraffin embedded, and then sectioned and stained with 1% Alcian Blue solution (pH 1.0) for 30 min at room temperature (Scytek Laboratories, Logan, UT, USA).

2.11. Quantitative Reverse Transcriptase Polymerase Chain Reaction (qRT-PCR)

ASC pellet cultured under the control or chondrogenic inductive conditions with either 10% FBS or 0.75% PL medium were frozen at −80 °C prior to isolation of total RNA using the RNeasy® Mini Kit (Qiagen, Valencai, CA, USA) according to the manufacturer's instructions. The resulting total RNA (1 µg) was reverse transcribed using the iScript™ cDNA Synthesis Kit (BioRad, Hercules, CA, USA) according to the manufacturer's instructions. Real time PCR was performed using a CFX96 Touch™ Real Time PCR Detection System (BioRad, Hercules, CA, USA) as follows: 1 cycle at 95 °C for 4 min, 40 cycles of 95 °C for 15 s followed by 60 °C for 1 min, followed by a melt curve of 55 to 95 °C with an increment of 0.5 °C. The amplification was performed in a 20 µL volume containing iQ™ SYBR Green Supermix (BioRad, Hercules, CA, USA) 2× concentrate (10 µL), each of two primers (4 µL from a 1 µM stock for a 200 nM final concentration), and cDNA template (25 ng). The following human primer sets were synthesized by Integrated DNA Technologies (Coralville, IA, USA) (Gene Bank Accession numbers are presented in parentheses):

Aggrecan Forward AAGTATCATCAGTCCCAGAATCTAGCA (NM_001135).
Aggrecan Reverse CGTGGAATGCAGAGGTGGTT.
Collagen I Forward CACCAATCACCTGCGTACAGAA (NM_000088).
Collagen I Reverse ACAGATCACGTCATCGCACAAC.
Collagen II Forward GGCAATAGCAGGTTCACGTACA (NM_001844).
Collagen II Reverse CGATAACAGTCTTGCCCCACTT.
GAPDH Forward TAAAAGCAGCCCTGGTGACC (NM_002046).
GAPDH Reverse CCACATCGCTCAGACACCAT.
Matrilin I Forward AGGGACTGCGTTTGCATTTTT (NM_002379).
Matrilin I Reverse TCAGTAAAGAAATTCACAGCACTCAGA.

The relative expression of each PCR product was normalized relative to the GAPDH (GlycerAldehyde 3 Phosphate DeHydrogenase) as a control.

2.12. Statistical Analysis

All values are reported as mean ± standard error. The student's T-test was performed on equivalent experiments between PL and FBS, with significance being defined as results with a p value < 0.05.

3. Results

3.1. Effect of Platelet Lysate Concentration in Culture Medium on ASC Proliferation

Initial studies evaluated the impact of platelet lysate concentration on ASC proliferation in vitro. ASC cultures were initiated in stromal media supplemented with increasing concentrations of HPLs (Figure 1). These displayed a concentration dependent change in cellular proliferation when compared to equivalent media prepared with 10% FBS. The FBS used in the study was lot characterized based on its reproducible ability to support robust human ASC proliferation and adipogenesis in vitro. An equivalent number of ASCs were plated in each experiment. Data indicated that increasing the concentration of HPL provided a growth advantage relative to 10% FBS at the 72 and 96 h time points. After comparing ASC proliferation in 0.1%, 0.33%, and 1.0% HPL versus 10% FBS, the experiment was repeated with 0.75% HPL.

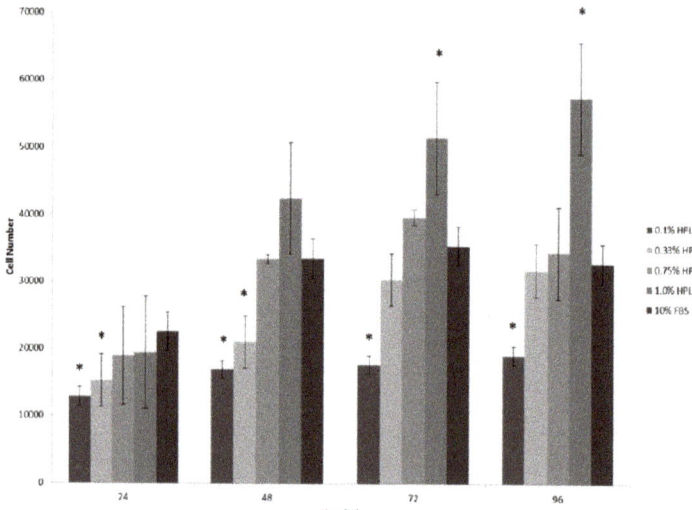

Figure 1. Effect of the concentration of HPL (Human Platelet Lysate) supplementation on ASC proliferation compared to 10% FBS. Stromal media containing 0.1%, 0.33%, 0.75%, 1.0% PL, and 10% FBS were tested for impact on ASC proliferation. Data is reported as the mean ± standard error. * Significant difference; $p < 0.05$.

3.2. ASC Surface Immunophenotype as a Function of Medium Composition

Successive studies evaluated the impact of 0.75% human platelet lysate as compared to 10% FBS supplementation on the surface immunophenotype of ASCs cultured in stromal medium. Flow cytometry analyses were performed focusing on phenotypic ASC surface antigens as recommended by the International Society for Cell Therapy (ISCT) and International Federation for Adipose Therapeutics and Science (IFATS) consensus [1]. The outcomes indicated that the ASCs displayed comparable levels of characteristic surface antigens CD29, CD31, CD34, CD45, CD70, CD90, and CD105 based on the percentage of positive staining cells independent of the nutrient supplement (Figure 2 and Table 2; mean of n = 4 ASC donors).

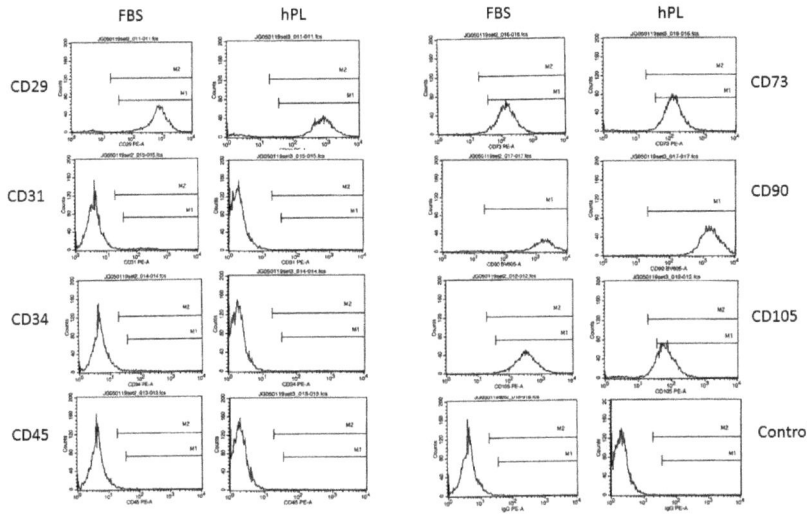

Figure 2. Histograms of flow cytometry detection of surface antigens. The ASCs were culture expanded in stromal media containing either 10% FBS or 0.75% PL and the expression determined for the following surface antigens by flow cytometry: CD29, CD31, CD34, CD45, CD73, CD90, and CD105, with IgG serving as a negative control. The histograms displayed are all derived from a single individual ASC donor and are representative of n = 3 donors. CD: cluster of differentiation.

Table 2. Immunophenotype of adipose derived stromal/stem cells following expansion in 10% FBS or 0.75% HPL.

Antibody	FBS	HPL
CD29 PE-A	93.97 ± 3.56	81.80 ± 29.50
CD105 PE-A	95.66 ± 3.66	90.47 ± 10.52
CD45 PE-A	−0.1 ± 0.82	0.02 ± 0.37
CD34 PE-A	2.98 ± 2.35	0.89 ± 0.47
CD31 PE-A	0.53 ± 1.19	0.23 ± 0.27
CD73 PE-A	93.69 ± 5.10	92.74 ± 6.44
CD90 BV605-A	93.66 ± 3.08	99.15 ± 0.75
IgG PE-A	0.32 ± 0.19	−0.10 ± 0.37
PE-A	0.74 ± 0.79	0.33 ± 0.65

3.3. Colony Forming as a Function of Medium Composition

A colony-forming unit-fibroblast assay was performed to assess ASCs' ability to form colonies in stromal media supplemented with 0.75% PL compared to 10% FBS at passage 1 (Figure 3). The observed morphology of colonies grown in both media was essentially equal, with representative images shown in Figure 3. There was no statistically significant difference in CFU-F numbers as a function of nutrient supplement (10% FBS: 6.65 ± 2.38, 0.75% HPL: 2.56 ± 1.15 colonies, n = 7, p value = 0.11).

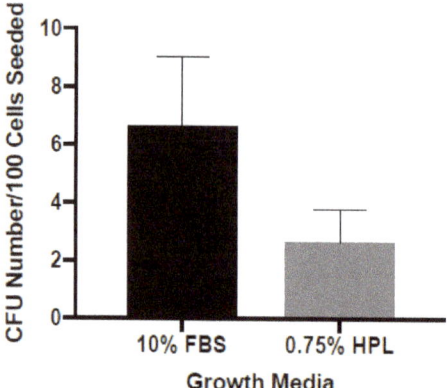

Figure 3. Effect of 0.75% HPL supplementation on the colony-forming unit-fibroblast assay compared to 10% FBS per 10^2 ASC. Stromal media containing 0.75% PL and 10% FBS were tested for impact on ASC colony-forming unit-fibroblast count. Data are reported as the mean ± standard error.; n = 7, one replicate.

3.4. Differentiation as a Function of Medium Nutrient Supplement Composition

Characterization of ASCs' ability to differentiate along mesenchymal lineages, specifically adipogenic, osteogenic, and chondrogenic, in differentiation media containing 0.75% PL compared to 10% FBS was qualitatively assessed using histochemical staining (Figure 4A,B). Adipogenesis was assessed based on Oil Red O staining of the intracellular neutral lipid droplets. Adipogenesis was observed in ASCs cultured in AdipoQual prepared with either 0.75% HPL or 10% FBS differentiation media. While both nutrient supplements supported differentiation, adipogenesis was more robust in the presence of FBS. Osteogenesis was assessed based on alizarin red staining of extracellular calcium phosphate deposition and mineralization. While OsteoQual prepared with both nutrient supplements supported differentiation, stain uptake was greater in the presence of 0.75% HPL. Chondrogenesis was assessed based on alcian blue staining of glycosaminoglycan deposition in 3-dimensional pellet cultures. ChondroQual prepared with either nutrient supplement supported chondrocyte formation based on histochemical detection of glycosaminoglycan. While the presence of ChondroQual appeared to increase the relative diameter of the pellet cultures relative to StromaQual, the actual percentage increase was not quantified. Additionally, ChondroQual prepared with either 0.75% HPL or 10% FBS induced a consistent qRT-PCR fold-expression profile for the chondrogenic associated mRNAs aggrecan, collagen type II, and matrilin 1 relative to StromaQual control medium. In contrast, the expression of collagen I was comparable regardless of whether pellets were cultured in the presence of medium with or without chondrogenic inductive agents.

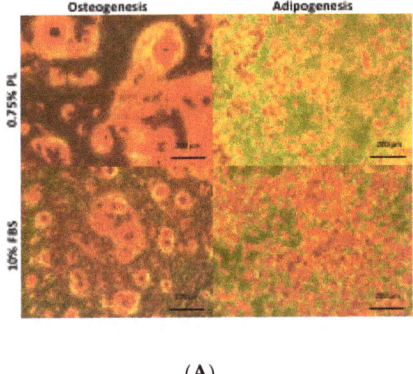

(A)

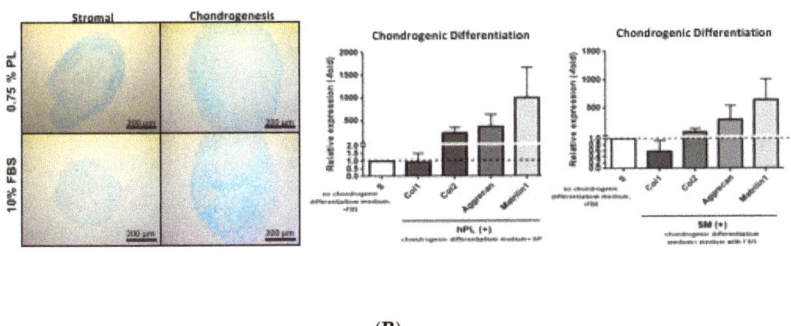

(B)

Figure 4. Adipogenic, chondrogenic, and osteogenic differentiation ability of ASCs cultured in 0.75% HPL or 10% FBS containing media. (A) Differentiation of ASCs confirmed by staining of two-dimensional cultures with Oil Red O (adipogenesis in the presence of AdipoQual) or Alizarin Red (osteogenesis in the presence of OsteoQual). (B) Differentiation of ASCs confirmed by staining with Alcian Blue (chondrogenesis in the presence of ChondroQual vs. StromaQual controls) and by qRT-PCR analysis of the transcribed total RNA for the mRNAs collagen I (Col I), collagen II (Col II), aggrecan, and matrilin 1 (qRT-PCR reactions were conducted in triplicate).

4. Discussion

The current study validates HPL as a potential nutrient substitute for FBS in the culture and differentiation of human ASCs. The HPL over a range of concentrations promotes enhanced ASC proliferation in a dose dependent manner. Indeed, the ASC proliferation in the presence of 0.75% HPL is approximately equal to that observed in the presence of 10% FBS. Nevertheless, the two supplements are not identical with respect to all outcomes. While the number of CFU-F tends to be greater in the presence of FBS compared to HPL, this did not reach statistical significance. Based on histochemical analyses, the ASC are capable of undergoing adipogenic, chondrogenic, and osteogenic differentiation in the presence of either FBS or HPL nutrient supplementation. This was further supported by qRT-PCR analysis of a select panel of chondrogenic mRNA biomarkers, which were induced to a comparable fold-expression level independent of the presence of either FBS or HPL. Nevertheless, further quantitative analyses of histochemical stain elution and more comprehensive qRT-PCR analysis of lineage specific mRNAs will be necessary to determine if the relative level of differentiation along any one lineage is favored by one or the other nutrient supplement.

These outcomes confirm findings reported by a growing body of literature. Platelet lysate was initially used as a cell culture supplement providing growth factors to promote CFU formation from breast cancers [17,18]. Likewise, the current study demonstrates that HPL supports CFU-F from ASCs in a manner comparable to FBS, consistent with prior observations reported by Chowela et al. [29]. Additional studies have further examined the utility of platelet lysate as an FBS substitute for the growth of bone marrow-derived mesenchymal stem/stromal cells (BM-MSCs) and ASCs [19–24,26–29,36–38]. Consistent with the current findings, HPL displayed support of ASC and BM-MSC proliferation in a concentration dependent manner [19,20,23,24,27,28,30,36,39]. Further analyses correlated the proliferative effects of HPL to the enriched presence of cytokines, including Acrp30 (Adiponectin), bFGF (basic Fibroblast Growth Factor), IL-6, MCP-1 (Monocyte Chemoattractant Protein-1), and PDGF, relative to FBS [39]. Additionally, mass spectroscopic analyses have determined that HPLs contains abundant levels of actin, fibrinogen, tropomyosin, and tubulin [36]. Both Cholewa et al. and Naaijkens et al. noted that HPLs significantly promoted ASC proliferation relative to FBS based on an increased number of population doublings and doubling times, respectively [26,29]. Additionally, they and Blande et al. noted that the size of individual ASCs was larger when cultured in FBS as compared to HPL [19,26,29]. Such observations are consistent with a recent cost analysis, which concluded that HPL is substantially more economical than FBS for clinical grade ASC expansion due to accelerated growth rates [14]. Comparable to the current analysis, Blande et al., Cholewa et al., and Naaijikens et al. independently demonstrated that the immunophenotype of ASCs cultured in FBS and HPL is comparable; however, Naaijikens et al. alone reported an increased intensity of the CD73, CD90, and CD166 surface antigens in the presence of HPL as compared to FBS [19,26,29]. Likewise, these same groups demonstrated that the ASCs cultured in either FBS or HPL continued to display adipogenic, chondrogenic, and/or osteogenic differentiation potential [19,26,29]. Based on this background, groups have begun adapting HPL supplements in the large scale production of human ASCs suitable for clinical applications [22,23].

While there are substantial advantages to the substitution of expired human platelet lysates for FBS in manufacturing protocols for clinical grade ASCs, there are potential issues remaining to be addressed. First is the question of how strong the supply chain will be for expired platelets from authorized blood centers. There is a need for careful consideration of the supply and demand for human platelets. It remains to be determined if an expanded outreach to the blood donor community will be necessary to ensure an appropriate balance between supply and demand. Second is a better understanding of the characterization of HPL expanded ASCs with respect to a wider range of clinical translational applications. Further studies will be necessary to evaluate the HPL expanded ASC product with respect to immunogenicity, immunosuppression, and exosome/secretome expression. Each of these outcomes may influence the utility of ASCs in the context of organ transplantation, immune regulation, and acute and chronic disease therapies [4,10,11]. Nevertheless, the current work and existing literature demonstrate the feasibility of substituting HPL for FBS as an alternative cell culture nutrient supplement and its practicality for in vitro and pre-clinical discovery research.

Funding: This research received no external funding.

Acknowledgments: The authors wish to thank James Wade and his patients and staff in Baton Rouge LA for their participation and support of this project.

Conflicts of Interest: M.H.M. is an employee of Obatala Sciences. T.F. is a co-owner, co-founder, CEO and President of Obatala Sciences and former employee of LaCell. X.W. is co-owner and co-founder of LaCell and Obatala and serves as Vice President for R & D at LaCell. J.M.G. is co-owner and co-founder of LaCell and Obatala Sciences, serves as Chief Scientific Officer of LaCell. T.F., X.W., and J.M.G. are inventors on patents relevant to this field. The remaining authors have no disclosures to declare.

References

1. Bourin, P.; Bunnell, B.A.; Casteilla, L.; Dominici, M.; Katz, A.J.; March, K.L.; Redl, H.; Rubin, J.P.; Yoshimura, K.; Gimble, J.M. Stromal cells from the adipose tissue-derived stromal vascular fraction and culture expanded adipose tissue-derived stromal/stem cells: A joint statement of the International Federation for Adipose Therapeutics and Science (IFATS) and the International Society for Cellular Therapy (ISCT). *Cytotherapy* **2013**, *15*, 641–648. [PubMed]
2. Gimble, J.M.; Katz, A.J.; Bunnell, B.A. Adipose-derived stem cells for regenerative medicine. *Circ. Res.* **2007**, *100*, 1249–1260. [CrossRef] [PubMed]
3. Kilroy, G.E.; Foster, S.J.; Wu, X.; Ruiz, J.; Sherwood, S.; Heifetz, A.; Ludlow, J.W.; Stricker, D.M.; Potiny, S.; Green, P.; et al. Cytokine profile of human adipose-derived stem cells: Expression of angiogenic, hematopoietic, and pro-inflammatory factors. *J. Cell. Physiol.* **2007**, *212*, 702–709. [CrossRef] [PubMed]
4. Salgado, A.J.; Reis, R.L.; Sousa, N.J.; Gimble, J.M. Adipose tissue derived stem cells secretome: Soluble factors and their roles in regenerative medicine. *Curr. Stem Cell Res. Ther.* **2010**, *5*, 103–110. [CrossRef] [PubMed]
5. Hu, L.; Wang, J.; Zhou, X.; Xiong, Z.; Zhao, J.; Yu, R.; Huang, F.; Zhang, H.; Chen, L. Exosomes derived from human adipose mensenchymal stem cells accelerates cutaneous wound healing via optimizing the characteristics of fibroblasts. *Sci. Rep.* **2016**, *6*, 32993. [CrossRef] [PubMed]
6. Ma, T.; Fu, B.; Yang, X.; Xiao, Y.; Pan, M. Adipose mesenchymal stem cell-derived exosomes promote cell proliferation, migration, and inhibit cell apoptosis via Wnt/beta-catenin signaling in cutaneous wound healing. *J. Cell. Biochem.* **2019**, *120*, 10847–10854. [CrossRef] [PubMed]
7. Maumus, M.; Jorgensen, C.; Noel, D. Mesenchymal stem cells in regenerative medicine applied to rheumatic diseases: Role of secretome and exosomes. *Biochimie* **2013**, *95*, 2229–2234. [CrossRef] [PubMed]
8. Wang, L.; Hu, L.; Zhou, X.; Xiong, Z.; Zhang, C.; Shehada, H.M.A.; Hu, B.; Song, J.; Chen, L. Exosomes secreted by human adipose mesenchymal stem cells promote scarless cutaneous repair by regulating extracellular matrix remodelling. *Sci. Rep.* **2017**, *7*, 13321. [CrossRef]
9. McIntosh, K.R.; Frazier, T.; Rowan, B.G.; Gimble, J.M. Evolution and future prospects of adipose-derived immunomodulatory cell therapeutics. *Expert Rev. Clin. Immunol.* **2013**, *9*, 175–184. [CrossRef]
10. Nordberg, R.C.; Loboa, E.G. Our Fat Future: Translating Adipose Stem Cell Therapy. *Stem Cells Transl. Med.* **2015**, *4*, 974–979. [CrossRef]
11. Bateman, M.E.; Strong, A.L.; Gimble, J.M.; Bunnell, B.A. Concise Review: Using Fat to Fight Disease: A Systematic Review of Nonhomologous Adipose-Derived Stromal/Stem Cell Therapies. *Stem Cells* **2018**, *36*, 1311–1328. [CrossRef] [PubMed]
12. Gottipamula, S.; Muttigi, M.S.; Kolkundkar, U.; Seetharam, R.N. Serum-free media for the production of human mesenchymal stromal cells: A review. *Cell Prolif.* **2013**, *46*, 608–627. [CrossRef] [PubMed]
13. World Health Organizatio. Medicinal and other products and human and animal transmissible spongiform encephalopathies: Memorandum from a WHO meeting. *Bull. World Health Organ.* **1997**, *75*, 505–513.
14. Bandeiras, C.; Cabral, J.M.; Finkelstein, S.N.; Ferreira, F.C. Modeling biological and economic uncertainty on cell therapy manufacturing: The choice of culture media supplementation. *Regen. Med.* **2018**, *13*, 917–933. [CrossRef] [PubMed]
15. McIntosh, K.R.; Lopez, M.J.; Borneman, J.N.; Spencer, N.D.; Anderson, P.A.; Gimble, J.M. Immunogenicity of allogeneic adipose-derived stem cells in a rat spinal fusion model. *Tissue Eng. Part A* **2009**, *15*, 2677–2686. [CrossRef] [PubMed]
16. Mesimaki, K.; Lindroos, B.; Tornwall, J.; Mauno, J.; Lindqvist, C.; Kontio, R.; Miettinen, S.; Suuronen, R. Novel maxillary reconstruction with ectopic bone formation by GMP adipose stem cells. *Int. J. Oral Maxillofac. Surg.* **2009**, *38*, 201–209. [CrossRef]
17. Cowan, D.H.; Graham, J. Stimulation of human tumor colony formation by platelet lysate. *J. Lab. Clin. Med.* **1983**, *102*, 973–986.
18. Cowan, D.H.; Graham, J.; Paskevich, M.C.; Quinn, P.G. Influence of platelet lysate on colony formation of human breast cancer cells. *Breast Cancer Res. Treat.* **1983**, *3*, 171–178. [CrossRef]
19. Blande, I.S.; Bassaneze, V.; Lavini-Ramos, C.; Fae, K.C.; Kalil, J.; Miyakawa, A.A.; Schettert, I.T.; Krieger, J.E. Adipose tissue mesenchymal stem cell expansion in animal serum-free medium supplemented with autologous human platelet lysate. *Transfusion* **2009**, *49*, 2680–2685. [CrossRef]

20. Castegnaro, S.; Chieregato, K.; Maddalena, M.; Albiero, E.; Visco, C.; Madeo, D.; Pegoraro, M.; Rodeghiero, F. Effect of platelet lysate on the functional and molecular characteristics of mesenchymal stem cells isolated from adipose tissue. *Curr. Stem Cell Res. Ther.* **2011**, *6*, 105–114. [CrossRef]
21. Dessels, C.; Durandt, C.; Pepper, M.S. Comparison of human platelet lysate alternatives using expired and freshly isolated platelet concentrates for adipose-derived stromal cell expansion. *Platelets* **2019**, *30*, 356–367. [CrossRef]
22. Glovinski, P.V.; Herly, M.; Mathiasen, A.B.; Svalgaard, J.D.; Borup, R.; Talman, M.M.; Elberg, J.J.; Kolle, S.T.; Drzewiecki, K.T.; Fischer-Nielsen, A. Overcoming the bottleneck of platelet lysate supply in large-scale clinical expansion of adipose-derived stem cells: A comparison of fresh versus three types of platelet lysates from outdated buffy coat-derived platelet concentrates. *Cytotherapy* **2017**, *19*, 222–234. [CrossRef] [PubMed]
23. Haack-Sorensen, M.; Juhl, M.; Follin, B.; Harary Sondergaard, R.; Kirchhoff, M.; Kastrup, J.; Ekblond, A. Development of large-scale manufacturing of adipose-derived stromal cells for clinical applications using bioreactors and human platelet lysate. *Scand. J. Clin. Lab. Investig.* **2018**, *78*, 293–300. [CrossRef] [PubMed]
24. Hildner, F.; Eder, M.J.; Hofer, K.; Aberl, J.; Redl, H.; van Griensven, M.; Gabriel, C.; Peterbauer-Scherb, A. Human platelet lysate successfully promotes proliferation and subsequent chondrogenic differentiation of adipose-derived stem cells: A comparison with articular chondrocytes. *J. Tissue Eng. Regen. Med.* **2015**, *9*, 808–818. [CrossRef] [PubMed]
25. Muller, A.M.; Davenport, M.; Verrier, S.; Droeser, R.; Alini, M.; Bocelli-Tyndall, C.; Schaefer, D.J.; Martin, I.; Scherberich, A. Platelet lysate as a serum substitute for 2D static and 3D perfusion culture of stromal vascular fraction cells from human adipose tissue. *Tissue Eng. Part A* **2009**, *15*, 869–875. [CrossRef]
26. Naaijkens, B.A.; Niessen, H.W.; Prins, H.J.; Krijnen, P.A.; Kokhuis, T.J.; de Jong, N.; van Hinsbergh, V.W.; Kamp, O.; Helder, M.N.; Musters, R.J.; et al. Human platelet lysate as a fetal bovine serum substitute improves human adipose-derived stromal cell culture for future cardiac repair applications. *Cell Tissue Res.* **2012**, *348*, 119–130. [CrossRef]
27. Shih, D.T.; Chen, J.C.; Chen, W.Y.; Kuo, Y.P.; Su, C.Y.; Burnouf, T. Expansion of adipose tissue mesenchymal stromal progenitors in serum-free medium supplemented with virally inactivated allogeneic human platelet lysate. *Transfusion* **2011**, *51*, 770–778. [CrossRef]
28. Trojahn Kolle, S.F.; Oliveri, R.S.; Glovinski, P.V.; Kirchhoff, M.; Mathiasen, A.B.; Elberg, J.J.; Andersen, P.S.; Drzewiecki, K.T.; Fischer-Nielsen, A. Pooled human platelet lysate versus fetal bovine serum-investigating the proliferation rate, chromosome stability and angiogenic potential of human adipose tissue-derived stem cells intended for clinical use. *Cytotherapy* **2013**, *15*, 1086–1097. [CrossRef]
29. Cholewa, D.; Stiehl, T.; Schellenberg, A.; Bokermann, G.; Joussen, S.; Koch, C.; Walenda, T.; Pallua, N.; Marciniak-Czochra, A.; Suschek, C.V.; et al. Expansion of adipose mesenchymal stromal cells is affected by human platelet lysate and plating density. *Cell Transplant.* **2011**, *20*, 1409–1422. [CrossRef]
30. Li, C.Y.; Wu, X.Y.; Tong, J.B.; Yang, X.X.; Zhao, J.L.; Zheng, Q.F.; Zhao, G.B.; Ma, Z.J. Comparative analysis of human mesenchymal stem cells from bone marrow and adipose tissue under xeno-free conditions for cell therapy. *Stem Cell Res. Ther.* **2015**, *6*, 55. [CrossRef]
31. Yu, G.; Wu, X.; Dietrich, M.A.; Polk, P.; Scott, L.K.; Ptitsyn, A.A.; Gimble, J.M. Yield and characterization of subcutaneous human adipose-derived stem cells by flow cytometric and adipogenic mRNA analyzes. *Cytotherapy* **2010**, *12*, 538–546. [CrossRef]
32. Yu, G.; Floyd, Z.E.; Wu, X.; Halvorsen, Y.D.; Gimble, J.M. Isolation of human adipose-derived stem cells from lipoaspirates. *Methods Mol. Biol.* **2011**, *702*, 17–27. [PubMed]
33. Yu, G.; Floyd, Z.E.; Wu, X.; Hebert, T.; Halvorsen, Y.D.; Buehrer, B.M.; Gimble, J.M. Adipogenic differentiation of adipose-derived stem cells. *Methods Mol. Biol.* **2011**, *702*, 193–200. [PubMed]
34. Hicok, K.C.; Du Laney, T.V.; Zhou, Y.S.; Halvorsen, Y.D.; Hitt, D.C.; Cooper, L.F.; Gimble, J.M. Human adipose-derived adult stem cells produce osteoid in vivo. *Tissue Eng.* **2004**, *10*, 371–380. [CrossRef] [PubMed]
35. Estes, B.T.; Diekman, B.O.; Gimble, J.M.; Guilak, F. Isolation of adipose-derived stem cells and their induction to a chondrogenic phenotype. *Nat. Protoc.* **2010**, *5*, 1294–1311. [CrossRef] [PubMed]
36. Kinzebach, S.; Dietz, L.; Kluter, H.; Thierse, H.J.; Bieback, K. Functional and differential proteomic analyses to identify platelet derived factors affecting ex vivo expansion of mesenchymal stromal cells. *BMC Cell Biol.* **2013**, *14*, 48. [CrossRef] [PubMed]
37. Bieback, K. Platelet lysate as replacement for fetal bovine serum in mesenchymal stromal cell cultures. *Transfus. Med. Hemother.* **2013**, *40*, 326–335. [CrossRef] [PubMed]

38. Doucet, C.; Ernou, I.; Zhang, Y.; Llense, J.R.; Begot, L.; Holy, X.; Lataillade, J.J. Platelet lysates promote mesenchymal stem cell expansion: A safety substitute for animal serum in cell-based therapy applications. *J. Cell. Physiol.* **2005**, *205*, 228–236. [CrossRef]
39. Bieback, K.; Hecker, A.; Kocaomer, A.; Lannert, H.; Schallmoser, K.; Strunk, D.; Kluter, H. Human alternatives to fetal bovine serum for the expansion of mesenchymal stromal cells from bone marrow. *Stem Cells* **2009**, *27*, 2331–2341. [CrossRef]

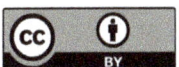 © 2019 by the authors. Licensee MDPI, Basel, Switzerland. This article is an open access article distributed under the terms and conditions of the Creative Commons Attribution (CC BY) license (http://creativecommons.org/licenses/by/4.0/).

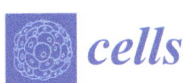

Article

Differences between the Proliferative Effects of Human Platelet Lysate and Fetal Bovine Serum on Human Adipose-Derived Stem Cells

Natsuko Kakudo *, Naoki Morimoto, Yuanyuan Ma and Kenji Kusumoto *

Department of Plastic and Reconstructive Surgery, Kansai Medical University, 2-5-1 Shin-machi, Hirakata, Osaka 573-1010, Japan; mnaoki22@kuhp.kyoto-u.ac.jp (N.M.); myy1002@163.com (Y.M.)
* Correspondence: kakudon@hirakata.kmu.ac.jp (N.K.); kusumoto@hirakata.kmu.ac.jp (K.K.);
 Tel.: +81-072-804-0101 (N.K.)

Received: 17 July 2019; Accepted: 6 October 2019; Published: 8 October 2019

Abstract: Background: Recently, human adipose-derived stem cells (hASCs) were discovered in the human subcutaneous adipose tissue. PLTMax Human Platelet Lysate (PLTMax), a supplement refined from human platelets, has been reported to have proliferative effects on bone marrow mesenchymal stem cells. The proliferative effects of PLTMax on ASCs were investigated in this study. Methods: The ASCs in DMEM (serum-free), DMEM+PLTMax (1%, 2%, 5%, and 10%), and DMEM+FBS (10%) were cultivated for two, five, and seven days. The cell growth rate was examined, BrdU incorporation, and the cell cycle and Ki-67 immunostaining were performed. The cell growth rate was investigated when each inhibitor (PD98059, SP600125, SB203580, and LY294002) was added and phosphorylation of ERK1/2, JNK, p38, and Akt were examined by western blotting. The cell surface marker of hASCs was also analyzed. Results: The cells in the PLTMax (5%) group showed significantly more proliferation compared to the cells in control (serum-free) and FBS (10%) groups, and a significant increase in the number of cells in the S phase and G2/M phase. The number of Ki-67 positive cells increased significantly in the DMEM+ PLTMax (5%) and the FBS (10%) groups. The addition of inhibitors PD98059, SP600125, SB203580, and LY294002 decreased the proliferative effects of PLTMax on ASCs. Phosphorylation of ERK1/2, JNK, p38, and Akt was observed in both the PLTMax (5%) and the FBS (10%) groups. Conclusions: For human adipose stem cells, 5% PLTMax was the optimum concentration, which showed a significantly higher proliferative effect than 10% FBS. PLTMax is a useful medium additive, which can substitute FBS. The proliferative effects of PLTMax are suggested to function via multiple signaling pathways, similar to FBS.

Keywords: human adipose-derived stem cells; human platelet lysate; stem cell proliferation; fetal bovine serum; signaling pathway

1. Introduction

Human adipose-derived stem cells (hASCs) have the potential to differentiate into adipose, bone, cartilage, tendons, nerves, and fat when cultivated under lineage-specific conditions [1,2]. The majority of ASCs exhibit fibroblastic morphological features and are easily grown under standard tissue culture conditions. Compared with bone marrow mesenchymal stem cells, hASCs are easier to obtain and carry a relatively lower donor site morbidity at harvest [3]. Due to their convenient isolation and extensive proliferative capacities in vitro, hASCs are a promising source of human stem cells for regenerative medicine.

Human platelet lysate (hPL), as prepared by repeated freeze/thaw cycles and sonication from fresh blood or outdated platelet concentrates, was found to support the proliferation of established cell lines, fibroblasts, and bone marrow mesenchymal stem cells [4–6]. Since our initial discovery of the enhanced proliferative effects of hPL on hASCs in 2008 [7], this phenomenon has been validated by Trojahn Kølle et al. [8] and Cervelli et al. [9]. However, the detailed mechanism of proliferation or its comparison with the effects of fetal bovine serum has not been elucidated yet. Although fetal bovine serum is the most commonly used culture supplement for hASCs at present, it has been found to increase the risk of xenogeneic infection and immune reactions as a side effect [10]. The risk of unknown infectious reagents in FBS is also a significant concern. Thus, alternatives to FBS are under investigation.

PLTMax® Human Platelet Lysate (PLTMax) was a kind of hPL that has been developed as a growth factor rich supplement that is a superior alternative to fetal bovine serum (FBS) for human cell expansion. PLTMax is derived from normal human donor platelets collected at U.S. blood centers. Multiple donor units are pooled in large batch sizes and manufactured to produce a consistent product. Each donor unit was approved for human use and has been tested for infectious diseases including HIV-1, HIV-2, HCV, HBsAg, and RPR for Syphilis. To date, although there are studies showing that PLTMax can be used in cell cultures for oral mucosal epithelial cells and human corneal epithelial cell lines [11], there are no reports on its proliferative effects on hASCs and its mechanism of action.

In this study, the proliferative effects of PLTMax on hASCs were investigated by evaluating the cell proliferation, BrdU incorporation, and cell cycle changes after the addition of PLTMax to the cells. In addition, the localization of Ki-67 was assessed using immunostaining as well as activation of ERK1/2, JNK, p38, and Akt by western blotting and compared these results with that obtained from FBS treated cells.

2. Materials and Methods

2.1. Reagents and Antibodies

PLTMax® Human Platelet Lysate was purchased from Merck (Darmstadt, Germany). Fetal bovine serum (FBS) was from Hyclone (Logan, UT, USA). PD98059 (an inhibitor of MEK), LY294002 (an inhibitor of phosphatidylinositol-3-kinase-AKT), and SB203580 (an inhibitor of p38) were all from Calbiochem-Novabiochem (San Diego, CA, USA). SP600125 (an inhibitor of JNK) was from Sigma (St. Louis, MO, USA). Rabbit anti-phospho-ERK1/2 was from Epitomics Inc. (Burlingame, CA, USA). Rabbit anti-phospho-AKT and rabbit anti-AKT were from Abcam (Cambridge, UK). Rabbit anti-ERK1/2 and rabbit anti-β-actin were from Cell Signaling Technology (Beverly, MA, USA). Heparin sodium injection-N was purchased from Mochida Pharmaceutical CO., LTD. (Tokyo, Japan). Antibodies of CD90, CD31, CD45, and CD34 were purchased from Beckton Dickinson Pharmingen (San Diego, CA, USA). All the other reagents, unless specified otherwise, were purchased from Sigma (St. Louis, MO, USA).

2.2. Isolation of hASCs

The study was approved by the Ethics Review Board of Kansai Medical University in accordance with the ethical guidelines of the Helsinki Declaration of 1975 (approval code: 2006106). All specimens were collected and used with informed consent from the volunteer donors. Adipose tissue was obtained from the patient through plastic surgery. Briefly, the adipose tissues used in this study were resected from fat mass, and not using liquid suction. The abdomen was defined as the donor site, where adipose tissues from disposed tissues from skin graft operations were extracted. hASCs were isolated using a method described previously [7,12,13]. After extensive washing with phosphate-buffered saline (PBS), the adipose tissues were cut into small pieces and then incubated with 3 volumes of 0.1% collagenase (Sigma-Aldrich, St. Louis, MO) solution with constant shaking at 40 °C for 40 min. After adding Dulbecco's Modified Eagle Medium (DMEM) containing 10% FBS and antibiotics, it was centrifuged at 400× g for 3 min. After removing cellular remains through a 100 μm nylon mesh (BD Falcon, Bedford, MA, USA), the cells were incubated with DMEM containing 10% FBS and antibiotics in a dish. The primary hASCs were cultured for 4 to 5 days until they reached confluence. For all experiments, cells from passage 7 through 9 were used for the culture.

2.3. Cell Proliferation Assay

For the cell proliferation assays, hASCs were seeded at a density of 1.0×10^4 cells/well in 24-well culture plates and incubated with the complete medium overnight. The cell medium was then replaced with serum-free DMEM. After 6 h incubation, hASCs were treated with various concentrations of PLTMax or FBS designated concentrations in serum-free DMEM for 2, 5, and 7 days. Heparin was added to the media at a final concentration of 2 U/mL for non-coagulation of medium with PLTMax. As the medium coagulated when PLTMax was added alone, the manufacturer's protocol specified that heparin should be added to the final concentration of 2 U/mL. When inhibitors were used, they were added at 1 h before the incubation with PLTMax. Cell proliferation was determined using the Cell Counting Kit-8 (Dojindo Molecular Technologies, Kumamoto, Japan), according to the manufacturer's instructions ($n = 4$). Absorbance was read at 450 nm on a multi-well plate reader (EnSpire 2300 Multilabel Reader; PerkinElmer, Inc., Waltham, MA, USA).

2.4. BrdU Incorporation Assay

The cells were seeded at a density of 2×10^3 cells/well in 96-well culture plates containing a complete medium. After overnight incubation, the hASCs were first starved in a serum-free DMEM for 6 h. These cells were then treated with PLTMax in the serum-free DMEM for 48 h. Inhibitors were added at 1 h before the incubation with PLTMax. Quantification of cell proliferation was determined using the Cell Proliferation ELISA BrdU kit (Roche), according to the manufacturer's instructions ($n = 4$).

2.5. Cell Cycle Assay

The MuseTM Cell Cycle reagent included propidium iodide (PI) as the binding reagent (intercalator) for DNA. Fluorescence intensity of an intercalated fluorescent substance represents the DNA amount and the cell cycle stage. Muse Cell Cycle Reagent was included in the Muse Cell Cycle Kit. hASCs (1×10^6) were seeded in a 10-cm culture dish containing complete medium and cultured overnight. The medium was then replaced with serum-free DMEM. After starvation for 6 h, the cells were then treated with the reagents with designated concentrations for 48 h. Treated cells were collected by trypsinization. After washing with ice-cold PBS twice, cells were fixed in 70% ethanol at −20 °C for 3 h. Based on the manufacturer's instructions, the fixed cells were then stained with MuseTM Cell Cycle reagent (200 µL) in the dark at room temperature for 30 min. Cell cycles were analyzed by flow cytometric quantification of their DNA by MuseTM Cell Analyzer (Millipore, Hayward, CA, USA) ($n = 6$ in each group).

2.6. Cell Surface Marker of hASCs

The phenotypical characterization of the ASCs was analyzed using BD FACSCalibur (Becton-Dickinson, Heidelberg, Germany) and accompanying software. At the 7th generation, the cells were detached with trypsin-EDTA, washed with phosphate-buffered saline (PBS), and immediately stained with the following labeled antibodies: CD90, CD31, CD45, CD34. Regarding ASCs after 48 h of PLTMax culturing, 1×10^6 cells were prepared per measurement, and the positive cell rate was analyzed ($n = 3$).

2.7. Immunofluorescence Confocal Microscopy

The cells were plated in Celldesk LF (Sumitomo Bakelite Co Ltd., Tokyo, Japan) with serum-free DMEM for 24 h before stimulation. Subsequently, cells were stimulated with PLTMax or FBS for 48 h. The cells were fixed with 4% formaldehyde solution for 15 min and then washed thrice with

PBS. Following that, 0.2% Triton X-100 was added to the cells, incubated for 5 min, and then washed thrice with PBS. Further, the cells were blocked using Protein Block Serum-Free solution (Dako Japan Inc., Tokyo, Japan) for 1 h, stained using Phalloidin, and conjugated using Rhodamine X (FUJIFILM Wako Pure Chemical Corporation, Osaka, Japan) for 30 min. Phalloidin is a bicyclic peptide belonging to a family of toxins isolated from the deadly Amanita phalloides mushroom, and it is commonly used in imaging applications to selectively label F-actin. In this study, rhodamine-labeled phalloidin was used. After washing thrice with PBS, the cells were incubated with the Ki-67 rabbit monoclonal antibody (Cell Signaling Technology) at a concentration in 1:400 at 4 °C overnight. Then, anti-rabbit IgG (H+L) and F(ab')2 fragment (Alexa Fluor® 488 Conjugate; Cell Signaling Technology) was added and incubated for 2 h. After washing thrice with PBS, ProLong® Gold Antifade Reagent with DAPI (Cell Signaling Technology) was added to the cells and enclosed. Cells were viewed using a laser scanning confocal microscope (LSM510-META, Carl Zeiss, Jena, Germany).

2.8. Western Blot Analysis

The cells were treated with indicated compounds and lysed. Extracted cellular proteins (20 μg) were separated by sodium dodecyl sulfate-polyacrylamide gel electrophoresis (SDS-PAGE) and then transferred to a polyvinylidene difluoride (PVDF) membrane. In the SDS-PAGE step of the Western blotting, the cellular protein was isolated under reducing conditions using β-mercaptoethanol. The membrane was first blocked with Blocking One-P reagent (Nacalai Tesque, Kyoto, Japan) for 30 min at room temperature, and then incubated with primary antibodies at 4 °C overnight. After washing with PBS (-), the membranes were incubated with a peroxidase-linked secondary antibody at room temperature for 30 min. The labeled proteins were detected with the enhanced chemiluminescence using the Prime Western blotting detection system (GE Healthcare).

2.9. Statistical Analysis

The Mann-Whitney U test was used for comparisons between groups, with $p < 0.05$ being regarded as significant. Data are presented as means ± S.D.

3. Results

3.1. PLTMax Stimulated Proliferation of hASCs

The cell growth stimulated by PLTMax was confirmed by observation with phase-contrast microscopy. Compared to the control (no serum) and FBS (10%) groups, the cells treated with PLTMax (5%) were slightly elongated, and the nucleus was visible (Figure 1A).

Cell proliferation was increased by treatment with the 1%, 3%, 5% PLAMax group, and the FBS (10%) group ($p < 0.01$ vs. control). Among them, the cells in the 5% PLTMax group showed the highest proliferation, even higher than the 10% FBS group (Figure 1B). When the cells were incubated in PLTMax (5%), FBS (10%), and control (no serum) conditions for 2 to 7 days, high proliferation in the PLTMax (5%) group and FBS (10%) group on the 5th and 7th days was observed, while no proliferation was observed in the control group, even on the 7th day (Figure 1C).

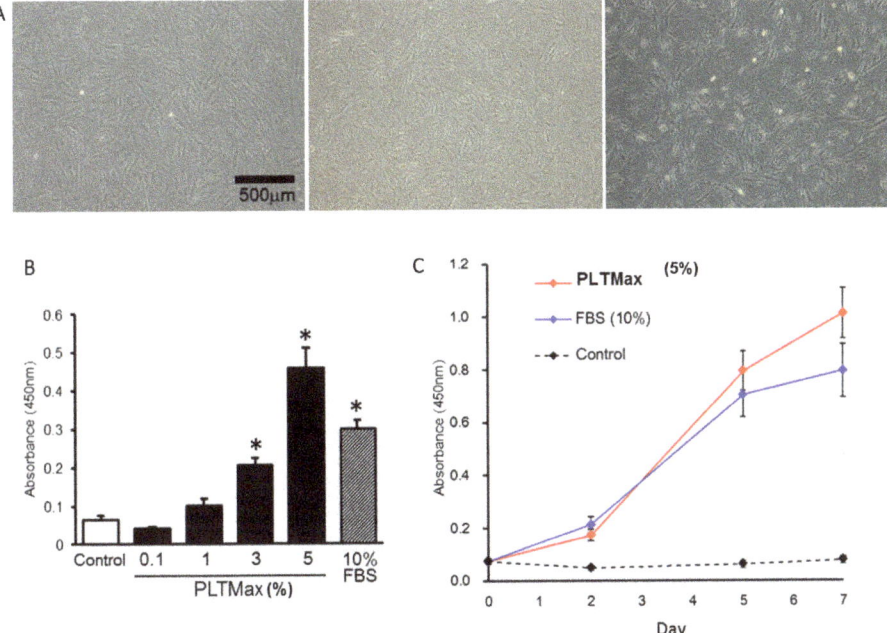

Figure 1. (**A**) The morphology of human adipose-derived stem cells (hASCs) observed by phase-contrast microscopy. Representative images of the cultures in the control group (no serum), fetal bovine serum (FBS) (10%), PLTMax (5%) after two days are shown. (**B**) The proliferation of hASCs cultured using 1%, 3%, and 5% PLTMax. The 3% PLTMax group showed significantly higher proliferation compared to the control group (no serum) and the 5% PLTMax group showed higher proliferation compared to the 10% FBS group. * $p < 0.05$ (**C**) The chronological changes in the proliferation of cells cultured on days 2, 5, and 7 in the control group, FBS-treated (10%), and PLTMax-treated (5%) cells. On days 5 and day 7, the cells treated with PLTMax (5%) showed higher proliferation compared to FBS (10%).

3.2. PLTMax Promoted Cell Cycle Transition from G0/G1 to S Phase

In the FBS (10%) group and the PLTMax (5%) group, a decrease in the percentage of cells in the G0/G1 period compared to that in the control group was observed. A histogram of the typical cell cycle, as evaluated by flow cytometry is shown in Figure 2A. The cells in the G0/G1 period were 62.87% ± 1.93% in the control group, 49.62% ± 2.60% in the FBS (10%) group, and 46.89% ± 2.72% in the PLTMax (5%) group, respectively. The cells in the S period were 5.41% ± 0.61% in the control group, 12.16% ± 1.77% in the FBS (10%) group, and 13.41% ± 1.44% in the PLTMax (5%) group, respectively. Further, the cells in the G2/M period were 31.71% ± 1.81% in the control group, 38.19% ± 3.11% in the FBS (10%) group, and 39.69% ± 3.05% in the PLTMax (10%) group, respectively. In the G0/G1 period, the FBS (10%) group and the PLTMax (5%) group showed significantly lower cell counts than the control group. In the S period and the G2/M period, the FBS (10%) group and the PLTMax (5%) group showed significantly higher cell counts than the control group, and among them, the cell count in the PLTMax (5%) group was the highest (Figure 2B).

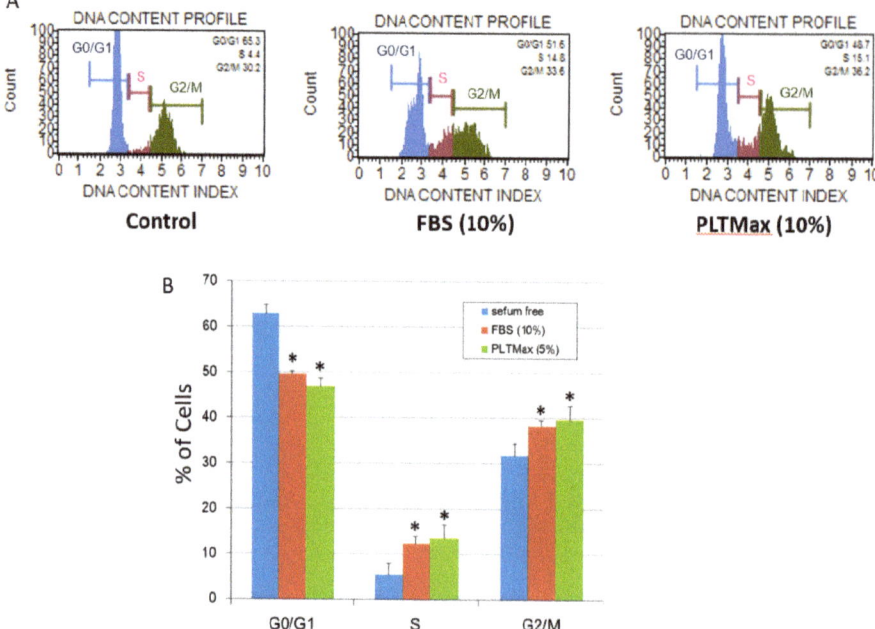

Figure 2. (**A**) Histogram of the typical cell cycle of hASCs from the control group (no serum), FBS (10%) group, and PLTMax (5%) group, as evaluated using flow cytometry. (**B**) The percentage of hASCs cultured in the PLTMax (5%) group in the G0/G1 phase, S phase, and G2/M phase. Compared to the control group (no serum), the cells in the FBS (10%) and PLTMax (5%) group showed a significantly increased percentage of cells in the S phase and G1/G2 phase. ($n = 6$) * $p < 0.05$.

3.3. Effect of PLTMax on the Number of Ki-67 Positive Cells

Fluorescent triple immunostaining was performed, which included Ki-67 fluorescent staining, Phalloidin staining, and DAPI nuclear staining, for the cells in the control group, the FBS (10%) group, and the PLTMax (5%) group. Ki-67 staining was found to be localized in the nucleus (Figure 3A). The percentage of Ki-67 positive cells was 7.46% ± 11.49% in the control (no serum) group, 63.33% ± 12.92% in the FBS (10%) group, and 85.19% ± 7.01% in the PLTMax (5%) group (Figure 3B), respectively. In the FBS (10%) group and the PLTMax (5%) group, the number of Ki-67 positive cells was significantly higher than that in the control group with the PLTMax (5%) group showing the highest number.

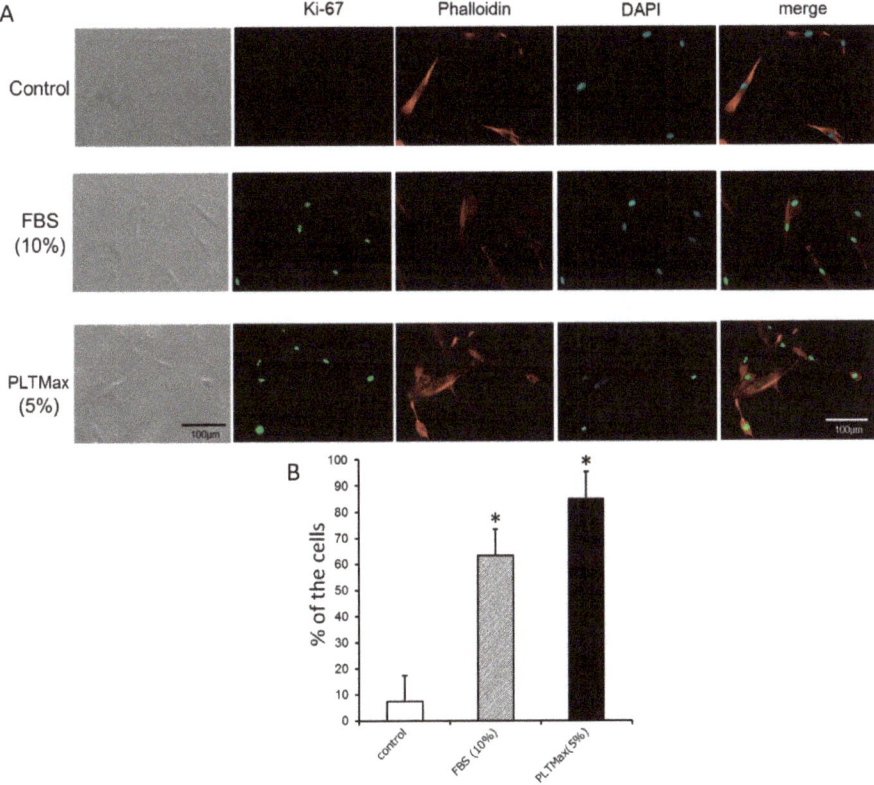

Figure 3. (**A**) Typical images of hASCs cultured without serum (control), with FBS (10%), and PLTMax (5%) immunostained for Ki-67, and with phalloidin and DAPI, or triple stained. Ki-67 staining was localized in the nucleus. (**B**) Percentage of Ki-67 positive cells. Compared to the control group, FBS (10%) and PLTMax (10%) showed a significantly increased percentage of Ki-67 positive cells. PLTMax (5%) showed the highest percentage among the 3 groups. * $p < 0.05$.

3.4. Effect of PLTMax on the Cell Surface Marker of hASCs

The effects of PLTMax on the cell surface marker of hASCs after 48 h of PLTMax culturing were analyzed. ASCs were CD90 (98.60% ± 0.99%), CD31 (0.20% ± 0.28%), CD45 (7.10% ± 3.77%), CD34 (5.77% ± 0.70%) at the seventh generation. After PLTMax culturing, they were CD90 (99.33% ± 1.15%), CD31 (0.33% ± 0.31%), CD45 (7.27% ± 7.64%), and CD34 (9.20% ± 4.69%). There was no significant difference between the cell surface markers before and after culturing.

3.5. PLTMax Activated ERK1/2, AKT, and JNK Signaling Pathways

The cells were treated with ERK1/2 inhibitor (PD98059, 50 µM), PI3K/AKT inhibitor (LY294002, 10 µM), JNK inhibitor (SP600125, 20 µM) and p38 inhibitor (SB203580, 20 µM), to examine the signaling pathways involved in the stimulation of hASCs by PLTMax. The PLTMax induced proliferation of cells was suppressed by PD98059, LY294002, SP600125, and SB203580 (Figure 4A). The PLTMax induced BrdU incorporation of cells was also suppressed by PD98059, LY294002, SP600125, and SB203580 (Figure 4B). The signaling pathways were further analyzed in the hASCs by Western blot. Phosphorylation of ERK1/2, JNK, p38, and AKT pathways was increased with the stimulation of either PLTMax or FBS. In the control group, phosphorylation of ERK1/2, JNK, p38, and AKT pathways did not occur. Thus, the stimulation of cell growth by PRP was mediated through multiple signal pathways (Figure 4C).

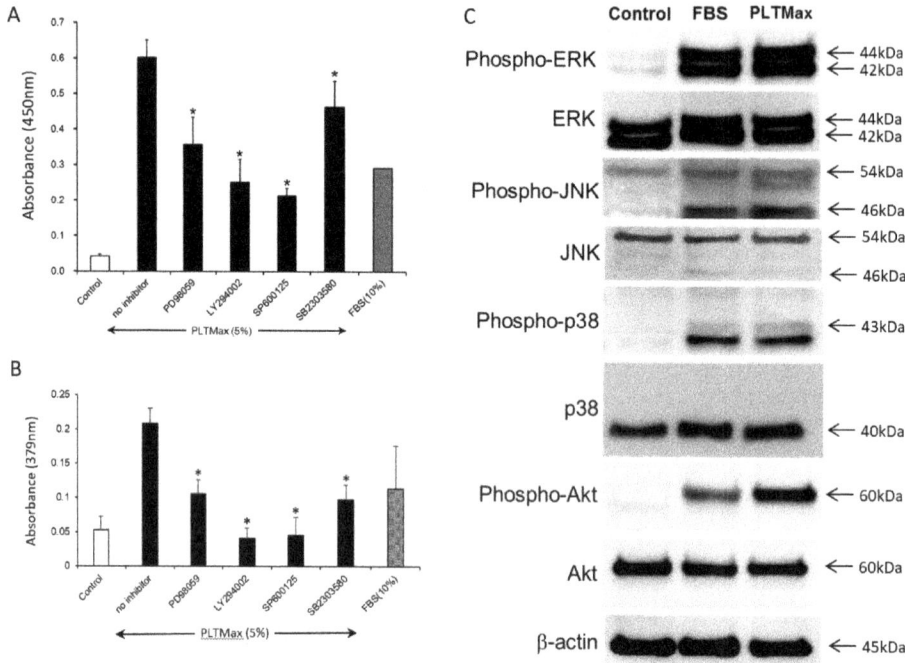

Figure 4. (**A**) The effect of various inhibitors (PD98059, LY294002, SP600125, and SB2303580) added in the presence of PLTMax (5%) on the proliferation of hASCs. The proliferative effect of PLTMax was partially inhibited by all the inhibitors. * $p < 0.05$ (**B**) The effect of various inhibitors (PD98059, LY294002, SP600125, and SB2303580) added in the presence of PLTMax (5%) on the BrdU incorporation of hASCs. The proliferative effect of PLTMax was partially inhibited by all the inhibitors. * $p < 0.05$ (**C**) MAP kinase-related proteins and phosphorylation seen in the hASCs in the control (no serum), FBS (10%) and PLTMax (5%) groups. The protein expressions of phospho-ERK, phospho-JNK, phospho-p38, and phospho-Akt were observed in FBS (10%) group and PLTMax (5%) group.

4. Discussion

PLTMax is a medium supplement that can be used as an FBS replacement. In this study, it was shown that 5% PLTMax is the optimal concentration and its proliferative effect was significantly higher compared to 10% FBS. PLTMax may have exerted its proliferative effect via multiple signaling pathways, similar to FBS.

Mesenchymal stromal stem cells (MSCs) can potentially differentiate into mesenchymal cells, including osteoblasts, adipocytes, muscle cells, and chondrocytes, and they have been considered for their application in regenerative medicine. Although the studies conducted with MSCs thus far have focused on the cells established from the bone marrow, recent studies have revealed that these cells can be established from several other tissues, such as cord blood, placenta, and adipose tissues [14]. Among them, adipose tissue contains a higher number of MSCs compared to the bone marrow, and the MSCs established from the adipose tissues proliferate rapidly [15]. Although the studies conducted with MSCs thus far have focused on the cells established from the bone marrow, recent studies have revealed that these cells can be established from several other tissues, such as cord blood, placenta, and adipose tissues. Among them, adipose tissues contain a higher number of MSCs compared to the bone marrow, and MSCs established from the adipose proliferate rapidly. Therefore, adipose-derived MSCs are garnering a lot of interest [16]. In order to clinically use hASCs in regenerative medicine, hASCs have to be prepared from a small number of adipose tissues and cultured ex vivo on a large scale to minimize invasiveness in the donor. To date, FBS has been generally used as a supplement to culture hASCs. However, concerns related to the use of FBS, such as bovine spongiform encephalopathy infection and certain other unidentified infections, risks of xeno-immunization against bovine antigens, the transmission of pathogens, and ethical issues associated with crude methods of FBS collection [17–22] have led to the exploration of supplements that can substitute FBS.

Platelets play an essential role not only in primary hemostasis but also in wound healing and tissue regeneration. The α-granules of the platelets contain several chemokines and growth factors, such as isoforms of platelet-derived growth factor (PDGF), transforming growth factor-β (TGF-β), insulin-like growth factor (IGF), vascular endothelial growth factor (VEGF), epidermal growth factor (EGF), and basic fibroblast growth factor (bFGF) [10]. To our knowledge, our study was the first to report that platelet-rich plasma prepared from whole blood contains high levels of PDGF and TGF-β and has a proliferative effect when added to hASCs. Human platelet lysate (hPL) is created from single or pooled donor-derived platelets isolated from the whole blood or by apheresis, and it is distributed in standard platelet collection bags. Several researchers have reported the proliferative effect of hPL on bone marrow MSCs. The proliferative effect of hPL (5% to 10%) on bone marrow MSCs was superior to that of FBS [6,23,24]. However, there are currently no studies investigating the mechanism underlying the effect of hPL on hASC proliferation.

PLTMax is a commercialized human platelet lysate product manufactured by Merck, created from the whole blood of American donors, which has been checked for infections. Studies on cell proliferation using PLTMax were recently conducted using human corneal epithelial cells [11,25] and oral mucosal epithelial cells [26]. Huang et al. reported that in human corneal epithelial cells, FBS seemed to have a higher proliferative effect compared to PLTMax. In addition, they reported that a higher concentration (10%) of PLTMax showed stronger inhibitory effects on cell proliferation compared to FBS [11]. In this study, the hASCs treated with 5% PLTMax showed significantly higher proliferation compared to those treated with 10% FBS. Different cell-types can show different reactions to PLTMax. PLTMax might be a better supplement for the mass cell culture of hASCs compared to FBS. Hsueh et al. reported that they succeeded in creating an oral mucosal epithelial cell sheet without animal-derived components with the addition of PLTMax instead of FBS [26]. Therefore, it is possible to create a cell sheet with hASCs using PLTMax.

In this study, it was found that PLTMax increased the percentage of cells in the S phase and G2/M phase of the cell cycle, as well as the Ki-67 positive cells. While Ki-67 is present in all cell cycle (G1, S, G2, and M) phases in proliferating cells, the G0 phase does not occur when cell proliferation is intermitotic. The cellular content of Ki-67 markedly increases during cell cycle progression throughout the synthetic phase (S phase) of the cell cycle [26]. Therefore, the high nuclear expression of Ki-67 in ASCs that were treated with PLTMax indicates an enhanced proliferative effect of the additive. This proliferative effect is suppressed by the addition of ERK, JNK, p38, and Akt inhibitors, suggesting the involvement of multiple signaling pathways. Studies conducted by both Chen et al. and Huang et al. revealed that PLTMax contains PDGF, TGF-β, and EGF. These factors might be involved in inducing the proliferative effect via several signal pathways in the treated hASCs [11,25]. Hence, in the future, it is necessary to investigate the proliferative factors and cytokines affected by the addition of PLTMax and to identify the factor that is most closely associated with cell proliferation.

Lensch M. et al. [27] published an article about the effect of commercially available synthetic media designed for adipose-derived stem cell expansion, including PLTMax Human Platelet Lysate (acquired from Sigma-Aldrich). Lensch M. et al. also performed immunophenotypic characterization of ASCs and evaluated their ability to differentiate into osteoblasts and adipocytes after treatment with PLTMax. They reported that PLTMax had a proliferative effect on the ASCs. In addition, they reported that cell culture using PLTMax up-regulated CD105, which is a cell surface marker, by 21%, while it has no effect on CD73 and CD90. However, the PLTMax that was used in the study by Lensch M. et al. [27] was manufactured by Sigma-Aldrich, while the PLTMax used in our study was manufactured by Merck. Thus, it is uncertain if their composition is similar due to the difference in manufacturers. Furthermore, they did not clearly mention the percentage concentration of PLTMax added to the medium in their report. On the other hand, other researchers have also reported the proliferative effect of PLTMax on ASCs. In a study by Morten et al., they added a 5% concentration of PLTMax to the ASCs and compared it with the FBS culture, similar to our study. They reported that while the levels of CD105 and CD90 hardly changed at P0, the expression of CD19 was higher (~30%) in the ASCs cultured in FBS medium at P0 and not in the PLAMax medium. They also reported that the expression of the secondary ASCs marker, CD 36 generally varied between 40% and 60% for PLTMax-supplemented ASC cultures, which decreased slightly after passaging. Interestingly, they investigated the genetic stability of ASCs till the 5th passage and they did not observe any imbalanced chromosomal rearrangements. These results are consistent with our study results. Moreover, recently it has been reported that the expression of ASC markers might be affected by the in vitro culture conditions and the passage number [16]. Therefore, the genetic stability and aging after culture with PLTMax should be investigated in the future for better understanding.

Previous studies have made efforts to develop serum-free products that can provide all the essential nutrients and the growth factors to maintain physiological function and to promote cell proliferation [28–31]. However, most of these serum replacements could not support cell growth [32]. Therefore, as an alternative to animal serum for cell proliferation, autoserum and allogeneic human serum have been investigated. On the one hand, few studies have reported that human serum improved cell growth, and on the other hand, some studies showed that it suppressed cell growth [33]. Our study showed that human serum promoted the proliferation of adipose-derived stem cells. However, certain concerns regarding the clinical applications, such as difficulty in collection and processing and the difference in the quality of autoserum from patient to patient, might hamper the standardization of culture conditions. In addition, the optimum amount of autoserum required for the expansion of cultures exceeds the amount that a single donor can provide [29]. In the future, we plan to investigate methods for collection and processing that can overcome these issues.

PLTMax has been suggested to be a more effective cell culture supplement for the culture of hASCs compared to FBS. If the culture of hASCs using hPL prepared from autologous platelets is successful, it would be possible to conduct an efficient mass cell culture without the risk of infection by unknown pathogens derived from animals. hPL is a supplement that might replace FBS in the future. Further studies need to be conducted to obtain the basic data for its application in regenerative medicine, particularly data regarding the changes in the cell surface markers, differentiation potency, and presence/absence of karyotype abnormality.

Author Contributions: Conceptualization, N.K. and K.K. Methodology, N.K., N.M. and Y.M., Writing—original draft preparation, N.K.

Funding: This research was partially funded by Grant-in-Aid for Scientific Research (C) 17K11558.

Acknowledgments: We wish to thank Shigeru Taketani for the advice and expertise. We also would like to thank Mikiyo Tokura and Mie Aoki for technical assistance.

Conflicts of Interest: The authors declare no conflict of interest.

References

1. Zuk, P.A.; Zhu, M.; Mizuno, H.; Huang, J.; Futrell, J.W.; Katz, A.J.; Benhaim, P.; Lorenz, H.P.; Hedrick, M.H. Multilineage Cells from Human Adipose Tissue: Implications for Cell-Based Therapies. *Tissue Eng.* **2001**, *7*, 211–228. [CrossRef] [PubMed]
2. Zuk, P.A.; Zhu, M.; Ashjian, P.; De Ugarte, D.A.; Huang, J.I.; Mizuno, H.; Alfonso, Z.C.; Fraser, J.K.; Benhaim, P.; Hedrick, M.H. Human Adipose Tissue Is a Source of Multipotent Stem Cells. *Mol. Boil. Cell* **2002**, *13*, 4279–4295. [CrossRef] [PubMed]

3. Mizuno, H. Adipose-derived stem and stromal cells for cell-based therapy: Current status of preclinical studies and clinical trials. *Curr. Opin. Mol. Ther.* **2010**, *12*, 442–449. [PubMed]
4. Hara, Y.; Steiner, M.; Baldini, M.G. Platelets as a source of growth-promoting factor(s) for tumor cells. *Cancer Res.* **1980**, *40*, 1212–1216. [PubMed]
5. Umeno, Y.; Okuda, A.; Kimura, G. Proliferative behaviour of fibroblasts in plasma-rich culture medium. *J. Cell Sci.* **1989**, *94*, 567–575. [PubMed]
6. Doucet, C.; Ernou, I.; Zhang, Y.; Begot, L.; Holy, X.; Llense, J.-R.; Lataillade, J.-J.; Llense, J.; Lataillade, J. Platelet lysates promote mesenchymal stem cell expansion: A safety substitute for animal serum in cell-based therapy applications. *J. Cell. Physiol.* **2005**, *205*, 228–236. [CrossRef] [PubMed]
7. Kakudo, N.; Minakata, T.; Mitsui, T.; Kushida, S.; Notodihardjo, F.Z.; Kusumoto, K. Proliferation-Promoting Effect of Platelet-Rich Plasma on Human Adipose–Derived Stem Cells and Human Dermal Fibroblasts. *Plast. Reconstr. Surg.* **2008**, *122*, 1352–1360. [CrossRef]
8. Trojahn Kolle, S.; Oliveri, R.S.; Glovinski, P.V.; Kirchhoff, M.; Mathiasen, A.B.; Elberg, J.J.; Andersen, P.S.; Drzewiecki, K.T.; Fischer-Nielsen, A. Pooled Human Platelet Lysate Versus Fetal Bovine Serum-Investigating the Proliferation Rate, Chromosome Stability and Angiogenic Potential of Human Adipose Tissue-Derived Stem Cells Intended for Clinical Use. *Cytotherapy* **2013**, *15*, 1086–1097. [CrossRef] [PubMed]
9. Cervelli, V.; Scioli, M.G.; Gentile, P.; Doldo, E.; Bonanno, E.; Spagnoli, L.G.; Orlandi, A. Platelet-Rich Plasma Greatly Potentiates Insulin-Induced Adipogenic Differentiation of Human Adipose-Derived Stem Cells Through a Serine/Threonine Kinase Akt-Dependent Mechanism and Promotes Clinical Fat Graft Maintenance. *Stem Cells Transl. Med.* **2012**, *1*, 206–220. [CrossRef]
10. Burnouf, T.; Strunk, D.; Koh, M.B.; Schallmoser, K. Human platelet lysate: Replacing fetal bovine serum as a gold standard for human cell propagation? *Biomaterials* **2016**, *76*, 371–387. [CrossRef]
11. Huang, C.-J.; Sun, Y.-C.; Christopher, K.; Pai, A.S.-I.; Lu, C.-J.; Hu, F.-R.; Lin, S.-Y.; Chen, W.-L. Comparison of corneal epitheliotrophic capacities among human platelet lysates and other blood derivatives. *PLoS ONE* **2017**, *12*, 0171008. [CrossRef] [PubMed]
12. Kakudo, N.; Kushida, S.; Suzuki, K.; Ogura, T.; Notodihardjo, P.V.; Hara, T.; Kusumoto, K. Effects of transforming growth factor-beta1 on cell motility, collagen gel contraction, myofibroblastic differentiation, and extracellular matrix expression of human adipose-derived stem cell. *Hum. Cell* **2012**, *25*, 87–95. [CrossRef] [PubMed]
13. Kakudo, N.; Morimoto, N.; Ogawa, T.; Taketani, S.; Kusumoto, K. Hypoxia Enhances Proliferation of Human Adipose-Derived Stem Cells via HIF-1a Activation. *PLoS ONE* **2015**, *10*, e0139890. [CrossRef] [PubMed]
14. Fraser, J.K.; Wulur, I.; Alfonso, Z.; Hedrick, M.H. Fat tissue: An underappreciated source of stem cells for biotechnology. *Trends Biotechnol.* **2006**, *24*, 150–154. [CrossRef] [PubMed]
15. Lai, F.; Kakudo, N.; Morimoto, N.; Taketani, S.; Hara, T.; Ogawa, T.; Kusumoto, K. Platelet-rich plasma enhances the proliferation of human adipose stem cells through multiple signaling pathways. *Stem Cell Res. Ther.* **2018**, *9*, 107. [CrossRef] [PubMed]
16. Palumbo, P.; Lombardi, F.; Siragusa, G.; Cifone, M.G.; Cinque, B.; Giuliani, M. Methods of Isolation, Characterization and Expansion of Human Adipose-Derived Stem Cells (ASCs): An Overview. *Int. J. Mol. Sci.* **2018**, *19*, 1897. [CrossRef]
17. Selvaggi, T.A.; Walker, R.E.; Fleisher, T.A. Development of antibodies to fetal calf serum with arthus-like reactions in human immunodeficiency virus-infected patients given syngeneic lymphocyte infusions. *Blood* **1997**, *89*, 776–779.
18. Mackensen, A.; Dräger, R.; Schlesier, M.; Mertelsmann, R.; Lindemann, A. Presence of IgE antibodies to bovine serum albumin in a patient developing anaphylaxis after vaccination with human peptide-pulsed dendritic cells. *Cancer Immunol. Immunother.* **2000**, *49*, 152–156. [CrossRef]
19. Horwitz, E.M.; Gordon, P.L.; Koo, W.K.K.; Marx, J.C.; Neel, M.D.; McNall, R.Y.; Muul, L.; Hofmann, T. Isolated allogeneic bone marrow-derived mesenchymal cells engraft and stimulate growth in children with osteogenesis imperfecta: Implications for cell therapy of bone. *Proc. Natl. Acad. Sci. USA* **2002**, *99*, 8932–8937. [CrossRef]
20. Rauch, C. Alternatives to the use of fetal bovine serum: Human platelet lysates as a serum substitute in cell culture media. *ALTEX* **2011**, *28*, 305–316. [CrossRef]
21. Schallmoser, K.; Strunk, D. Preparation of pooled human platelet lysate (pHPL) as an efficient supplement for animal serum-free human stem cell cultures. *J. Vis. Exp.* **2009**, *32*, e1523. [CrossRef]

22. Schallmoser, K.; Strunk, D. Generation of a pool of human platelet lysate and efficient use in cell culture. *Methods Mol. Biol.* **2013**, *946*, 349–362. [PubMed]
23. Carrancio, S.; Lopez-Holgado, N.; Sanchez-Guijo, F.M.; Villaron, E.; Barbado, V.; Tabera, S.; Diez-Campelo, M.; Blanco, J.; Miguel, J.F.S.; Del Cañizo, M.C. Optimization of mesenchymal stem cell expansion procedures by cell separation and culture conditions modification. *Exp. Hematol.* **2008**, *36*, 1014–1021. [CrossRef] [PubMed]
24. Azouna, N.B.; Jenhani, F.; Regaya, Z.; Berraeis, L.; Othman, T.B.; Ducrocq, E.; Domenech, J. Phenotypical and functional characteristics of mesenchymal stem cells from bone marrow: Comparison of culture using different media supplemented with human platelet lysate or fetal bovine serum. *Stem Cell Res. Ther.* **2012**, *3*, 6. [CrossRef] [PubMed]
25. Chen, L.W.; Huang, C.-J.; Tu, W.-H.; Lu, C.-J.; Sun, Y.-C.; Lin, S.-Y.; Chen, W.-L. The corneal epitheliotrophic abilities of lyophilized powder form human platelet lysates. *PLoS ONE* **2018**, *13*, e0194345. [CrossRef] [PubMed]
26. Hsueh, Y.-J.; Huang, S.-F.; Lai, J.-Y.; Ma, S.-C.; Chen, H.-C.; Wu, S.-E.; Wang, T.-K.; Sun, C.-C.; Ma, K.S.-K.; Chen, J.-K.; et al. Preservation of epithelial progenitor cells from collagenase-digested oral mucosa during ex vivo cultivation. *Sci. Rep.* **2016**, *6*, 36266. [CrossRef]
27. Lensch, M.; Muise, A.; White, L.; Badowski, M.; Harris, D. Comparison of Synthetic Media Designed for Expansion of Adipose-Derived Mesenchymal Stromal Cells. *Biomedicines* **2018**, *6*, 54. [CrossRef] [PubMed]
28. Parker, A.; Shang, H.; Khurgel, M.; Katz, A. Low serum and serum-free culture of multipotential human adipose stem cells. *Cytotherapy* **2007**, *9*, 637–646. [CrossRef]
29. Mizuno, N.; Shiba, H.; Ozeki, Y.; Mouri, Y.; Niitani, M.; Inui, T.; Hayashi, H.; Suzuki, K.; Tanaka, S.; Kawaguchi, H. Human autologous serum obtained using a completely closed bag system as a substitute for foetal calf serum in human mesenchymal stem cell cultures. *Cell Boil. Int.* **2006**, *30*, 521–524. [CrossRef] [PubMed]
30. Nimura, A.; Muneta, T.; Koga, H.; Mochizuki, T.; Suzuki, K.; Makino, H.; Umezawa, A.; Sekiya, I. Increased proliferation of human synovial mesenchymal stem cells with autologous human serum: Comparisons with bone marrow mesenchymal stem cells and with fetal bovine serum. *Arthritis Rheum.* **2008**, *58*, 501–510. [CrossRef] [PubMed]
31. Shahdadfar, A.; Frønsdal, K.; Haug, T.; Reinholt, F.P.; Brinchmann, J.E. In Vitro Expansion of Human Mesenchymal Stem Cells: Choice of Serum Is a Determinant of Cell Proliferation, Differentiation, Gene Expression, and Transcriptome Stability. *Stem Cells* **2005**, *23*, 1357–1366. [CrossRef] [PubMed]
32. Hemeda, H.; Giebel, B.; Wagner, W. Evaluation of human platelet lysate versus fetal bovine serum for culture of mesenchymal stromal cells. *Cytotherapy* **2014**, *16*, 170–180. [CrossRef] [PubMed]
33. Haack-Sorensen, M.; Friis, T.; Bindslev, L.; Mortensen, S.; Johnsen, H.E.; Kastrup, J. Comparison of different culture conditions for human mesenchymal stromal cells for clinical stem cell therapy. *Scand. J. Clin. Lab. Investig.* **2008**, *68*, 192–203. [CrossRef] [PubMed]

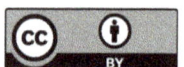

© 2019 by the authors. Licensee MDPI, Basel, Switzerland. This article is an open access article distributed under the terms and conditions of the Creative Commons Attribution (CC BY) license (http://creativecommons.org/licenses/by/4.0/).

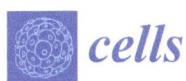

Article

Metformin Increases Proliferative Activity and Viability of Multipotent Stromal Stem Cells Isolated from Adipose Tissue Derived from Horses with Equine Metabolic Syndrome

Agnieszka Smieszek [1,*], Katarzyna Kornicka [1], Jolanta Szłapka-Kosarzewska [1], Peter Androvic [2,3], Lukas Valihrach [2], Lucie Langerova [4], Eva Rohlova [2,5], Mikael Kubista [2,6] and Krzysztof Marycz [1,7]

1. Department of Experimental Biology, The Faculty of Biology and Animal Science, University of Environmental and Life Sciences, 50375 Wroclaw, Poland; kornicka.katarzyna@gmail.com (K.K.); jolanta.szlapka@upwr.edu.pl (J.S.-K.); krzysztof.marycz@upwr.edu.pl (K.M.)
2. Laboratory of Gene Expression, Institute of Biotechnology CAS, Biocev, 25250 Vestec, Czech Republic; peter.androvic@ibt.cas.cz (P.A.); lukas.valihrach@ibt.cas.cz (L.V.); eva.rohlova@ibt.cas.cz (E.R.); mikael.kubista@ibt.cas.cz or mikael.kubista@tataa.com (M.K.)
3. Laboratory of Growth Regulators, Faculty of Science, Palacky University, 78371 Olomouc, Czech Republic
4. Gene Core BIOCEV, Průmyslová 595, 25250 Vestec, Czech Republic; lucie.langerova@ibt.cas.cz
5. Department of Anthropology and Human Genetics, Faculty of Science, Charles University, 12843 Prague, Czech Republic
6. TATAA Biocenter AB, 41103 Gothenburg, Sweden
7. Faculty of Veterinary Medicine, Equine Clinic-Equine Surgery, Justus-Liebig-University, 35392 Giessen, Germany
* Correspondence: agnieszka.smieszek@upwr.edu.pl; Tel.: +48-71-320-5202

Received: 5 December 2018; Accepted: 21 January 2019; Published: 22 January 2019

Abstract: In this study, we investigated the influence of metformin (MF) on proliferation and viability of adipose-derived stromal cells isolated from horses (EqASCs). We determined the effect of metformin on cell metabolism in terms of mitochondrial metabolism and oxidative status. Our purpose was to evaluate the metformin effect on cells derived from healthy horses (EqASC$_{HE}$) and individuals affected by equine metabolic syndrome (EqASC$_{EMS}$). The cells were treated with 0.5 µM MF for 72 h. The proliferative activity was evaluated based on the measurement of BrdU incorporation during DNA synthesis, as well as population doubling time rate (PDT) and distribution of EqASCs in the cell cycle. The influence of metformin on EqASC viability was determined in relation to apoptosis profile, mitochondrial membrane potential, oxidative stress markers and *BAX/BCL-2* mRNA ratio. Further, we were interested in possibility of metformin affecting the Wnt3a signalling pathway and, thus, we determined mRNA and protein level of *WNT3A* and β-catenin. Finally, using a two-tailed RT-qPCR method, we investigated the expression of *miR-16-5p*, *miR-21-5p*, *miR-29a-3p*, *miR-140-3p* and *miR-145-5p*. Obtained results indicate pro-proliferative and anti-apoptotic effects of metformin on EqASCs. In this study, MF significantly improved proliferation of EqASCs, which manifested in increased synthesis of DNA and lowered PDT value. Additionally, metformin improved metabolism and viability of cells, which correlated with higher mitochondrial membrane potential, reduced apoptosis and increased *WNT3A*/β-catenin expression. Metformin modulates the miRNA expression differently in EqASC$_{HE}$ and EqASC$_{EMS}$. Metformin may be used as a preconditioning agent which stimulates proliferative activity and viability of EqASCs.

Keywords: adipose-derived stromal cells; equine metabolic syndrome; metformin

1. Introduction

Currently, equine metabolic syndrome (EMS) is considered as a burning issue in veterinary medicine, affecting more and more horses. By definition, EMS is related to insulin resistance (IR), insulin dysregulation and obesity, as well as hyperleptinemia and past or chronic laminitis. Until recently, it was thought that only primitive-type horses, such as ponies and cold-bloods, suffer from EMS, but recent findings suggest that also non-obese and even sport horses might be affected by EMS—mainly due to a high starch and high energy diet [1]. Although obesity was excluded as a sine qua non condition in the course of the diagnostic procedure of EMS, specific local accumulation of adipose tissue, i.e., adiposity (cresty neck) is considered a diagnostic marker. Moreover, it is thought that EMS horses that are not overweight might accumulate abdominal adipose tissue, which is not without physiological significance for the other organs, including liver. Adipose tissue produces a number of factors, including cytokines, adipokines, as well as hormones, all influencing the clinical picture of EMS horses. It was shown that adipocytes isolated from subcutaneous adipose tissue of EMS horses produce pro-inflammatory cytokines, i.e., tumour necrosis factor-alpha (TNF-α), interleukin 1 (IL-1) and interleukin 6 (IL-6), which all may lead to the development of local inflammation [2]. Our previous studies indicate that subcutaneous adipose tissue inflammation is mediated by tissue resident immune cells, including macrophages that, under EMS condition, are characterised by elevated activity. This unfavourable pro-inflammatory microenvironment of adipose tissue has an adverse effect on residing progenitor cells, i.e., adipose-derived multipotent stromal stem cells (ASCs). Equine ASCs are characterised by the presence of mesenchymal specific surface antigens, including CD73, CD90 and CD105, and lack of expression of hematopoietic markers, i.e., CD45 [3–5]. Additionally, this population of cells is endowed with self-renewal properties regulated by the expression of *OCT4* (octamer binding transcription factor-4), *SOX2* (sex-determining region Y-box 2) and homeobox protein Nanog [6]. Furthermore, it was shown that ASCs possess immunomodulatory properties and secrete anti-inflammatory cytokines, such as IL-4 and IL-13. The increased proliferative activity and immunomodulatory properties of ASC, along with low immunogenicity, makes them promising a therapeutic tool for the treatment of various musculoskeletal diseases in horses [7]. ASCs, in general, are also characterised by unique ability for multilineage differentiation, including osteogenic, adipogenic and chondrogenic, which is crucial for their clinical use. Our own previous clinical research showed a positive effect of ASCs in horses with particular musculoskeletal system disorders [8,9]. In general, the pro-regenerative properties of ASCs are explained by their autocrine and paracrine activity [10]. For example, it was shown that application of ASCs in injured Achilles tendons is more efficient than the application of growth differentiation factor 5 (GDF-5). The transplantation of ASCs increased the expression of several genes (including *TGFβ*), which improved collagen fibre organisation and tendon biomechanics [11]. Additionally, it was demonstrated that equine ASCs are able to synthesise and secrete extracellular microvesicles (ExMVs), rich in broad range of growth factors, including bone morphogenetic protein isoform 2 (BMP-2) and vascular endothelial growth factor (VEGF) [12]. Various studies, including ours, demonstrated that regenerative potential of ASCs depends strictly on donor age or its physiological status [13–16]. Importantly, in our previous research, we have shown that ASCs derived from EMS horses (EqASC$_{EMS}$) show impaired proliferative and metabolic activity, reduced clonogenic potential, as well as lowered expression of KI-67, a widely known proliferation marker. Furthermore, when determining the multipotency of EqASC$_{EMS}$, we noticed that their chondrogenic and osteogenic differentiation potential had declined, which was associated with the reduced expression of transcripts such as *BMP-2*, *SOX-9*, *COL-1/2* and vimentin [5]. Moreover, in EqASC$_{EMS}$, we have observed deterioration of mitochondrial dynamics, which is related to lowered mitochondrial metabolism and induced macroautophagy process. The results question the utility of EqASC$_{EMS}$ in terms of autologous transplants, that are considered as well-established therapeutic strategies for the treatment of tendon and joint diseases [8,9,17,18]. Bearing in mind these facts, we see great need for the development of new preconditioning regimens to enhance the regenerative potential of EqASC$_{EMS}$. Most recently, our group has shown that EqASC$_{EMS}$ displayed anti-inflammatory properties and decreasing activity of TNF-α, IL-1 and IL-6 when preconditioned with a combination of 5-azatacidine and resveratrol (AZA/RES). The preconditioned cells were able to regulate and activate the anti-inflammatory response related to regulatory T lymphocytes (T$_{REG}$) [19]. Additionally, we have shown that AZA/RES may rejuvenate EqASC$_{EMS}$ by modulating mitochondrial dynamics and increasing their viability [20]. Our previous studies indicate that metformin and biguanide, both anti-diabetic drugs, can be considered as promising candidates in terms of improving progenitor cells' viability and their proliferative potential. Using the ex vivo model, we showed that metformin is able to increase the proliferative activity and viability of mice ASCs (mASCs). The pro-proliferative effect of metformin towards mASCs was manifested by increased proliferation ratio, lowered population doubling time and enhanced clonogenic potential [21]. Moreover, our other studies have shown that metformin may also improve viability and stabilise the phenotype of mouse glial progenitor cells, i.e., olfactory ensheathing cells (mOECs), without influence on their proliferative status [22]. Our studies showed that increased viability of progenitor cells after metformin treatment may be associated with its antioxidant effect and improved metabolism of mitochondria [21,22]. Additionally, it was shown that metformin suppresses proinflammatory responses of adipocyte and improves the balance of brown/white adipose acting upon obesity effects [23–25]. Furthermore, some clinical studies showed the beneficial effect of metformin in terms of insulin resistance treatment in horses. For example, it was shown that metformin can reduce glycaemic and insulinaemic responses both in healthy horses and in horses with experimentally induced insulin resistance [26]. There is also data indicating that metformin reverses insulin resistance and decreases serum insulin concentration during the first 6 to 14 days of treatment, however, this effect diminishes by 220 days [27]. The clinical efficacy of metformin in terms of EMS treatment has not been proven, due to some questions concerning its bioavailability [28,29]. Still, being aware of pro-regenerative effects of metformin towards progenitor cells [21,22] and its pro-aging activities [30], we decided to characterise metformin influence on viability and proliferative potential of EqASC$_{EMS}$. We determined the effect of metformin on cells morphology, apoptosis profile and mitochondrial membrane activity. We analysed the antioxidative and anti-apoptotic effect of metformin in terms of expression of several markers both on mRNA and miRNA level. We tested the expression of *BAX* and *BCL-2*, as well as *miR-16-5p*, *miR-21-5p*, *miR-29a-3p*, *miR-140-3p* and *miR-145-5p*. The specificity of miRNA measurement was assured by highly sensitive two-tailed RT-qPCR method [31]. It is well known that metformin acts through AMP-activated protein kinase (AMPK) which regulates lipid, cholesterol and glucose metabolism in various metabolic tissues, including adipose tissue, yet, it was also shown that metformin may improve cells survival through WNT/β-catenin signalling [32]. Therefore, we were also interested in whether *WNT* signalling is activated in EqASC$_{EMS}$ after metformin treatment. The obtained results show promise for the potential application of metformin as a preconditioning agent, improving cellular health of adipose-derived multipotent stromal cells isolated from horses with equine metabolic syndrome (EqASC$_{EMS}$).

2. Materials and Methods

2.1. Characterisation of Equine Multipotent Stromal Cells (EqASCs)

Cells derived from healthy horses ($n = 6$) and horses affected by metabolic syndrome ($n = 6$) were used in the study. The method to classify the animals has been detailed previously [1–4]. Subcutaneous adipose tissue collected from horses' tail base was used for isolation of EqASCs. The procedure of tissue collection was performed with the standard surgical protocols in compliance with ethical standards and approved by the II Local Ethics Committee of Environmental and Life Sciences University (Chelmonskiego 38C, 51–630 Wroclaw, Poland; decision No. 84/2012; extension No. 84/2018). The multipotent stromal cells were isolated from the stromal vascular fraction obtained by enzymatic digestion of adipose tissue using collagenase type I. The precise protocol of EqASC isolation was previously described in detail [3–5,33,34]. Primary cultures of EqASCs were maintained in Dulbecco's Modified Eagle's Medium (DMEM) with F-12 Ham nutrient. The medium was supplemented with

10% foetal bovine serum (FBS) and 1% of antibiotic solution containing penicillin, streptomycin and amphotericin B (PSA). Constant and aseptic growth conditions were assured by maintaining the cells in CO_2 incubator at 37 °C and 95% humidity. Cultures were passaged using trypsin solution (TrypLE Express; Life Technologies, Warsaw, Poland) after reaching 80% confluence. Complete growth medium (CGM) used for the subsequent EqASC cultures consisted of DMEM containing 4500 mg/L glucose supplemented with 10% FBS and 1% of PSA. The media were changed every two days. The cells used for experiments were passaged three times and were characterised as multipotent stromal cells based on a specific phenotype and ability to differentiate into adipocytes, chondrocytes and osteocytes [3–5].

2.2. The Experimental Cultures

The multipotent stromal cells isolated from adipose tissue derived from healthy horses ($EqASC_{HE}$) and horses with equine metabolic syndrome ($EqASC_{EMS}$) were inoculated in a 24-well plates. The initial inoculum was 30,000 cells per well. The cells were cultivated for 72 h in CGM containing metformin at a final concentration equal to 500 µM. The control for the experiment was EqASCs maintained in CGM without metformin.

2.3. The Analysis of Metformin Influence on Morphology of EqASCs and Metabolic and Proliferative Activity

The morphology of cells was evaluated using an epifluorescence microscope (EpiFM). For the analysis, cultures were fixed using 4% paraformaldehyde and stained with atto-488-labeled phalloidin (1:800) and with diamidino-2-phenylindole (DAPI; 1:1000). The observations were performed using Axio Observer A.1 microscope (Zeiss, Oberkochen, Germany). The metabolic activity of cells was monitored every 24 h using Alamar Blue assay and, additionally, population doubling time was determined accordingly to the method described previously [22,35]. The distribution of cells in the cell cycle was determined using Muse™ Cell Analyzer (Merck KGaA, Darmstadt, Germany) using the Cell Cycle Assay Kit (Merck, Warszawa, Poland). The assay was performed following manufacturer's instructions. Each analysis was performed in triplicate.

2.4. The Analysis of Metformin Influence on Mitochondrial Metabolism of EqASCs

The mitochondrial membrane potential was assessed with Muse™ Cell Analyzer. After culture, cells were harvested with trypsin solution and counted with trypan blue solution using a standard protocol [36]. For the assay, 100,000 cells were stained with MitoPotential kit (Merck, Warszawa, Poland). Staining was performed according to the protocol provided by manufacturer (Merck, Warszawa, Poland). Each measurement was performed at least three times. The ultrastructural analyses of EqASC mitochondria were performed using focused ion beam microscope (FIB, Cobra, AURIGA 60, Zeiss, Oberkochen, Germany). The protocol of preparing the material for FIB imaging was previously described by Marycz et al. [5,37]. The analysis was conducted using an SE2 detector (Zeiss, Oberkochen, Germany) at 2 kV of electron beam voltage. Moreover, the influence of metformin on mitochondrial metabolism was determined based on oxidative stress factors accumulation. The supernatants after 72 h of culture were collected in order to evaluate the activity of intracellular reactive oxygen species (ROS), nitric oxide (NO) and superoxide dismutase (SOD). ROS were measured using H2DCF-DA solution, while NO activity was measured using Griess reagent kit (both reagents from Thermo Fisher Scientific, Warszawa, Poland). SOD was determined using a commercially available SOD determination kit (Sigma Aldrich, Munich, Germany).

2.5. The Analysis of Metformin Influence on the Viability of EqASC

The apoptosis and necrosis were quantified using Muse™ Cell Analyzer. For this purpose, 100,000 cells were stained with Muse® Annexin V and Dead Cell Assay Kit (Merck, Warszawa, Poland). The procedure of staining was performed following the manufacturer's protocol. The analysis was performed three times. Moreover, the viability of cultures was investigated using a well-established staining method [33,38] with a two-colour fluorescence live/dead assay according to the manufacturer's instructions (Double Staining Kit: Sigma Aldrich, Munich, Germany). The cultures were analysed using an epifluorescence microscope (Axio Observer A.1; Zeiss, Oberkochen, Germany) and images were captured using a PowerShot camera (Canon, Warszawa, Poland).

2.6. Influence of Metformin on Endogenous Levels of WNT3A and β-Catenin

The expression of endogenous WNT3A and β-catenin was determined using Western blot technique. After harvesting, cells were lysed with ice-cold RIPA extraction buffer. The extraction buffer contained 1% of protease and phosphatase inhibitor cocktail (Sigma Aldrich, Munich, Germany). To normalise the amount of protein loaded onto the gel, the total concentration of protein in the samples was determined using the Bicinchoninic Acid Assay Kit (Sigma Aldrich, Munich, Germany). The cell extracts containing 50 µg of protein were separated using 10% sodium dodecyl sulphate-polyacrylamide gel electrophoresis (SDS-PAGE; 30 mA ~80 min) and transferred to nitrocellulose membrane at 100 V for 1 h at 4 °C in Tris/glycine buffer using the Mini Trans-Blot® system (Bio-Rad, Hercules, CA, USA). After transfer, the membranes were washed with Tris/NaCl/Tween buffer (TBST) and blocked overnight at 4 °C with 5% bovine serum albumin (BSA). Membranes were then washed twice with TBST, and three times with TBS. Each rinsing lasted 5 min and was performed at room temperature under agitation (15 rpm). Next, the membranes were incubated for 2 h at room temperature with primary antibodies detecting Wnt-3a (SAB2105736), phospho-β-catenin (SAB4300630) and β-actin (A2066) that were prepared at a dilution of 1:200 in 5% of BSA in TBST. After incubation with primary antibody, the membranes were washed again as described above. After rinsing, membranes were incubated with secondary antibody conjugated with alkaline phosphatase (A9919) for 1.5 h at room temperature. All antibodies were from Sigma Aldrich (Munich, Germany). The membranes were washed and incubated with BCIP®/NBT-Purple Liquid Substrate (Sigma Aldrich, Munich, Germany) for 10 min. The reaction was stopped by washing the membrane with distilled water. The Western blot analysis was repeated twice. The blots were analysed using Bio-Rad ChemiDoc™ XRS system. The signals were captured from the bands and the intensity was quantified using Image Lab™ Software (Bio-Rad).

2.7. The Analysis of Metformin Influence on Expression of Genes Associated with Apoptosis

The cultures were washed with Hanks' Balanced Salt solution (HBSS) and homogenised directly in culture dishes using TRI Reagent® (Sigma Aldrich, Munich, Germany). The isolation of total RNA was performed accordingly to the protocol published by Chomczynski and Sacchi [39]. The quantity of RNA was measured using NanoDrop 8000 (ThermoFisher Scientific, Waltham, MA, USA).

2.7.1. The Analysis of mRNA Expression

The cDNA used for the qPCR was obtained from 1 µg of RNA and was synthesised accordingly to a method described previously [40]. SensiFast SYBR & Fluorescein Kit (Bioline Reagents Ltd., London, United Kingdom) was used for the detection of specific amplicons. The total volume of PCR was 10 µL, and cDNA did not exceed 10% of the final PCR mix volume, while the concentration of the primers was 400 nM. The primer sequences have been published previously [41,42]. All primers were synthesised by Sigma Aldrich (Sigma Aldrich, Munich, Germany). The qPCR was performed applying CFX Connect Real-Time PCR Detection System (Bio-Rad Polska Sp. z.o.o., Warszawa, Poland) using a protocol described elsewhere [43]. The transcript levels were normalised to the expression of reference gene housekeeping gene, i.e., glyceraldehyde 3-phosphate dehydrogenase (*GAPDH*).

2.7.2. The Analysis of miRNA Expression

The quality of RNA was tested using capillary electrophoresis (Fragment Analyser, Agilent Technologies, Inc., BioVendor, Brno, Czech Republic). Only fully intact RNA was used for further analysis. The RT was performed from 10 ng of RNA using qScript Flex cDNA Kit (QuantaBio; Beverly, MA, USA). For the reaction, target-specific primers were used, designed according to principles described previously [31]. The primers are listed in Table S1. The final concentration of primers in each reaction was 50 nM. To monitor the technical aspects of the experiment, a mix of artificial spike-in miRNA molecules was added into each sample prior to RNA extraction and RT. The RT reaction was performed in accordance to the protocol provided by the producer. Obtained cDNA was 10-times diluted and used in subsequent qPCR reactions measuring the expression of miRNAs, reference gene (snU6) and 5 spike assays. Each reaction was performed in triplicates. The reaction mix was composed of TATAA SYBR® GrandMaster® Mix (TATAA), 400 nM of primers (ThermoFisher Scientific), 2.6 µL nuclease free water (ThermoFisher Scientific) and 2 µL of diluted cDNA. qPCR was performed in CFX384 instrument (Biorad, Hercules, California USA). The following temperature profile was used: 95 °C for 30 s, 45 cycles of amplification (95 °C for 5 s and 60 °C for 15 s). The specificity of products was determined based on melting curve analysis. The primer sequences used for qPCR are shown in Table S1. RT-qPCR data were processed and analysed with GenEx software (MultiD, Sweden). Cq values were normalised to a reference gene (snU6), transformed into relative quantities (scaled to the sample having the lowest expression), and converted into log2 scale as described previously [44,45]. Significant differences between data were tested by analysis of variance (ANOVA).

3. Results

3.1. Metformin Improves Metabolic Activity and Proliferation of EqASCs

Obtained results revealed that metformin may act as an agent that increases the proliferative activity of EqASCs derived both from healthy and EMS horses (Figure 1). Microscopic evaluation of EqASC$_{HE}$ and EqASC$_{EMS}$ cultures showed that metformin does not affect the cells' morphology—the cells maintain proper fibroblast-like morphotype. However, the distribution of cells and the growth pattern indicated on increased confluency of cultures treated with metformin (Figure 1a). Direct evidence of pro-proliferative activity of metformin towards EqASCs was found in shortened population doubling time (PDT). The PDT decreased after metformin treatment in ASC cultures derived from both healthy and EMS horses (Figure 1b,c). The metformin influenced the metabolic activity of cells, which was visible, in particular, in significant improvement of metabolic activity in cultures after 48 h of propagation. The increased metabolic activity of cells maintained for 72 h of culture is shown in Figure 1d,e.

The analysis of cell cycle showed that metformin treatment may change the distribution of EqASCs and induce their shift towards S-phase. Simultaneously, we observed the decrease of percentage of cells in G0/G1-phase. Moreover, the metformin significantly ($p < 0.05$) increased the number of EqASC$_{HE}$ in G2/M-phase (Figure 2).

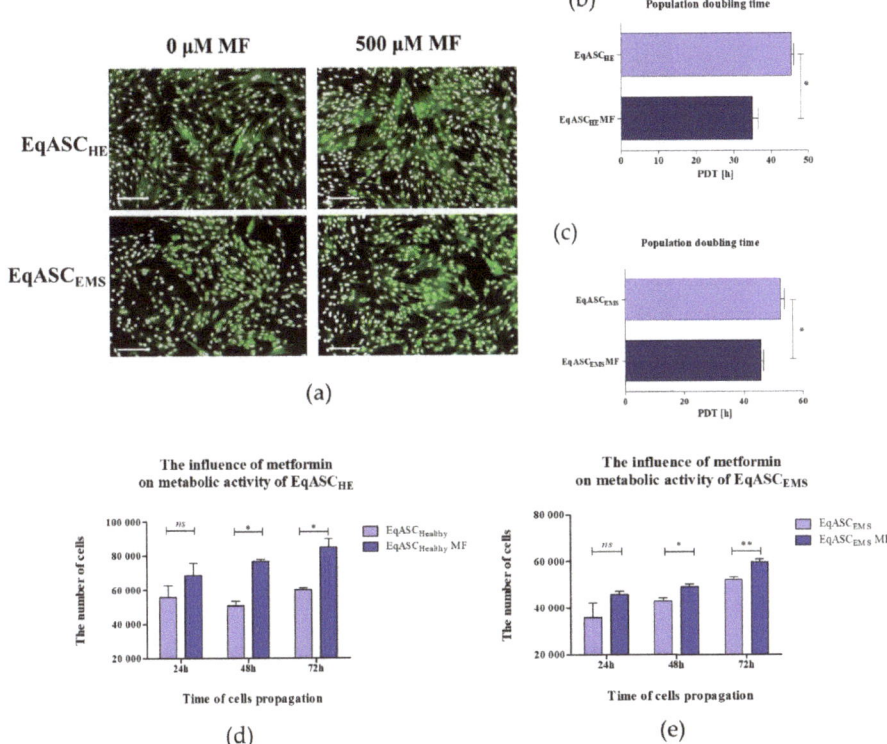

Figure 1. The influence of metformin on proliferative and metabolic activity of adipose-derived stromal cells isolated from horses (EqASCs). The proliferative activity was evaluated based on microphotographs obtained with epifluorescence microscope—scale bar 250 μm (**a**) population doubling time ratio (**b,c**) and metabolic activity (**d,e**). The statistically significant changes were indicated with asterisks; * $p < 0.05$; ** $p < 0.01$, while non-significant differences are marked as *ns*.

3.2. Metformin Enhances Mitochondrial Potential and Improves Oxidative Status in EqASCs

The analysis of mitochondrial membrane potential confirmed that metformin improves the metabolic activity of EqASCs isolated both from healthy and from EMS individuals (Figure 3a). The number of cells with improved mitochondrial potential increased significantly, both in $EqASC_{HE}$ and $EqASC_{EMS}$ cultures, after metformin treatment (Figure 3c). Simultaneously, the percentage of total depolarised cells decreased in cultures treated with metformin (Figure 3d). Nevertheless, the impairment of mitochondrial function in $EqASC_{EMS}$ remained significant when compared to $EqASC_{HE}$, and metformin did not reverse mitochondrial deterioration due to EMS. We did not observe significant changes of mitochondria morphology in $EqASC_{HE}$ treated with metformin; in these cells, mitochondria had proper shape and morphology as well as visible cristae (Figure 3b). Analysis of $EqASC_{EMS}$ ultrastructure showed that, in cultures treated with metformin, the number of mitochondria increased. Additionally, elongated mitochondria were noted (Figure 3b). These ultrastructural features, along with the lowered activity of reactive oxygen species (ROS, Figure 3e) and nitric oxide (NO, Figure 3f), may indicate that metformin may improve the elimination of dysfunctional mitochondria by autophagy, enhancing mitochondrial dynamics. Additionally, in $EqASC_{EMS}$ cultures treated with metformin, we observed increased levels of superoxide dismutase (SOD, Figure 3g).

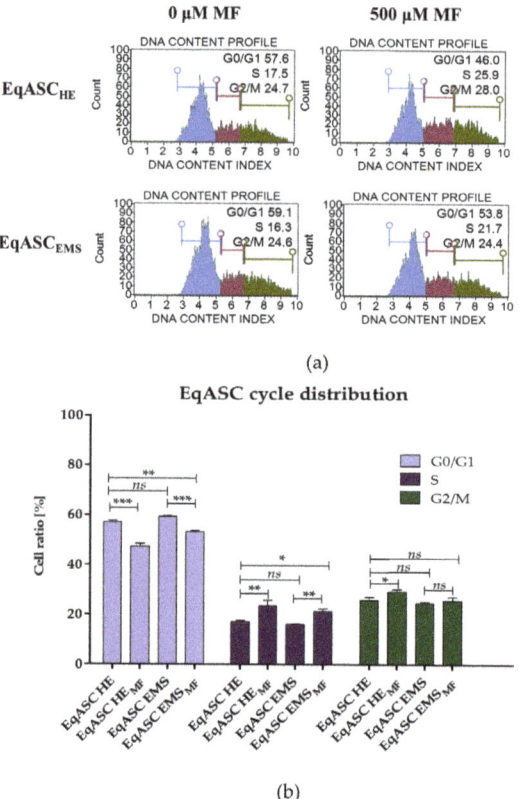

(a)

(b)

Figure 2. The influence of metformin on the distribution of EqASCs during the cell cycle, with representative histograms (**a**) and results of statistical analysis (**b**). The statistically significant changes are indicated with asterisks; * $p < 0.05$; ** $p < 0.01$ and *** $p < 0.001$. Non-significant differences are marked as *ns*.

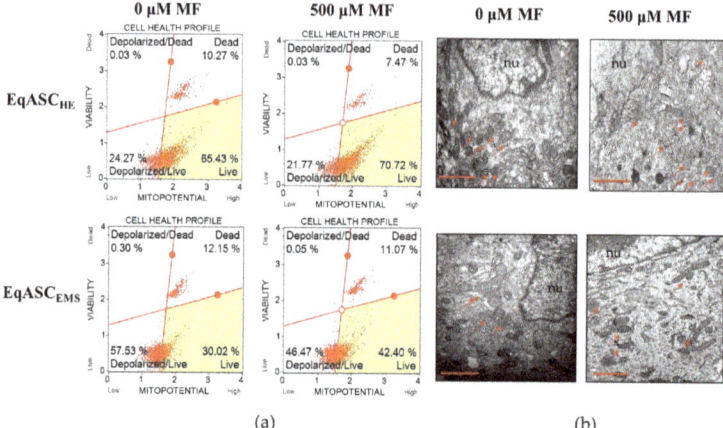

(a) (b)

Figure 3. *Cont.*

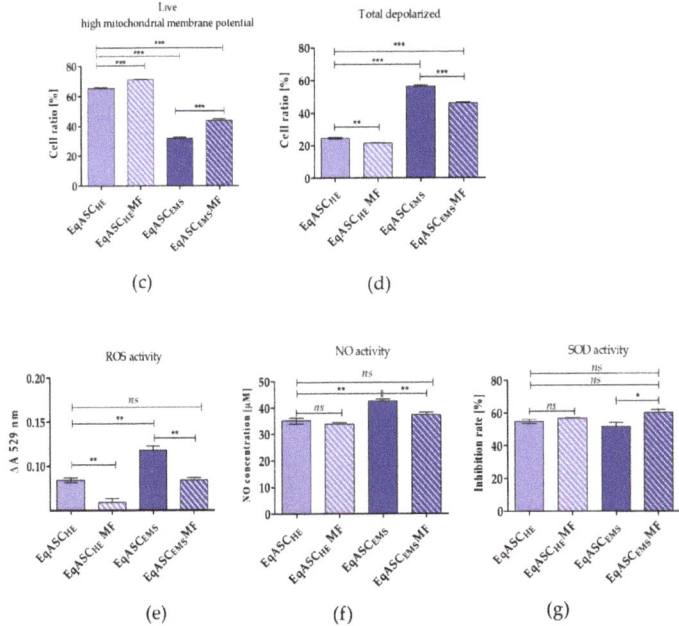

Figure 3. The influence of metformin on mitochondrial membrane potential and oxidative. Representative dot plots indicating distribution of cells accordingly to the mitochondrial membrane potential (**a**). The ultrastructure of EqASC$_{HE}$ and EqASC$_{EMS}$ without metformin treatment and after metformin treatment. Mitochondria are indicated with red arrows, and nuclei with *nu* symbol, scale bar: 2 μm (**b**). Analysis of cell viability based on mitochondrial potential (**c**). Comparison of total depolarised cells in tested experiments (**d**). Evaluation of reactive oxygen species (**e**), nitric oxide (**f**) and superoxide dismutase activity (**g**). Significant changes are indicated with asterisks: * $p < 0.05$; ** $p < 0.01$ and *** $p < 0.001$, while non-significant differences are marked as *ns*.

3.3. Metformin Increases Viability of EqASC Cultures

Quantification of apoptosis and necrosis by annexin V binding and propidium iodide uptake revealed that metformin exerts an anti-apoptotic effect on EqASC$_{EMS}$ cultures (Figure 4a). The cellular viability of EqASC$_{EMS}$ was significantly restored following metformin treatment. The percentage of early and late apoptotic cells decreased after metformin administration, not only in EqASC$_{EMS}$ but also in EqASC$_{HE}$ (Figure 4c,d). Additionally, the viable cells were visualised with calcein-AM staining, while dead cells were counterstained with propidium iodide. The images confirmed the previous observations that metformin increases confluency of EqASCs in cultures. Nevertheless, based on the pictures, it was difficult to ascertain the influence of metformin on cells viability, because dead cells were dimly fluorescent in analysed cultures (Figure 4b). The anti-apoptotic effect of metformin towards EqASCs was confirmed using RT-qPCR. We determined that metformin decreases mRNA expression of *BAX* in EqASC$_{EMS}$ cultures, while increasing the mRNA expression of anti-apoptotic *BCL-2*. Further, the *BAX* transcript level increased following metformin treatment in EqASC$_{HE}$ cultures, however, the *BAX/BCL-2* ratio decreased, indicating an anti-apoptotic effect correlating with low ROS activity in those cultures (Figure 4e–g).

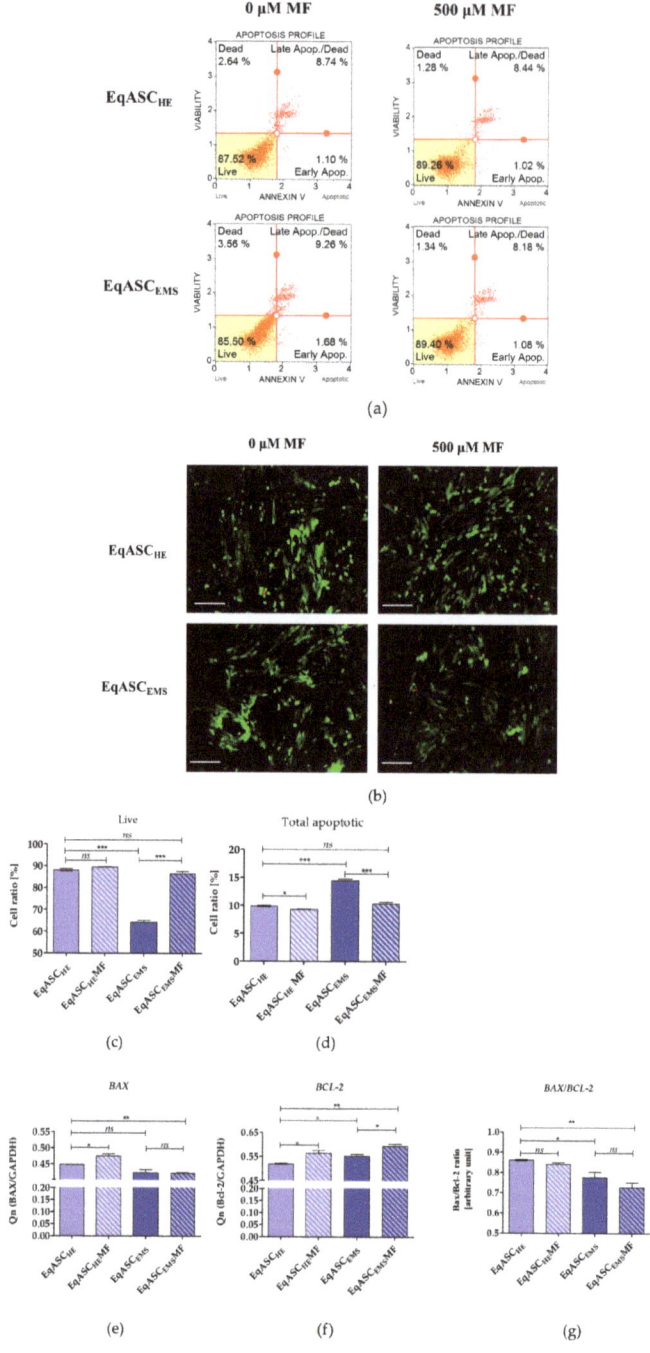

Figure 4. The influence of metformin on the apoptosis profile. Representative dot plots indicating distribution of cells after annexin V/ propidium iodide staining (**a**) Representative images obtained after calcein/PI staining, scale bar—250 µm. (**b**) Analysis of cell viability (**c**) and apoptosis (**d**). Measured transcript levels for *BAX* (**e**) *BCL-2* (**f**) and their ratio (**g**) Statistically significant changes are indicated with asterisks: * $p < 0.05$; ** $p < 0.01$ and *** $p < 0.001$, while non-significant differences are marked as *ns*.

3.4. Metformin Induces Intracellular Accumulation of β-Catenin and Wnt-3a, However, Only in EqASCs Derived from EMS Horses

The expression of WNT-3a and β-catenin was analysed on mRNA and protein levels. The mRNA level for β-catenin increased following metformin treatment both in EqASC$_{HE}$ and EqASC$_{EMS}$. We also noted that metformin increases the transcript level of *WNT-3A*, however, only significantly in EqASC$_{EMS}$ cultures. The intracellular accumulation of Wnt-3a and β-catenin was also significantly higher in EqASC$_{EMS}$ (Figure 5).

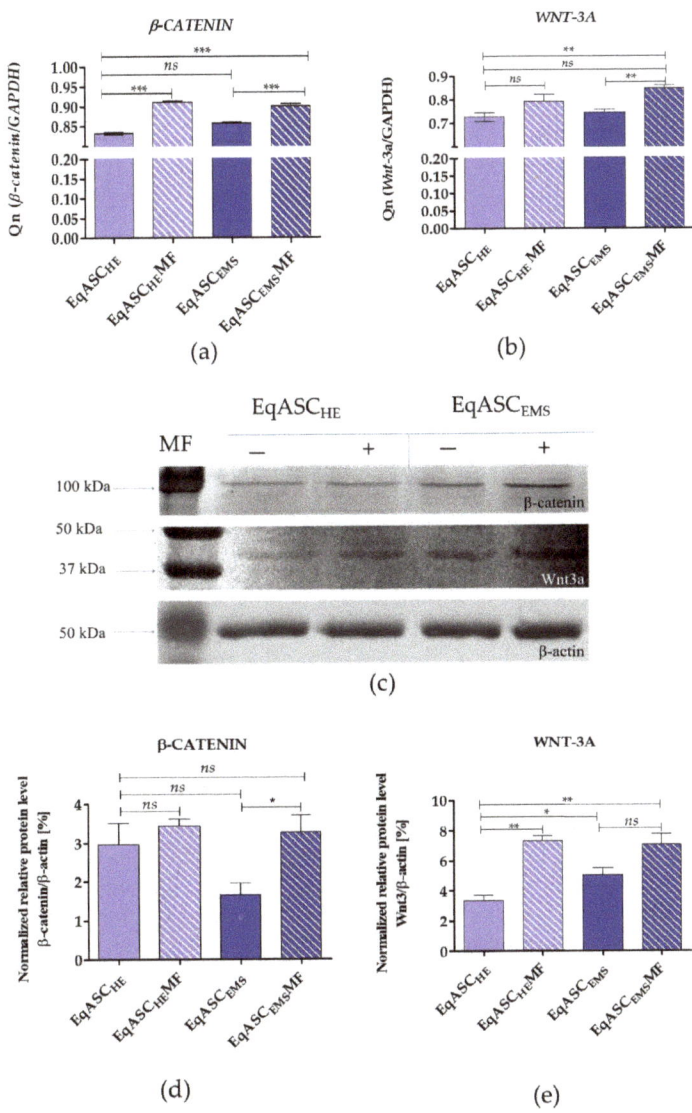

Figure 5. Determination of Wnt-3/β-catenin expression (**a,b**) and corresponding intracellular accumulation of protein (**c–e**). Statistically significant changes are indicated with asterisks: * $p < 0.05$; ** $p < 0.01$ and *** $p < 0.001$, while non-significant differences are marked as *ns*.

3.5. Metformin Decreases miR-16-5p, miR-21-5p, miR-29a-3p, miR-140-3p and miR-145-5p Levels in EqASCs Derived from EMS Horses

miRNA analysis showed that metformin does not influence *miR-16-5p*, *miR-21-5p* and *miR-29a-3p* levels in EqASC$_{HE}$, while the levels of *miR-140-3p* and *miR-145-5p* in those cultures were increased. All tested miRNAs were significantly downregulated in EqASC$_{EMS}$ cultures (Figure 6).

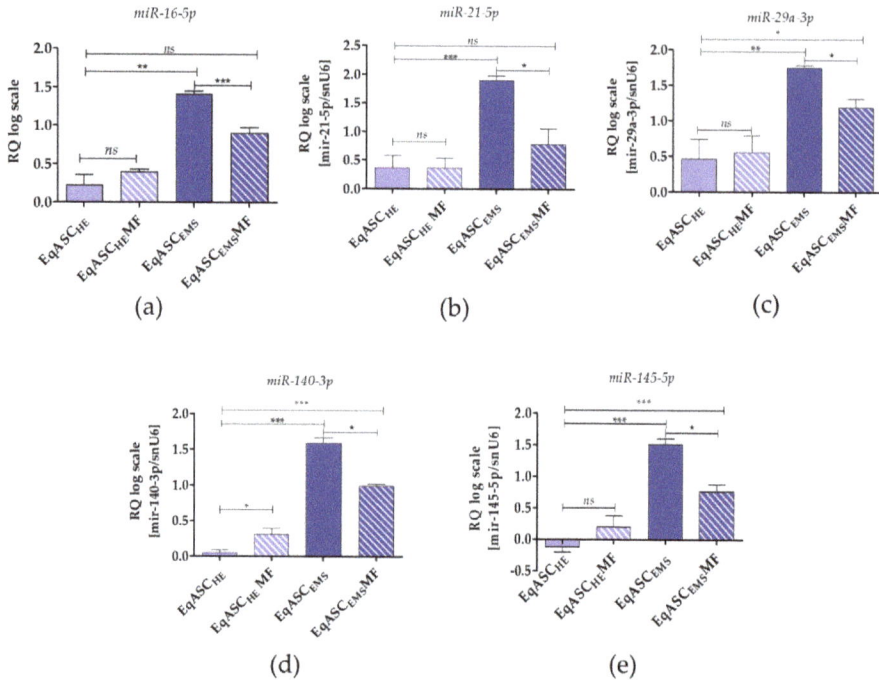

Figure 6. miRNA expression measured with two-tailed RT-qPCR. The following miRNAs were tested: miR-16-5p (**a**), miR-21-5p (**b**), miR-29a-3p(**c**), miR-140-3p (**d**) and miR-145-5p (**e**). Data are normalised to U6 snRNA levels and expressed as fold changes compared to the sample with the lowest level. Statistically significant changes are indicated with asterisks: * $p < 0.05$; ** $p < 0.01$ and *** $p < 0.001$, while non-significant differences are marked as *ns*.

4. Discussion

Adipose tissue is defined by heterogenous cellular composition that may be altered during disease conditions, such as diabetes and equine metabolic syndrome [46–49]. The morphology of mature adipocytes is also influenced by physiological conditions and might change under specific medication treatment, e.g., metformin was shown to reduce the diameter of adipocytes as well as to induce a greater heterogeneity of the tissue [50]. Currently, much attention is paid to the cellular composition of stromal vascular fraction (SVF) obtained from adipose tissue. This fraction contains a plethora of cells, including endothelial cells, fibroblasts, B- and T-lymphocytes, macrophages, myeloid cells, pericytes, pre-adipocytes, smooth muscle cells and, finally, culture-adherent adipose stromal cells (ASCs) [51]. Due to high cellular plasticity and enhanced self-renewal, ASCs are considered an excellent therapeutic tool in cell-based therapies for various disorders, including diabetes and the metabolic syndrome [46]. Moreover, the great pro-regenerative potential of ASCs also relies on their paracrine activity and immunomodulatory properties [52,53].

We have previously shown that EMS affects various aspects of ASC cellular activity and limits their clinical application. Generally, ASCs derived from horses with EMS (EqASC$_{EMS}$) exhibit lower proliferative and metabolic potential. Moreover, cultures of EqASC$_{EMS}$ are characterised by increased senescence and cell death. Further, we noticed imbalance of the oxidative status in that EqASC$_{EMS}$ was related to endoplasmic reticulum (ER) stress and deterioration of mitochondrial dynamics [2–5,41]. Currently, various pretreatment conditions and culture strategies are applied in terms of improvement of the regenerative potential of multipotent stromal cells residing in different tissue niches [52,54]. We previously found that combination of 5-azacytydine and resveratrol (AZA/RES) has a favourable influence on the proliferation, viability and multipotency of EqASC$_{EMS}$ [20]. The mechanism of 5-azacitidine (5-AZA) is related to inhibition of DNA methyltransferase (DNMT), while resveratrol was recognised, inter alia, as an activator of AMPK/PGC-1α signalling, improving mitochondrial biogenesis and dynamics [20]. The anti-aging and senolytic action of AZA/RES combination has been demonstrated towards progenitor cells of adipose origin. In the experiment, we focused on another AMPK activator, i.e., metformin, and its potential effect on the basic cytophysiological features of ASCs, including proliferation, metabolism and viability. The metformin was described as an agent with pleiotropic activity, which also includes anti-aging and senolytic activity [55]. Recently, we have observed growing interest in metformin and its application as a pro-regenerative molecule [56].

Our current research shows that metformin exerts pro-proliferative effect towards EqASCs derived from both healthy and EMS-affected horses (EqASC$_{HE}$ and EqASC$_{EMS}$, respectively). We noted increased proliferation and metabolic activity after metformin treatment, as well as shift of EqASCs to the S-phase of the cell cycle. The results are consistent with our previous studies applying an ex vivo model and showing the pro-proliferative effect of metformin on mouse ASC (mASCs) and progenitor cells isolated from olfactory bulb [21,22]. Previously, recognising the pro-regenerative potential of metformin, we used it as a bioactive molecule for functionalisation of sol–gel coatings covering metallic implants. We tested cytocompatibility of the obtained biomaterials using a model of human ASCs (hASCs) [57]. In this experiment, we found that metformin may enhance proliferation of cells, shorten the population doubling time, and improve metabolic activity. Earlier, the pro-proliferative effect of metformin was also established in terms of MSCs derived from bone marrow (BMSC) and osteoblast progenitors [58,59], as well as adipose-derived stromal cells [60]. Metformin generally acts in dose- and time-dependent manner, therefore, consideration of proper metformin dosage is crucial in terms of obtaining a desirable effect [50,61]. Metformin is also known as an anticancer drug. We previously tested metformin at concentrations that inhibited proliferation of various cancer cell lines, including breast, ovarian and pancreatic [62]. Our results showed that metformin in higher concentrations exerts an anti-proliferative effect towards mASCs [50] and mBMSCs [61].

We also indicated an improved oxidative status of mASCs derived from animals treated with metformin. This was correlated with reduction of reactive oxygen species (ROS) and nitric oxide (NO), and increase of SOD (superoxide dismutase) activity [21]. In the current study of EqASCs, we have confirmed the antioxidant effect of metformin. We also show that metformin improves mitochondrial membrane activity. The ultrastructural observations of metformin indicated enhanced dynamics of mitochondria in cultures derived from EMS horses. In EqASC$_{EMS}$, we have observed elongated mitochondria. Mitochondria elongation occurs during macroautophagy, which is a mechanism allowing to sustain cellular ATP production and viability of cells [63]. These results correlate with increased viability of EqASCs in cultures treated with metformin, and are in agreement with studies performed by Wang et al., who showed that metformin can protect H9c2 cells against hyperglycaemia-induced apoptosis and Cx43 downregulation through the induction of the autophagy pathway [64].

Analysis of the apoptosis profile revealed that metformin may act as anti-apoptotic agent towards EqASCs derived both from healthy and EMS horses. The results correlate with our previous findings, showing increased viability of mouse progenitor cells derived from animals treated with metformin [21,22]. However, the results are in contradiction to data presented by He et al. [65], who showed that metformin significantly induces apoptosis of MSCs isolated from human umbilical cord, even at 0.1 mM concentration. He et al. showed that metformin induces apoptosis in cells in dose- and time-dependent manner, and indicated that metformin at 2 mM concentration induced a sub-G1 peak, which is a suggestive marker of apoptosis [65]. We confirmed the anti-apoptotic activity of metformin in EqASC cultures at different levels. Firstly, by the distribution of cells in the cell cycle, showing a reduced percentage of cells in G0/G1-phase; secondly, by depicting increased mitochondrial membrane potential following metformin treatment; and, finally, determining the apoptosis profile using annexin V/PI and calcein/PI staining. Our results clearly indicate that metformin improves EqASC viability. Additionally, we noted increased transcript levels of the anti-apoptotic *BCL-2* gene, in contrast to the findings of He et al. [65]. The discrepancy between our findings and those of He et al. may be due to the model used, as well as different metformin concentrations. He et al. performed a comprehensive analysis of the pro-apoptotic effect of metformin using dosages above 1 mM, which is in agreement with our previous studies [50,61].

Due to the fact that Wnt/β-catenin signalling was indicated as a crucial pathway in terms of modulating MSC self-renewal and differentiation, we were interested in its expression profile after metformin treatment. It has been shown that fine-tuning of Wnt/β-catenin signalling coordinates MSC function [66]. Particularly, Kim et al. (2015) revealed that low levels of β-catenin in MSCs result in increased expression of genes involved in cell cycle control and DNA metabolism, while high levels of β-catenin were linked to increased expression of genes crucial for development and metabolism [66]. Additionally, Subramaniam et al. [32] tested the influence of AICAR and metformin on hepatic stellate cells (HSCs). The study showed that both agents activate AMPK signalling in quiescent HSCs, but elicit distinct effects on cells function. Interestingly, AICAR rapidly induced cell death of HSCs, while the cells remained viable after metformin treatment. Metformin induced activin membrane-bound inhibitor (Bambi) and activated a pro-survival Wnt/β-catenin signalling pathway [32]. Wnt pathway can also be regulated by ROS levels, which indicates crosstalk between Wnt and redox signalling. It has been shown that low levels of ROS activate Wnt signalling and improve differentiation of MSCs towards osteogenic cells [67]. Our results confirm that lowered levels of ROS may induce intracellular accumulation of WNT. Increased expression of WNT in cells treated with metformin may also explain the pro-osteogenic action of the drug towards ASCs, which was emphasised in our previous studies [21,57].

Metformin was also found to modulate microRNA levels. The miRNA profile following metformin treatment has previously mainly been established for cancer cell lines [68,69]. Here, we measured the levels of the following miRNAs: *miR-16-5p*, *miR-21-5p*, *miR-29a-3p*, *miR-140-3p* and *miR-145-5p*, that previously have been reported relevant for self-renewal and differentiation of mesenchymal stem cells [70,71]. We found that, in EqASC$_{EMS}$ cultures, expression of *miR-16-5p*, *miR-21-5p* and *miR-29a-3p* decreased following metformin treatment. miR-16-1 level has been reported inversely correlated to BCL-2 expression in chronic lymphocytic leukaemia (CLL) [72]. Indeed, our data indicate increased expression of *BCL-2* in cultures treated with metformin. Further, it has been reported that miR-16 controls myoblast proliferation and apoptosis via coordinated regulation of BCL-2 activation [72]. It has also been shown that overexpression of mir-21 is related to increased proliferation activity of BMSCs [73]. This also correlated to increased expression of BCL-2 and vascular endothelial growth factor (VEGF), and decreased expression of BAX. This is different to the profiles observed in our model. Firstly, we observe constitutive expression of miR-21-5p in EqASCs derived from healthy horses. Secondly, native cultures of EqASC$_{EMS}$ are characterised by increased occurrence of apoptosis and increased expression of *BAX* transcripts, which is associated to accumulation of *mir-21-5p*. Upon metformin treatment, the pattern was reversed: we found reduced levels of *mir-21-5p* and *BAX*, while *BCL-2* level was increased. It seems that regulation of mir-21-5p is complex, and it may influence the differentiation process of BMSCs [74]. Contradictory data exist concerning mir-21 function as a regulator of MSC fate and lineage commitment. For example, it has been shown that overexpression of mir-21 is related to osteoclastogenesis [75], adipogenesis [76], and osteolysis [77]. Nevertheless, it was also reported that rat BMSCs overexpressing mir-21 accelerate fracture healing in a rat closed femur fracture model [74].

Further, miR-29a-3p, in EqASCs, was found to have the same expression pattern as what we observed for miR-21-5p. Overexpression of miR-29a was correlated to reduced levels of Slit glycoprotein 2 (SLIT2) and its receptor Roundabout 1 (ROBO1) which, in turn, resulted in inhibition of mesenchymal stem cell viability and proliferation [78]. Moreover, it was shown that transfection of miR-29 family members at an early stage of somatic cell reprogramming may decrease the number of colonies expressing pluripotent markers, such as *Oct4* [79]. These results may explain the mir-29a-3p expression profile observed in EqASC$_{EMS}$ treated with metformin. These cultures were characterised by higher proliferative activity and viability when compared to non-treated cells characterised by increased levels of *mir-29a-3b*.

miR-140-3p and miR-145-5p in EqASC$_{HE}$ and EqASC$_{EMS}$ were differentially modulated by metformin. Following treatment, we observed increased levels of both transcripts in EqASC$_{HE}$, while miR-140-3p and miR-145-5 levels in EqASC$_{EMS}$ cultures were lower. mir-140 has been reported to modulate proliferation and differentiation of human dental pulp stem cells (DPSCs) [80]. Overexpression of miR-140-5p improved proliferation of DPSCs and aggravated their differentiation, whereas suppression of miR-140-5p had the opposite effect. Similarly, higher level of mir-145-5p was related to the lower ability of MSCs to undergo chondrogenic differentiation. mir-145-5p is generally considered suppressor of cell growth, and its reduced level in EqASC$_{EMS}$ cultures may explain their increased proliferative activity. Moreover, we have previously shown that microvesicles isolated from EMS contained high levels of mir-140 [5]. mir-140 has been reported marker for type II diabetes (T2D) [81]. Individuals with T2D have mir-140-3p levels upregulated compared to individuals with gestational diabetes mellitus, and downregulated compared to individuals with type I diabetes mellitus [82].

Today, miRNA is in focus, and has been proposed to serve as new biomarker for the diagnosis and treatment of metabolic syndrome in horses [81]. Identification of useful miRNA signatures in horses is an emerging field [83], and highly specific and sensitive methods, such as the two-tailed RT-qPCR used here, are vital to establish their usefulness as biomarkers for various horse diseases, including EMS.

5. Conclusions

Our results indicate that metformin improves proliferative activity of EqASCs derived from healthy and EMS horses. Metformin enhances mitochondrial metabolism reducing the percentage of cells with low mitochondrial membrane potential, which was related to the increased viability of EqASCs. Following metformin treatment, accumulation of WNT-3A and β-catenin was observed in EqASC$_{EMS}$. Metformin also modulates the expression of several miRNAs associated with cell proliferation, viability and differentiation. Bearing in mind that metformin may also promote differentiation of MSCs, it may be reasonable to test this drug as a preconditioning agent in osteogenic, chondrogenic, as well as adipogenic cultures of EqASCs.

Supplementary Materials: The supplementary materials are available online at http://www.mdpi.com/2073-4409/8/2/80/s1.

Author Contributions: Conceptualisation, A.S. and K.M.; Methodology, A.S., K.K., J.S.-K., P.A., L.L., E.R. and L.V.; Software, A.S., P.A. and L.V.; Validation, A.S., K.K., J.S.-K., P.A. and L.V.; Formal Analysis, A.S., K.M., P.A., L.V. and M.K.; Investigation, A.S., K.K., P.A., L.L., E.R. and L.V.; Resources, A.S., K.M., L.V. and M.K.; Data Curation, A.S., K.M., P.A. and L.V.; Writing—Original Draft Preparation, A.S., K.M., P.A., L.V. and M.K.; Writing—Review & Editing, A.S., K.M., P.A., L.V and M.K.; Visualisation, A.S.; Supervision, A.S., K.M., L.V. and M.K.; Project Administration, A.S. and K.M.; Funding Acquisition, A.S., K.M., L.V. and M.K.

Funding: This project is financed in the framework of grant entitled "Modulation mitochondrial metabolism and dynamics and targeting DNA methylation of adipose derived mesenchymal stromal stem cell (ASC) using RES and 5-azacytydin as a therapeutic strategy in the course of EMS" (Grant no. 2016/21/B/NZ7/01111) and "Inhibition of tyrosine phosphatase as a strategy to enhance insulin sensitivity through activation of chaperone mediated autophagy and amelioration of inflammation and cellular stress in the liver of equine metabolic syndrome (EMS) horses" (Grant no. 2018/29/B/NZ7/02662) financed by The National Science Centre in Poland. The project is financed under the program of the Minister of Science and Higher Education "Strategy of Excellence—University of Research" in 2018–2019 project number 0019/SDU/2018/18 in the amount of PLN 700000. This study is supported by following grants: Czech Science Foundation P303/18/21942S; RVO 86652036; BIOCEV CZ.1.05/1.1.00/02.0109.

Acknowledgments: Authors are grateful to Justyna Trynda, Martyna Murat and Joanna Szydlarska for technical support. The authors are grateful to PORT Polski Ośrodek Rozwoju Technologii/Polish Center for Technology Development for ability to perform visualisation of cells ultrastructure.

Conflicts of Interest: M.K. has shares in TATAA Biocenter. The authors declare no conflict of interest.

References

1. Pagan, J.D.; Martin, O.A.; Crowley, N.L. Relationship Between Body Condition and Metabolic Parameters in Sport Horses, Pony Hunters and Polo Ponies. *J. Equine Vet. Sci.* **2009**, *29*, 418–420. [CrossRef]
2. Basinska, K.; Marycz, K.; Śmieszek, A.; Nicpoń, J. The production and distribution of IL-6 and TNF-α in subcutaneous adipose tissue and their correlation with serum concentrations in Welsh ponies with equine metabolic syndrome. *J. Vet. Sci.* **2015**, *16*, 113–120. [CrossRef] [PubMed]
3. Marycz, K.; Kornicka, K.; Basinska, K.; Czyrek, A. Equine Metabolic Syndrome Affects Viability, Senescence, and Stress Factors of Equine Adipose-Derived Mesenchymal Stromal Stem Cells: New Insight into EqASCs Isolated from EMS Horses in the Context of Their Aging. *Oxid. Med. Cell. Longev.* **2016**, *2016*, 4710326. [CrossRef] [PubMed]
4. Marycz, K.; Weiss, C.; Śmieszek, A.; Kornicka, K. Evaluation of Oxidative Stress and Mitophagy during Adipogenic Differentiation of Adipose-Derived Stem Cells Isolated from Equine Metabolic Syndrome (EMS) Horses. *Stem Cells Int.* **2018**, *2018*, 5340756. [CrossRef] [PubMed]
5. Marycz, K.; Kornicka, K.; Grzesiak, J.; Śmieszek, A.; Szłapka, J. Macroautophagy and Selective Mitophagy Ameliorate Chondrogenic Differentiation Potential in Adipose Stem Cells of Equine Metabolic Syndrome: New Findings in the Field of Progenitor Cells Differentiation. *Oxid. Med. Cell. Longev.* **2016**, *2016*, 3718468. [CrossRef] [PubMed]
6. Ranera, B.; Remacha, A.R.; Álvarez-Arguedas, S.; Romero, A.; Vázquez, F.J.; Zaragoza, P.; Martín-Burriel, I.; Rodellar, C. Effect of hypoxia on equine mesenchymal stem cells derived from bone marrow and adipose tissue. *BMC Vet. Res.* **2012**, *8*, 142. [CrossRef] [PubMed]
7. Del Bue, M.; Riccò, S.; Ramoni, R.; Conti, V.; Gnudi, G.; Grolli, S. Equine adipose-tissue derived mesenchymal stem cells and platelet concentrates: Their association in vitro and in vivo. *Vet. Res. Commun.* **2008**, *32*, 51–55. [CrossRef] [PubMed]
8. Nicpoń, J.; Marycz, K.; Grzesiak, J. Therapeutic effect of adipose-derived mesenchymal stem cell injection in horses suffering from bone spavin. *Pol. J. Vet. Sci.* **2013**, *16*, 753–754. [CrossRef] [PubMed]
9. Marycz, K.; Toker, N.Y.; Grzesiak, J.; Wrzeszcz, K. The Therapeutic Effect of Autogenic Adipose Derived Stem Cells Combined with Autogenic Platelet Rich Plasma in Tendons Disorders in Horses In Vitro and In Vivo Research. *J. Anim. Vet. Adv.* **2012**, *11*, 4324–4331.
10. Gnecchi, M.; Zhang, Z.; Ni, A.; Dzau, V.J. Paracrine mechanisms in adult stem cell signaling and therapy. *Circ. Res.* **2008**, *103*, 1204–1219. [CrossRef]
11. De Aro, A.A.; Carneiro, G.D.; Teodoro, L.F.R.; da Veiga, F.C.; Ferrucci, D.L.; Simões, G.F.; Simões, P.W.; Alvares, L.E.; de Oliveira, A.L.R.; Vicente, C.P.; et al. Injured Achilles Tendons Treated with Adipose-Derived Stem Cells Transplantation and GDF-5. *Cells* **2018**, *7*, 127. [CrossRef] [PubMed]
12. Marędziak, M.; Marycz, K.; Lewandowski, D.; Siudzińska, A.; Śmieszek, A. Static magnetic field enhances synthesis and secretion of membrane-derived microvesicles (MVs) rich in VEGF and BMP-2 in equine adipose-derived stromal cells (EqASCs)-a new approach in veterinary regenerative medicine. *In Vitro Cell. Dev. Biol. Anim.* **2015**, *51*, 230–240. [CrossRef] [PubMed]

13. Kornicka, K.; Marycz, K.; Tomaszewski, K.A.; Marędziak, M.; Śmieszek, A. The Effect of Age on Osteogenic and Adipogenic Differentiation Potential of Human Adipose Derived Stromal Stem Cells (hASCs) and the Impact of Stress Factors in the Course of the Differentiation Process. *Oxid. Med. Cell. Longev.* **2015**, *2015*, 309169. [CrossRef] [PubMed]
14. Nawrocka, D.; Kornicka, K.; Szydlarska, J.; Marycz, K. Basic Fibroblast Growth Factor Inhibits Apoptosis and Promotes Proliferation of Adipose-Derived Mesenchymal Stromal Cells Isolated from Patients with Type 2 Diabetes by Reducing Cellular Oxidative Stress. *Oxid. Med. Cell. Longev.* **2017**, *2017*, 3027109. [PubMed]
15. Wu, W.; Niklason, L.; Steinbacher, D.M. The effect of age on human adipose-derived stem cells. *Plast. Reconstr. Surg.* **2013**, *131*, 27–37. [CrossRef] [PubMed]
16. Liu, M.; Lei, H.; Dong, P.; Fu, X.; Yang, Z.; Yang, Y.; Ma, J.; Liu, X.; Cao, Y.; Xiao, R. Adipose-Derived Mesenchymal Stem Cells from the Elderly Exhibit Decreased Migration and Differentiation Abilities with Senescent Properties. *Cell Transplant.* **2017**, *26*, 1505–1519. [CrossRef] [PubMed]
17. Geburek, F.; Roggel, F.; van Schie, H.T.M.; Beineke, A.; Estrada, R.; Weber, K.; Hellige, M.; Rohn, K.; Jagodzinski, M.; Welke, B.; et al. Effect of single intralesional treatment of surgically induced equine superficial digital flexor tendon core lesions with adipose-derived mesenchymal stromal cells: A controlled experimental trial. *Stem Cell Res. Ther.* **2017**, *8*, 129. [CrossRef] [PubMed]
18. De Mattos Carvalho, A.; Alves, A.L.G.; de Oliveira, P.G.G.; Cisneros Álvarez, L.E.; Amorim, R.L.; Hussni, C.A.; Deffune, E. Use of Adipose Tissue-Derived Mesenchymal Stem Cells for Experimental Tendinitis Therapy in Equines. *J. Equine Vet. Sci.* **2011**, *31*, 26–34. [CrossRef]
19. Kornicka, K.; Śmieszek, A.; Węgrzyn, A.S.; Röcken, M.; Marycz, K. Immunomodulatory Properties of Adipose-Derived Stem Cells Treated with 5-Azacytydine and Resveratrol on Peripheral Blood Mononuclear Cells and Macrophages in Metabolic Syndrome Animals. *J. Clin. Med.* **2018**, *7*, 383. [CrossRef] [PubMed]
20. Kornicka, K.; Szłapka-Kosarzewska, J.; Śmieszek, A.; Marycz, K. 5-Azacytydine and resveratrol reverse senescence and ageing of adipose stem cells via modulation of mitochondrial dynamics and autophagy. *J. Cell. Mol. Med.* **2018**, *23*, 237–259. [CrossRef] [PubMed]
21. Marycz, K.; Tomaszewski, K.A.; Kornicka, K.; Henry, B.M.; Wroński, S.; Tarasiuk, J.; Maredziak, M. Metformin Decreases Reactive Oxygen Species, Enhances Osteogenic Properties of Adipose-Derived Multipotent Mesenchymal Stem Cells In Vitro, and Increases Bone Density In Vivo. *Oxid. Med. Cell. Longev.* **2016**, *2016*, 9785890. [CrossRef] [PubMed]
22. Śmieszek, A.; Stręk, Z.; Kornicka, K.; Grzesiak, J.; Weiss, C.; Marycz, K. Antioxidant and Anti-Senescence Effect of Metformin on Mouse Olfactory Ensheathing Cells (mOECs) May Be Associated with Increased Brain-Derived Neurotrophic Factor Levels—An Ex Vivo Study. *Int. J. Mol. Sci.* **2017**, *18*, 872. [CrossRef] [PubMed]
23. Qi, T.; Chen, Y.; Li, H.; Pei, Y.; Woo, S.-L.; Guo, X.; Zhao, J.; Qian, X.; Awika, J.; Huo, Y.; et al. A role for PFKFB3/iPFK2 in metformin suppression of adipocyte inflammatory responses. *J. Mol. Endocrinol.* **2017**, *59*, 49–59. [CrossRef] [PubMed]
24. Kim, E.K.; Lee, S.H.; Jhun, J.Y.; Byun, J.K.; Jeong, J.H.; Lee, S.-Y.; Kim, J.K.; Choi, J.Y.; Cho, M.-L. Metformin Prevents Fatty Liver and Improves Balance of White/Brown Adipose in an Obesity Mouse Model by Inducing FGF21. *Mediat. Inflamm.* **2016**, *2016*. [CrossRef] [PubMed]
25. Schosserer, M.; Grillari, J.; Wolfrum, C.; Scheideler, M. Age-Induced Changes in White, Brite, and Brown Adipose Depots: A Mini-Review. *Gerontology* **2018**, *64*, 229–236. [CrossRef] [PubMed]
26. Rendle, D.I.; Rutledge, F.; Hughes, K.J.; Heller, J.; Durham, A.E. Effects of metformin hydrochloride on blood glucose and insulin responses to oral dextrose in horses. *Equine Vet. J.* **2013**, *45*, 751–754. [CrossRef]
27. Durham, A.E.; Rendle, D.I.; Newton, J.R. The effect of metformin on measurements of insulin sensitivity and β cell response in 18 horses and ponies with insulin resistance. *Equine Vet. J.* **2008**, *40*, 493–500. [CrossRef]
28. Tinworth, K.D.; Edwards, S.; Noble, G.K.; Harris, P.A.; Sillence, M.N.; Hackett, L.P. Pharmacokinetics of metformin after enteral administration in insulin-resistant ponies. *Am. J. Vet. Res.* **2010**, *71*, 1201–1206. [CrossRef]
29. Tinworth, K.D.; Boston, R.C.; Harris, P.A.; Sillence, M.N.; Raidal, S.L.; Noble, G.K. The effect of oral metformin on insulin sensitivity in insulin-resistant ponies. *Vet. J.* **2012**, *191*, 79–84. [CrossRef]
30. Barzilai, N.; Crandall, J.P.; Kritchevsky, S.B.; Espeland, M.A. Metformin as a Tool to Target Aging. *Cell Metab.* **2016**, *23*, 1060–1065. [CrossRef]

31. Androvic, P.; Valihrach, L.; Elling, J.; Sjoback, R.; Kubista, M. Two-tailed RT-qPCR: A novel method for highly accurate miRNA quantification. *Nucleic Acids Res.* **2017**, *45*, e144. [CrossRef] [PubMed]
32. Subramaniam, N.; Sherman, M.H.; Rao, R.; Wilson, C.; Coulter, S.; Atkins, A.R.; Evans, R.M.; Liddle, C.; Downes, M. Metformin-mediated Bambi expression in Hepatic Stellate Cells induces pro-survival Wnt/β-catenin signaling. *Cancer Prev. Res.* **2012**, *5*, 553–561. [CrossRef] [PubMed]
33. Nawrocka, D.; Kornicka, K.; Śmieszek, A.; Marycz, K. Spirulina platensis Improves Mitochondrial Function Impaired by Elevated Oxidative Stress in Adipose-Derived Mesenchymal Stromal Cells (ASCs) and Intestinal Epithelial Cells (IECs), and Enhances Insulin Sensitivity in Equine Metabolic Syndrome (EMS) Horses. *Mar. Drugs* **2017**, *15*, 237. [CrossRef] [PubMed]
34. Marędziak, M.; Marycz, K.; Śmieszek, A.; Lewandowski, D.; Toker, N.Y. The influence of static magnetic fields on canine and equine mesenchymal stem cells derived from adipose tissue. *In Vitro Cell. Dev. Biol. Anim.* **2014**, *50*, 562–571. [CrossRef] [PubMed]
35. Marycz, K.; Krzak-Roś, J.; Donesz-Sikorska, A.; Śmieszek, A. The morphology, proliferation rate, and population doubling time factor of adipose-derived mesenchymal stem cells cultured on to non-aqueous SiO_2, TiO_2, and hybrid sol-gel-derived oxide coatings. *J. Biomed. Mater. Res. A* **2014**, *102*, 4017–4026. [CrossRef] [PubMed]
36. Nowak, U.; Marycz, K.; Nicpoń, J.; Śmieszek, A. Chondrogenic potential of canine articular cartilage derived cells (cACCs). *Open Life Sci.* **2016**, *11*, 151–165. [CrossRef]
37. Marycz, K.; Michalak, I.; Kocherova, I.; Marędziak, M.; Weiss, C. The Cladophora glomerata Enriched by Biosorption Process in Cr(III) Improves Viability, and Reduces Oxidative Stress and Apoptosis in Equine Metabolic Syndrome Derived Adipose Mesenchymal Stromal Stem Cells (ASCs) and Their Extracellular Vesicles (MV's). *Mar. Drugs* **2017**, *15*, 385. [CrossRef] [PubMed]
38. Marycz, K.; Sobierajska, P.; Smieszek, A.; Maredziak, M.; Wiglusz, K.; Wiglusz, R.J. Li+ activated nanohydroxyapatite doped with Eu3+ ions enhances proliferative activity and viability of human stem progenitor cells of adipose tissue and olfactory ensheathing cells. Further perspective of nHAP: Li+, Eu3+ application in theranostics. *Mater. Sci. Eng. C* **2017**, *78*, 151–162. [CrossRef] [PubMed]
39. Chomczynski, P.; Sacchi, N. Single-step method of RNA isolation by acid guanidinium thiocyanate-phenol-chloroform extraction. *Anal. Biochem.* **1987**, *162*, 156–159. [CrossRef]
40. Lis-Bartos, A.; Smieszek, A.; Frańczyk, K.; Marycz, K.; Lis-Bartos, A.; Smieszek, A.; Frańczyk, K.; Marycz, K. Fabrication, Characterization, and Cytotoxicity of Thermoplastic Polyurethane/Poly(lactic acid) Material Using Human Adipose Derived Mesenchymal Stromal Stem Cells (hASCs). *Polymers* **2018**, *10*, 1073. [CrossRef]
41. Marycz, K.; Kornicka, K.; Szlapka-Kosarzewska, J.; Weiss, C. Excessive Endoplasmic Reticulum Stress Correlates with Impaired Mitochondrial Dynamics, Mitophagy and Apoptosis, in Liver and Adipose Tissue, but Not in Muscles in EMS Horses. *Int. J. Mol. Sci.* **2018**, *19*, 165. [CrossRef] [PubMed]
42. Marycz, K.; Kornicka, K.; Marędziak, M.; Golonka, P.; Nicpoń, J. Equine metabolic syndrome impairs adipose stem cells osteogenic differentiation by predominance of autophagy over selective mitophagy. *J. Cell. Mol. Med.* **2016**, *20*, 2384–2404. [CrossRef] [PubMed]
43. Marycz, K.; Marędziak, M.; Grzesiak, J.; Lis, A.; Śmieszek, A.; Marycz, K.; Marędziak, M.; Grzesiak, J.; Lis, A.; Śmieszek, A. Biphasic Polyurethane/Polylactide Sponges Doped with Nano-Hydroxyapatite (nHAp) Combined with Human Adipose-Derived Mesenchymal Stromal Stem Cells for Regenerative Medicine Applications. *Polymers* **2016**, *8*, 339. [CrossRef]
44. Dzamba, D.; Valihrach, L.; Kubista, M.; Anderova, M. The correlation between expression profiles measured in single cells and in traditional bulk samples. *Sci. Rep.* **2016**, *6*, 37022. [CrossRef] [PubMed]
45. Pivonkova, H.; Hermanova, Z.; Kirdajova, D.; Awadova, T.; Malinsky, J.; Valihrach, L.; Zucha, D.; Kubista, M.; Galisova, A.; Jirak, D.; et al. The Contribution of TRPV4 Channels to Astrocyte Volume Regulation and Brain Edema Formation. *Neuroscience* **2018**, *394*, 127–143. [CrossRef] [PubMed]
46. Kornicka, K.; Houston, J.; Marycz, K. Dysfunction of Mesenchymal Stem Cells Isolated from Metabolic Syndrome and Type 2 Diabetic Patients as Result of Oxidative Stress and Autophagy may Limit Their Potential Therapeutic Use. *Stem Cell Rev.* **2018**, *14*, 337–345. [CrossRef] [PubMed]
47. Gallagher, D.; Kelley, D.E.; Yim, J.-E.; Spence, N.; Albu, J.; Boxt, L.; Pi-Sunyer, F.X.; Heshka, S. Adipose tissue distribution is different in type 2 diabetes123. *Am. J. Clin. Nutr.* **2009**, *89*, 807–814. [PubMed]

48. Lee, M.-J.; Wu, Y.; Fried, S.K. Adipose Tissue Heterogeneity: Implication of depot differences in adipose tissue for Obesity Complications. *Mol. Aspects Med.* **2013**, *34*, 1–11. [CrossRef] [PubMed]
49. Dev, R.; Bruera, E.; Dalal, S. Insulin resistance and body composition in cancer patients. *Ann. Oncol.* **2018**, *29*, ii18–ii26. [CrossRef] [PubMed]
50. Śmieszek, A.; Basińska, K.; Chrząstek, K.; Marycz, K. In Vitro and In Vivo Effects of Metformin on Osteopontin Expression in Mice Adipose-Derived Multipotent Stromal Cells and Adipose Tissue. *J. Diabetes Res.* **2015**, *2015*, 814896. [CrossRef] [PubMed]
51. Baer, P.C.; Geiger, H. Adipose-Derived Mesenchymal Stromal/Stem Cells: Tissue Localization, Characterization, and Heterogeneity. *Stem Cells Int.* **2012**, *2012*, 812693. [CrossRef] [PubMed]
52. Schäfer, R.; Spohn, G.; Baer, P.C. Mesenchymal Stem/Stromal Cells in Regenerative Medicine: Can Preconditioning Strategies Improve Therapeutic Efficacy? *Transfus. Med. Hemother.* **2016**, *43*, 256–267. [CrossRef] [PubMed]
53. Gimble, J.M.; Bunnell, B.A.; Frazier, T.; Rowan, B.; Shah, F.; Thomas-Porch, C.; Wu, X. Adipose-derived stromal/stem cells. *Organogenesis* **2013**, *9*, 3–10. [CrossRef] [PubMed]
54. Baer, P.C.; Overath, J.M.; Urbschat, A.; Schubert, R.; Koch, B.; Bohn, A.A.; Geiger, H. Effect of Different Preconditioning Regimens on the Expression Profile of Murine Adipose-Derived Stromal/Stem Cells. *Int. J. Mol. Sci.* **2018**, *19*, 1719. [CrossRef] [PubMed]
55. The Pleiotropic Effects of Metformin: Time for Prospective Studies | Cardiovascular Diabetology | Full Text. Available online: https://cardiab.biomedcentral.com/articles/10.1186/s12933-015-0273-5 (accessed on 19 November 2018).
56. Fatt, M.; Hsu, K.; He, L.; Wondisford, F.; Miller, F.D.; Kaplan, D.R.; Wang, J. Metformin Acts on Two Different Molecular Pathways to Enhance Adult Neural Precursor Proliferation/Self-Renewal and Differentiation. *Stem Cell Rep.* **2015**, *5*, 988–995. [CrossRef] [PubMed]
57. Śmieszek, A.; Szydlarska, J.; Mucha, A.; Chrapiec, M.; Marycz, K. Enhanced cytocompatibility and osteoinductive properties of sol-gel-derived silica/zirconium dioxide coatings by metformin functionalization. *J. Biomater. Appl.* **2017**, *32*, 570–586. [CrossRef] [PubMed]
58. Cortizo, A.M.; Sedlinsky, C.; McCarthy, A.D.; Blanco, A.; Schurman, L. Osteogenic Actions of the Anti-Diabetic Drug Metformin on Osteoblasts in Culture. *Eur. J. Pharmacol.* **2006**, *536*, 38–46. [CrossRef] [PubMed]
59. Molinuevo, M.S.; Schurman, L.; McCarthy, A.D.; Cortizo, A.M.; Tolosa, M.J.; Gangoiti, M.V.; Arnol, V.; Sedlinsky, C. Effect of metformin on bone marrow progenitor cell differentiation: In vivo and in vitro studies. *J. Bone Miner. Res.* **2010**, *25*, 211–221. [CrossRef] [PubMed]
60. Smieszek, A.; Tomaszewski, K.A.; Kornicka, K.; Marycz, K. Metformin Promotes Osteogenic Differentiation of Adipose-Derived Stromal Cells and Exerts Pro-Osteogenic Effect Stimulating Bone Regeneration. *J. Clin. Med.* **2018**, *7*, 482. [CrossRef] [PubMed]
61. Śmieszek, A.; Czyrek, A.; Basinska, K.; Trynda, J.; Skaradzińska, A.; Siudzińska, A.; Marędziak, M.; Marycz, K. Effect of Metformin on Viability, Morphology, and Ultrastructure of Mouse Bone Marrow-Derived Multipotent Mesenchymal Stromal Cells and Balb/3T3 Embryonic Fibroblast Cell Line. *BioMed Res. Int.* **2015**, *2015*, 769402. [CrossRef]
62. Kheirandish, M.; Mahboobi, H.; Yazdanparast, M.; Kamal, W.; Kamal, M.A. Anti-cancer Effects of Metformin: Recent Evidences for its Role in Prevention and Treatment of Cancer. *Curr. Drug Metab.* **2018**, *19*, 793–797. [CrossRef]
63. Gomes, L.C.; Di Benedetto, G.; Scorrano, L. During autophagy mitochondria elongate, are spared from degradation and sustain cell viability. *Nat. Cell Biol.* **2011**, *13*, 589–598. [CrossRef]
64. Wang, G.-Y.; Bi, Y.-G.; Liu, X.-D.; Zhao, Y.; Han, J.-F.; Wei, M.; Zhang, Q.-Y. Autophagy was involved in the protective effect of metformin on hyperglycemia-induced cardiomyocyte apoptosis and Connexin43 downregulation in H9c2 cells. *Int. J. Med. Sci.* **2017**, *14*, 698–704. [CrossRef] [PubMed]
65. He, X.; Yao, M.-W.; Zhu, M.; Liang, D.-L.; Guo, W.; Yang, Y.; Zhao, R.-S.; Ren, T.-T.; Ao, X.; Wang, W.; et al. Metformin induces apoptosis in mesenchymal stromal cells and dampens their therapeutic efficacy in infarcted myocardium. *Stem Cell Res. Ther.* **2018**, *9*, 306. [CrossRef] [PubMed]
66. Kim, J.-A.; Choi, H.-K.; Kim, T.-M.; Leem, S.-H.; Oh, I.-H. Regulation of mesenchymal stromal cells through fine tuning of canonical Wnt signaling. *Stem Cell Res.* **2015**, *14*, 356–368. [CrossRef] [PubMed]

67. Visweswaran, M.; Pohl, S.; Arfuso, F.; Newsholme, P.; Dilley, R.; Pervaiz, S.; Dharmarajan, A. Multi-lineage differentiation of mesenchymal stem cells—To Wnt, or not Wnt. *Int. J. Biochem. Cell Biol.* **2015**, *68*, 139–147. [CrossRef] [PubMed]
68. Zhou, J.Y.; Xu, B.; Li, L. A New Role for an Old Drug: Metformin Targets MicroRNAs in Treating Diabetes and Cancer. *Drug Dev. Res.* **2015**, *76*, 263–269. [CrossRef]
69. Avci, C.B.; Harman, E.; Dodurga, Y.; Susluer, S.Y.; Gunduz, C. Therapeutic potential of an anti-diabetic drug, metformin: Alteration of miRNA expression in prostate cancer cells. *Asian Pac. J. Cancer Prev.* **2013**, *14*, 765–768. [CrossRef]
70. Tan, K.; Peng, Y.T.; Guo, P. MiR-29a Promotes Osteogenic Differentiation of Mesenchymal Stem Cells via Targeting HDAC4. *Eur. Rev. Med. Pharmacol. Sci.* **2018**, *22*, 3318–3326.
71. Guo, L.; Zhao, R.C.H.; Wu, Y. The role of microRNAs in self-renewal and differentiation of mesenchymal stem cells. *Exp. Hematol.* **2011**, *39*, 608–616. [CrossRef]
72. Cimmino, A.; Calin, G.A.; Fabbri, M.; Iorio, M.V.; Ferracin, M.; Shimizu, M.; Wojcik, S.E.; Aqeilan, R.I.; Zupo, S.; Dono, M.; et al. miR-15 and miR-16 induce apoptosis by targeting BCL2. *Proc. Natl. Acad. Sci. USA* **2005**, *102*, 13944–13949. [CrossRef]
73. Zeng, Y.-L.; Zheng, H.; Chen, Q.-R.; Yuan, X.-H.; Ren, J.-H.; Luo, X.-F.; Chen, P.; Lin, Z.-Y.; Chen, S.-Z.; Wu, X.-Q.; et al. Bone marrow-derived mesenchymal stem cells overexpressing MiR-21 efficiently repair myocardial damage in rats. *Oncotarget* **2017**, *8*, 29161–29173. [CrossRef] [PubMed]
74. Sun, Y.; Xu, L.; Huang, S.; Hou, Y.; Liu, Y.; Chan, K.-M.; Pan, X.-H.; Li, G. mir-21 Overexpressing Mesenchymal Stem Cells Accelerate Fracture Healing in a Rat Closed Femur Fracture Model. *BioMed Res. Int.* **2015**, *2015*, 412327. [CrossRef]
75. Sugatani, T.; Vacher, J.; Hruska, K.A. A microRNA expression signature of osteoclastogenesis. *Blood* **2011**, *117*, 3648–3657. [CrossRef] [PubMed]
76. Mei, Y.; Bian, C.; Li, J.; Du, Z.; Zhou, H.; Yang, Z.; Zhao, R.C.H. miR-21 modulates the ERK-MAPK signaling pathway by regulating SPRY2 expression during human mesenchymal stem cell differentiation. *J. Cell. Biochem.* **2013**, *114*, 1374–1384. [CrossRef] [PubMed]
77. Zhou, Y.; Liu, Y.; Cheng, L. miR-21 expression is related to particle-induced osteolysis pathogenesis. *J. Orthop. Res.* **2012**, *30*, 1837–1842. [CrossRef] [PubMed]
78. Zhang, Y.; Zhou, S. MicroRNA-29a inhibits mesenchymal stem cell viability and proliferation by targeting Roundabout 1. *Mol. Med. Rep.* **2015**, *12*, 6178–6184. [CrossRef]
79. Fráguas, M.S.; Eggenschwiler, R.; Hoepfner, J.; Schiavinato, J.L.; Haddad, R.; Oliveira, L.H.B.; Araújo, A.G.; Zago, M.A.; Panepucci, R.A.; Cantz, T. MicroRNA-29 impairs the early phase of reprogramming process by targeting active DNA demethylation enzymes and Wnt signaling. *Stem Cell Res.* **2017**, *19*, 21–30. [CrossRef]
80. Sun, D.-G.; Xin, B.-C.; Wu, D.; Zhou, L.; Wu, H.-B.; Gong, W.; Lv, J. miR-140-5p-mediated regulation of the proliferation and differentiation of human dental pulp stem cells occurs through the lipopolysaccharide/toll-like receptor 4 signaling pathway. *Eur. J. Oral Sci.* **2017**, *125*, 419–425. [CrossRef]
81. Da Costa Santos, H.; Hess, T.; Bruemmer, J.; Splan, R. Possible Role of MicroRNA in Equine Insulin Resistance: A Pilot Study. *J. Equine Vet. Sci.* **2018**, *63*, 74–79. [CrossRef]
82. Raitoharju, E.; Seppälä, I.; Oksala, N.; Lyytikäinen, L.-P.; Raitakari, O.; Viikari, J.; Ala-Korpela, M.; Soininen, P.; Kangas, A.J.; Waldenberger, M.; et al. Blood microRNA profile associates with the levels of serum lipids and metabolites associated with glucose metabolism and insulin resistance and pinpoints pathways underlying metabolic syndrome: The cardiovascular risk in Young Finns Study. *Mol. Cell. Endocrinol.* **2014**, *391*, 41–49. [CrossRef] [PubMed]
83. Van der Kolk, J.H.; Pacholewska, A.; Gerber, V. The role of microRNAs in equine medicine: A review. *Vet. Q.* **2015**, *35*, 88–96. [CrossRef]

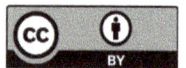

© 2019 by the authors. Licensee MDPI, Basel, Switzerland. This article is an open access article distributed under the terms and conditions of the Creative Commons Attribution (CC BY) license (http://creativecommons.org/licenses/by/4.0/).

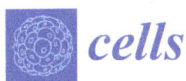

Article

Valproic Acid Promotes Early Neural Differentiation in Adult Mesenchymal Stem Cells Through Protein Signalling Pathways

Jerran Santos [1,*], Thibaut Hubert [1,2] and Bruce K Milthorpe [1]

1. Advanced Tissue Regeneration & Drug Delivery Group, School of Life Sciences, University of Technology Sydney, P.O. Box 123, Broadway, NSW 2007, Australia; tibo.hubert@gmail.com (T.H.); Bruce.Milthorpe@uts.edu.au (B.K.M.)
2. Ecole Nationale Supérieure D'agronomie et des Industries Alimentaires (ENSAIA), Université de Lorraine, 2 Avenue de la Forêt de Haye, 54505 Vandœuvre-lès-Nancy, France
* Correspondence: Jerran.Santos@uts.edu.au; Tel.: +61-(2)-9514-1353

Received: 23 January 2020; Accepted: 26 February 2020; Published: 4 March 2020

Abstract: Regenerative medicine is a rapidly expanding area in research and clinical applications. Therapies involving the use of small molecule chemicals aim to simplify the creation of specific drugs for clinical applications. Adult mesenchymal stem cells have recently shown the capacity to differentiate into several cell types applicable for regenerative medicine (specifically neural cells, using chemicals). Valproic acid was an ideal candidate due to its clinical stability. It has been implicated in the induction of neural differentiation; however, the mechanism and the downstream events were not known. In this study, we showed that using valproic acid on adult mesenchymal stem cells induced neural differentiation within 24 h by upregulating the expression of suppressor of cytokine signaling 5 (SOCS5) and Fibroblast growth factor 21 (FGF21), without increasing the potential death rate of the cells. Through this, the Janus Kinase/Signal Transducer and Activator of Transcription (JAK/STAT) pathway is downregulated, and the mitogen-activated protein kinase (MAPK) cascade is activated. The bioinformatics analyses revealed the expression of several neuro-specific proteins as well as a range of functional and structural proteins involved in the formation and development of the neural cells.

Keywords: adipose derived stem cells; valproic acid; protein interactions; MAPK pathway; JAK/STAT pathway

1. Introduction

Regenerative and translational medicine is a rapidly expanding area made possible by the availability of an abundant source of stem cells, particularly autologous adult mesenchymal stem cells acquired from lipoaspirates termed adipose derived stem cells (ADSCs). The application of autologous ADSCs to neural regeneration and repair therapies is of great interest due to the potential to reverse or limit the exacerbation of injuries that have severe effects on the quality of life while avoiding rejection [1].

Several studies have explored the effect of small molecule chemical inducers on the potential to drive neurogenic differentiation in stem cells. At optimized concentrations and short treatment times, chemicals such as beta-mercaptoethanol (BME) and dimethylsulfoxide (DMSO), have shown the potential to induce a structural and molecular phenotype in stem cells that resemble differentiating neural cells [2,3]. Not surprisingly, these molecules had negative effects inducing a range of stress and apoptotic markers with an increasing treatment time frame. Alternatively, less harsh chemicals with similar actions, such as butylated hydroxyanisole (BHA), retinoic acid (RA) and other chemical derivatives, have also shown a marked capacity for improving neural differentiation while decreasing cellular stress and death [4–7]. Valproic acid (VPA), as a focus molecule, has garnered some attention in neurogenic differentiation research, and was previously explored in certain stem cell types; however, the extent of the differentiation was not completely elucidated [8,9].

Valproic acid (VPA) is a short-chain fatty acid that is well known as a histone deacetylase (HDAC) inhibitor [10]. It is an established drug in epilepsy therapy and can be used clinically as an anticonvulsant and a mood stabilizer [11]. Its proprieties on adult neuron cells are known and its actions on transcription have been previously studied at variable concentrations in vitro [12]. Studies have proven that VPA can affect the proliferation and the differentiation of neural crest progenitors and hippocampal neural stem cells [13]. Furthermore, VPA was shown to increase white matter repair and neurogenesis after a stroke by supporting the survival and new growth of oligodendrocytes, as well as myelination and axonal density [14]. The effect of VPA inducing differentiation in other stem cell types has been studied to a lesser extent.

VPA is minimally cytotoxic and biologically relevant. The induction by VPA of placental mesenchymal stem cells toward neuronal differentiation has been analysed using the criteria of altered cell morphology, reduced proliferation, and the expression of marker genes [13]. VPA treatment for up to ten days induced profound changes in cell morphology, which were characterized by less tightly packed cells within the colonies and the generation of long filamentous structures [8]. VPA has a definite effect on stem cells and induced morphological changes that progressed to a stage of preneuronal-like cell.

Further studies showed that VPA influences the proliferation and differentiation of neuronal cells by expressing a small set of specific markers [15]. However, little is known about the downstream events. The role of VPA in protein expression involved in the cell cycle and neuronal differentiation was also investigated. It was shown that treatment with VPA during the progenitor stages resulted in the strong inhibition of cell proliferation and the induction of neuronal differentiation, accompanied by increases in the expression of pro-neural transcription factors and in neuronal cell numbers [15]. Furthermore, it was previously demonstrated that VPA initiated catecholaminergic neuronal differentiation. VPA launches differentiation mechanisms in sympathoadrenal progenitor cells that result in increased generation of functional neurons [9]. However, the target of VPA on the neuronal differentiation pathways is also largely unknown. A research void exists in the molecular mechanisms that play a role in ADSCs differentiation toward neuronal phenotypes.

Previous studies on how VPA affects the neural differentiation are largely based on the impact of the VPA on the transcription through inhibition of the histone deacetylases (HDACs). This study focuses on the VPA effects on ADSCs as analysed by a proteomics approach, with the aim to compare the effects of the neural induction by VPA to controls and the effects of neurobasal media B27. Media B27 supports the neural differentiation of stem cells [16,17]. Using microscopy analysis, the morphological changes of the ADSCs after induction with VPA may be tracked photographically and at specific chosen time points. The proteomic analysis provides a broader data pool of the global effect of the VPA, not only on the transcription but also directly on the different neural differentiation pathways by inducing critical interactions. Furthermore, investigation of the proteins critical in VPA induction of the cascade pathways such as MAPK/ERK and JAK/STAT may be undertaken. In addition to proteomics, a BioPlex analysis allows for the investigation of the roles of chemokines and cytokines as a complementary analytical technique. This provides more specific information on the secreted cytokines and their role in the induction of differentiation pathways in the cells [18].

2. Methods

2.1. Cell Culture

The procedures of adult human ADSCs isolation and expansion were used from Santos et al. [3] utilising cells that were cryo-stored from UTS-HREC Santos-2013000437. All donor participants volunteered through informed consent for waste lipoaspirate donation as per ethics guidelines and were de-identified for research purposes (Ethical Code: UTS-HREC Santos-2013000437, Committee: University of Technology Sydney (UTS) Human Research Ethics Committee, Date: 02/07/2013). Generally, ADSCs were cultured in T175 (Nunc, ThermoScientific, Carlsbad, CA, USA) in DMEM Glutmax/F12 Gibco, Life Technologies, Carlsbad, CA, USA) with 10% foetal bovine serum (FBS, Gibco, Life Technologies, Carlsbad, CA, USA) incubated at 37 °C at 5% CO_2 ADSCs were passaged three to five times post isolation by stripping the cells with TrypLE Express (12604 Gibco) before being used in differentiation experiments. The cells were seeded on to 6-well plates (Nunc, ThermoScientific, Carlsbad, CA, USA) at approximately 20,000 cells/mL in 5 mL of DMEM Glutmax/F12 with FBS and maintained till 80% prior to commencing chemical induction for differentiation.

2.2. Chemical Induction for Differentiation

Sub-confluent ADSCs were washed twice in pre-warmed sterile DMEM Glutmax/F12 (Invitrogen). The cells were then cultured for a further 24 h in a serum-free pre-induction medium consisting of DMEM/F12 (Invitrogen), and 10% of the final concentration of the added VPA. The media was then replaced after 24 h with the neuronal inducing media consisting of DMEM/F12 (Invitrogen), and the final optimised concentrations of 0.2 mM VPA. The control cells were maintained in DMEM Glutmax/F12 Gibco, Life Technologies, Carlsbad, CA, USA) with 10% foetal bovine serum (FBS, Gibco, Life Technologies, Carlsbad, CA, USA) and a further control of ADSCs in B27 for 24 h was also maintained for further comparative analysis.

2.3. Cell Harvesting Sample Preparation

The cells were harvested for proteomic analysis by liquid chromatography-tandem mass spectrometry (LC-MS/MS), at the selected time points of 0, 3, 6, and 24 h post-treatment, were completed in biological and technical triplicates. Culture media was collected from each well in 2 mL Eppendorf tubes and stored at −80 °C for later Bioplex, alkaline phosphatase, and Reazurin assays. Cells were rinsed twice in 5 mL of 1× phosphate buffered saline (PBS, Merck KGaA, Darmstadt, Germany) for 5 min each at 37 °C and aspirated. Cells were then scraped into 1 mL of 1× PBS using a cell scraper (Sarstedt, Numbrecht, Germany) liberated cells were collected into an Eppendorf tube and centrifuged at 4000× g for 10 min. The supernatant was then discarded, and the cell pellets were stored at −80 °C till processing.

2.4. Alkaline Phosphatase Activity Assay

Alkaline phosphatase (ALP) is widely used as a measure of stem cell proliferative capacity as well as a marker to show pluripotency [19] and a substantial expression increase from basal states is a measure of osteoblastic differentiation [20]. From the collected conditioned media at the chosen time points, 50 µL of media was combined with 50 µL of 4-nitrophenol phosphate (p-NNP), the substrate for the colorimetric assay, and the absorbance was measured at 405 nm and recorded on a Tecan spectrophotometer. As ALP is continuously expressed in dividing stem cells, a relative abundance of secreted ALP can be utilized to determine the cell population proliferation in the presence of cell culture additives. Student's t-test was used for statistical analysis, and p-values less than 0.05 were considered to be significant.

2.5. Cytotoxicity Assay

Similarly, the cytotoxicity assay was completed in triplicate using 100 µL aliquots of the collected conditioned media from the chosen time points combined with 10 µL of Reazurin from the Alamar blue kit and incubated for 2 h at 37 °C in a clear flat bottom 96-well plate. The plate was then scanned on a Tecan spectrophotometer at a measurement wavelength of 575 nm with a 9 nm bandwidth and a reference wavelength scan at 600 nm with a 9 nm bandwidth. Absorbance vs. time graphs were generated to examine the relative cytotoxicity for each time point. Student's t-test was used for statistical analysis, p-values less than 0.05 are considered to be significant.

2.6. Cytokine and Chemokine Bioplex Analysis

Bioplex analysis was performed as per Santos et al. [3] with 500 µL aliquots collected at timepoints and controls as follows: DMEM control, starve, B27 control, 0, 3, 6, and 24 h. The assay was performed with Bioplex human 27-plex (M50-0KCAF0Y Bio-Rad Laboratories, Hercules, CA, USA). The data analysis was completed in DanteR software (DanteR version 1.0.0.10. R version 2.12.0 The R Foundation for Statistical Computing, Auckland, New Zealand) [21].

2.7. Cell Lysate Protein Extraction Sample Preparation

The cell pellets were resuspended in 100 µL 8 M urea (Merck KGaA, Darmstadt, Germany) and 100 mM ammonium bicarbonate (Merck KGaA, Darmstadt, Germany), sonicated for 10 min at 50% power at three 10 s intervals. The samples were then heated to 95 °C on a heat block for 10 min, then centrifuged for 1 min at 5000× g. The solution was then reduced and alkylated by adding a final concentration of 10 mM tributyl-phosphate (TBP, Merck KGaA, Darmstadt, Germany) and 20 mM acrylamide (Merck KGaA, Darmstadt, Germany), then vortexed and spun down on a mini-centrifuge (Qik Spin QS7000 Edwards Instruments) at 2000× g for 2 s. The samples were incubated for 90 min at room temperature then quenched with a final concentration of 50 mM dithiothreitol (DTT, Merck KGaA, Darmstadt, Germany)) and again vortexed and spun down on a mini-centrifuge at 2000× g for 2 s. The samples were then diluted 1:8 in 100 mM ammonium bicarbonate. We then added 0.5 µg of trypsin to digest at 37 °C for a minimum of 12 h. The samples were then desalted using SiliaprepX SCX SPE solid phase extraction columns (Silicycle, Quebec City, Canada). The peptide concentration was determined using the Pierce quantitative colorimetric peptide assay (Thermofisher Scientific, NSW, Australia) and prepared for LC-MS/MS analysis.

2.8. Liquid Chromatography-Tandem Mass Spectrometry

An Acquity M-class nanoLC system (Waters, USA) was used, loading 5 µL of the sample (1 mg) at a rate of 15 mL/min for 3 min onto a nanoEase Symmetry C18 trapping column (180 mm × 20 mm). It was then washed onto a PicoFrit column (75 mm ID × 250 mm; New Objective, Woburn, MA, USA) packed with Magic C18AQ resin (Michrom Bioresources, Auburn, CA, USA). The column was then eluted of peptides into the Q Exactive Plus mass spectrometer (Thermofisher Scientific, NSW, Australia) using the following program: 5%–30% MS buffer B (98% Acetonitrile +0.2% Formic Acid) over 90 min, 30%–80% MS buffer B over 3 min, 80% MS buffer B for 2 min, 80%–5% for 3 min. The peptides that were eluted were ionised at 2000 V. A data dependant MS/MS (dd-MS2) experiment was performed, with a 350–1500 Da survey scan was performed at a resolution of 70,000 m/z for peptides of charge state 2+ or higher with an Automatic Gain Control (AGC) target of 3×10^6 and a 50 ms maximum injection time. The top 12 peptides were selectively fragmented in the Higher-energy collisional dissociation (HCD) cell using a 1.4 m/z isolation window, an AGC target of 1×10^5 and a 100 ms maximum injection time. The fragments were scanned in the Orbitrap analyser at a resolution of 17,500 and the product ion fragment masses were measured over a 120–2000 Da mass range. The mass of the precursor peptide was then excluded for 30 s.

2.9. Mass Spectrometry, Protein Identification and Data Analysis

The MS/MS data files were searched against the Human Proteome Database and against common contaminants using Peaks Studio version 8.5 with the following parameter settings: fixed modifications: none; variable modifications: propionamide, oxidised methionine, deamidated asparagine; enzyme: semi-trypsin; number of allowed missed cleavages: three; peptide mass tolerance: 30 ppm; MS/MS mass tolerance: 0.1 Da; charge states: 2+, 3+, and 4+. The search results were filtered to include peptides with a −log10P score (related to P-value) determined by the false discovery rate (FDR) of less than 1%, where the score indicates that the decoy database search matches were less than 1% of the total matches. Each condition was made up of the biological replicates that were treated at the same time, run in triplicate. Data analysis was completed in Microsoft Excel 365, Peaks version 8.5, DanteR (DanteR version 1.0.0.10. R version 2.12.0 The R Foundation for Statistical Computing, Auckland, New Zealand) [21], Cytoscape (version 3.7.1, Cytoscape Consortium, Seattle, WA, USA) [22].

3. Results

3.1. Live Cell Temporal Microscopy during Neurogenic Induction Differentiation of Human ADSCs

Live cell microscopy is a vital procedure to track cellular morphologies over time during differentiation. The physical attributes in the cell shape and formation of substructures on cells can specify the health status and stage of differentiation relative to the treatment [23]. The ADSC control (Figure 1A) shows non-induced cells at passage 3 at 0 h with a typical morphology and diffuse growth with wide cell bodies. Figure 1B–D shows the same field of view through time points 3, 6, and 24 h, respectively, displaying the temporal changes occurring in the identical field of view. The treatment with VPA induced morphological and phenotypical changes in the ADSCs resembling differentiating or pre-neural cells. Generally, over time, the cells structural rearrangement shows an adopted bipolar stretched out shape displaying a condensed cell membrane around the nuclear region within the first 3 h. Furthermore, the appearance of dendrite-like structures is also increasingly more apparent from the 6 h time point and are marked with arrows.

By 24 h, the majority of the cells now display signs of morphological shifts from the control, with a large majority of cells displaying uniform structural changes producing long-extensions between cells and neurite-like outgrowth on some cells. The cell population has remained relatively unchanged across all time points compared to the control, as shown in the average cell counts in Figure 1E. This indicates that minimal to no damage or death due to stress and apoptosis is present in the treated cells.

Supporting the observation of minimal to no damage or death are the graphs in Figure 2 displaying alkaline phosphatase activity on y-axis Figure 2A and Reazurin cytotoxicity assay on y-Figure 2B. The ALP column graphs show that the ALP activity decreases marginally in the serum starved cells and for the post VPA treated cells, the similar expression range of ALP confirms the cells are not experiencing osteogenic differentiation secretion levels and that the ALP secretion is maintained within basal levels. The Reazurin cytotoxicity assay line graph shows that the levels at 3 h post treatment are similar to the pre-treatment values. The stress is marginally increased at 6 and 24 h however this is lower than the ADSC media change at 24 h, confirming that the VPA treatment has a minimal stress and cytotoxic effect on ADSCs at the treated concentrations relative to controls. Student's t-test analysis revealed no significant change in cell numbers.

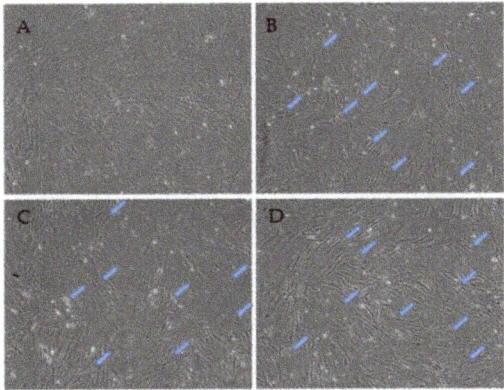

Figure 1. *Cont.*

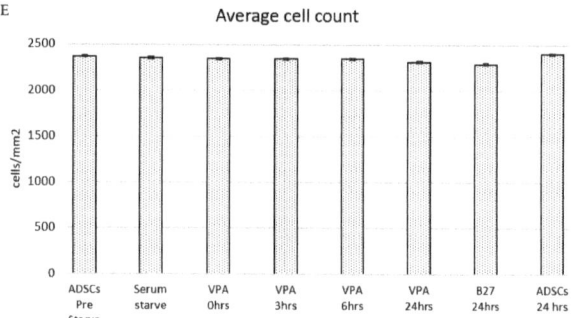

Figure 1. Live cell images of the temporal differentiation of human adipose derived stem cells (ADSCs) induced with 0.2 mM valproic acid (VPA) at (**A**) 0 h, (**B**) 3 h, (**C**) 6 h, and (**D**) 24 h at 10× magnification. The cellular morphology changes rapidly through the time points, with cells adopting a more slender and bipolar orientation with neurite extensions (arrows). (**E**) Average cell count across the treatments including all controls with standard error bars. Relatively minimal changes in numbers are shown across all treatments. A Student's t-test revealed no significant change in cell numbers.

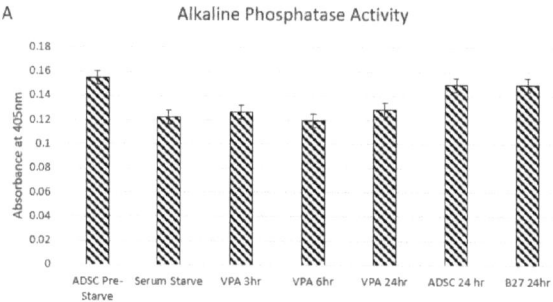

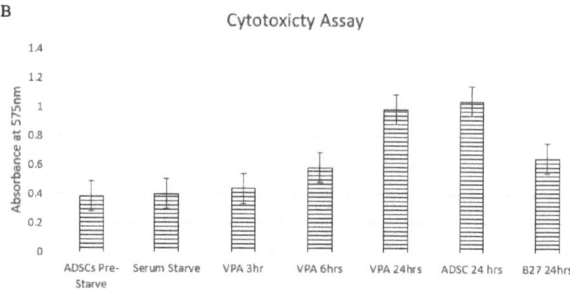

Figure 2. (**A**) shows the alkaline phosphatase (ALP) activity of cells in each treatment over time. ALP activity decreases marginally after serum starve and remains at relative levels through the treatment time points with standard error bars. There was no significant change seen in the t-test of data. (**B**) shows the cytotoxicity assay over time as cellular stress was detected by the Reazurin level with standard error bars. Early treatment time points are equivalent to the pre-starved ADSCs prior to treatment. The levels increase from 6 h and 24 h; however, they remain below ADSCs control at 24 h and B27 control at 24 h post media change. There is no statistical significance determined by the t-test.

3.2. Cytokine and Chemokine Bioplex Analysis

Cytokines and chemokines are multifunctional molecules with a plethora of roles based on their cellular location. Briefly, some of their roles include, pro-inflammation, anti-inflammation, intracellular signalling, intercellular signalling, response to external stimuli, induction or response to protein cascades, and response or guidance of differentiation in cells. Their importance in stem cell differentiation and their response to external stimulation is paramount to clarifying their role in response to VPA. To investigate the relative quantitative changes in the expression and secretion of cytokines and chemokines, the Bioplex multiplex immunoassay was used to simultaneously quantify the molecules in each sample collected from controls and VPA induced time points at 0, 3, 6, and 24 h (Figure 3). The molecules measured were Eotaxin, Granulocyte-colony stimulating factor (G-CSF), Interferon gamma (IFN-γ), Interleukin IL-1β, IL-1ra, IL-2, IL-4, IL-6, IL-7, IL-8, IL-10, IL-12 (p70), IL-13, IL-15, Interferon gamma-induced protein 10 (IP-10), Monocyte Chemoattractant Protein-1 (MCP-1), Macrophage Inflammatory Proteins1 alpha (MIP-1α), MIP-1β, Tumor necrosis factor alpha (TNF-α) and Vascular endothelial growth factor (VEGF). From the 3 h time point post VPA treatment of the ADSCs, there were lower concentrations of all measured molecules with no expression levels of IP-10 and MIP-1b detected through any successive time points. While most of the other molecules regain some cumulative presence post VPA treatment; IL-1β, IL-6, and TNF-α demonstrate a marked decrease in levels below the non-treated samples and remain low through all time points with relatively closer levels to the B27 treated cells.

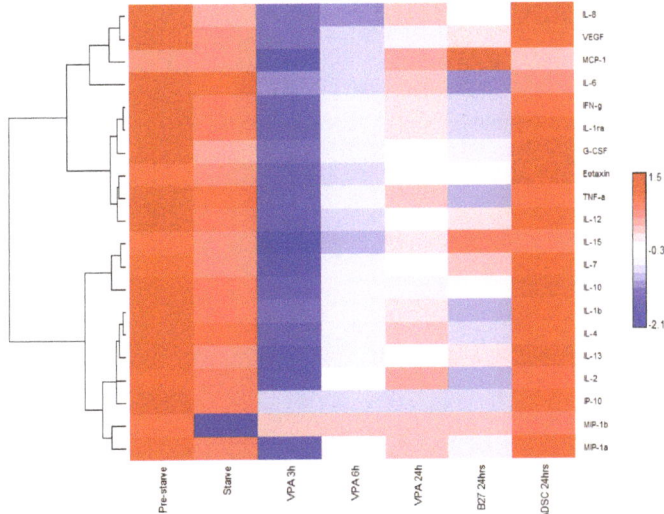

Figure 3. A Bioplex heat map of the log10 measure of cytokines and interleukins expressed in ADSCs in control DMEM media pre FBS starved; starved and in DMEM after 24 h or treated with B27 or VPA over time. Hierarchical clustering software and a Euclidean test. Red: expression above median; Blue: expression below the median; White: median expression across sample.

3.3. Proteome Comparisons of VPA Treated Cells

Each cell treatment was conducted in biological duplicates of tissue cultures. Subsequently, each sample was analysed in technical triplicates by mass spectrometry. This allowed for up to six analysis points for each treatment. This was completed for an increased stringency identification and analysis. Mass spectrometry data compilation (Table 1) identified, at the 95% confidence cutoff, 2067 unique proteins matched from 20,011 distinct peptides derived from a 344,510 total spectra count (Table 1). There was an average of 2.51 peptides matched per protein with an average of 10% sequence coverage. Proteins were removed from the analysis if they were identified by less than two quantifiable peptides per protein. The proteins analyzed were uniquely detected per time point or expressed successively through two or more treatment time points.

Table 1. The number of proteins and peptides identified after liquid chromatography-tandem mass spectrometry analysis of ADSCs and ADSCs treated with VPA.

Confidence Cut-off	Proteins Detected	Proteins Before Grouping	Distinct Peptides	Spectra Identified	%Total Spectra
>2.0 (99)	622	765	8286	313,119	66.8
>1.3 (95)	2067	2269	20,011	344,510	67.7
>0.47 (66)	2334	2460	34,492	406,322	68.5

Interaction network analysis (Figure 4A) using the Cytoscape overlays, the 0, 3, 6 and 24 h VPA treatment time points combining duplicates and removing proteins with less than two peptides, and post colour-coding for unique and shared proteins, the network displays 1256 proteins with 12,771 interactions. This was completed to locate the date interaction hubs between time points and to visualize the protein pathways. In Figure 4A, the nodes are Blue—ADSC unique, Violet-occurs in two or more time points, Red—3 h unique expression, Orange—6 h unique expression, and Green—24 h unique expression. The Venn diagram breakdown (Figure 4B) displays the number of proteins that are unique and shared between each time point as well as percentage of total proteins analysed in the network. The proteins expressed in the ADSC VPA treated time points overlap with only the VPA treated ADSCs total to 3 h—221 proteins, 6 h—200 proteins, and 24 h—243 proteins. The gene ontology analysis of the proteins expressed in the VPA treated ADSCs is graphed in Figure 4C. There are 150 proteins involved across several biological process ontologies aligned with neuron and axon development, projection, differentiation, and cell body morphogenesis.

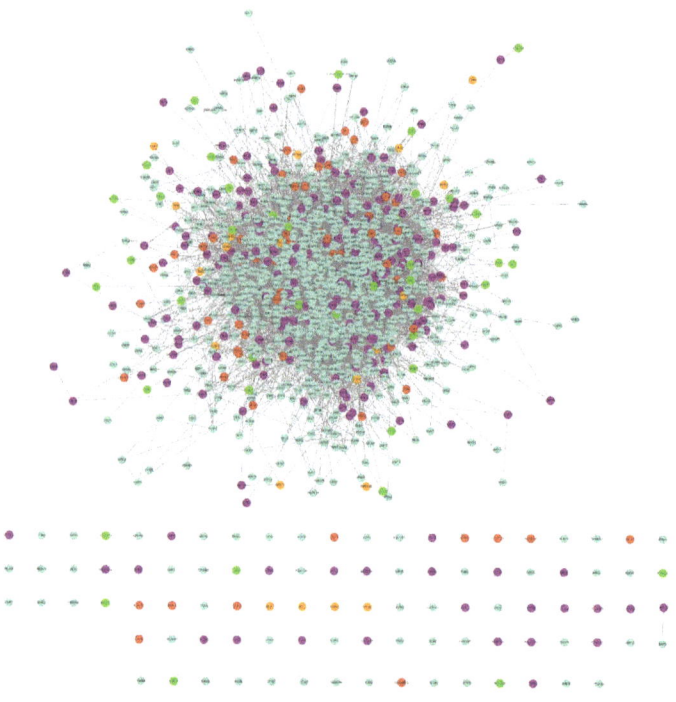

Figure 4. *Cont.*

B

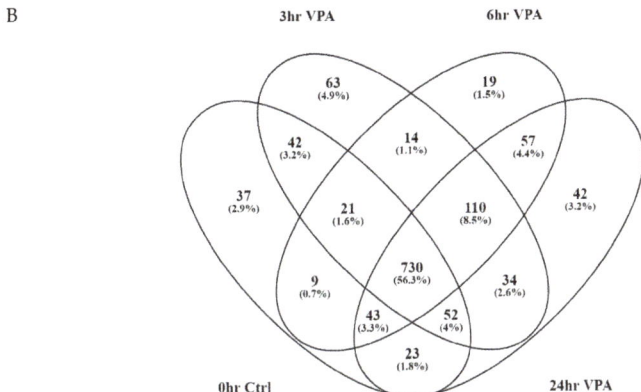

C

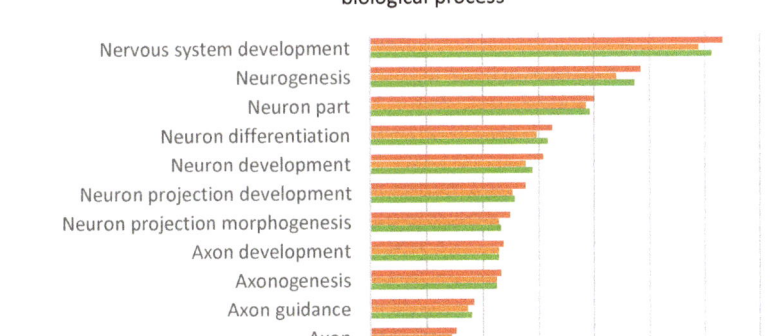

Figure 4. (**A**) Cytoscape protein interaction network graph of proteins identified by mass spectrometry. Blue—ADSC unique, Violet—occurs in two or more time points, Red—3 h unique expression, Orange—6 h unique expression, and Green—24 h unique expression. (**B**) Venn diagram displays breakdown of protein numbers unique and shared between time points. (**C**) Gene ontology biological process analysis of the proteins expressed in Red—3 h, Orange—6 h, and Green—24 h shows a high percentage of proteins linked to neural, neuron, or axon development.

3.4. Pathway Analysis of Gene Ontology Clustered Proteins

The above-mentioned neural-related proteins identified in gene ontology biological process categories were analysed in ClueGO (version 2.5.4) for group clustering and interaction pathway process analysis (Figure 5). Graphing only the neural-related proteins allowed for a concise interaction map of the probable roles played in the differentiated process as well as links in the signalling pathways. Table 2 breaks down the gene ontology type, number of proteins identified in this dataset as well as the GO term *p*-value Bonferroni step down to validate multiple pair wise tests.

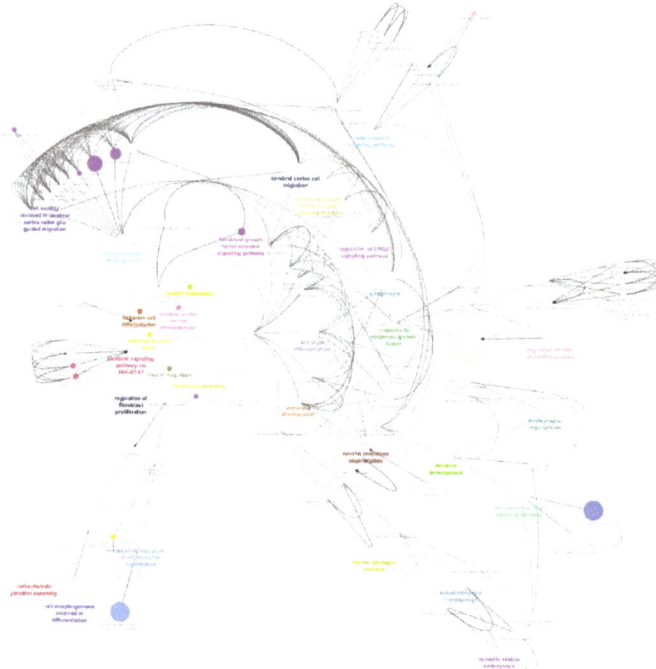

Figure 5. The ClueGo analysis of clustered proteins within each GO node for biological process interaction and signalling pathway analysis involved in the VPA treated cells. Node sizes are relative to number of proteins in dataset identified in that GO. Coloured nodes and labels represent important GO terms in the network.

Figure 6 is a reductive schematic derived from the previous ClueGO graph; it presents the proposed key proteins (summarized in Table 3) and possible summary pathway involved in VPA's action in directing signalling and differentiation in the treated ADSCs. VPA is known to be an HDAC inhibitor, by this direct interaction, HDAC secondary interaction with H1 and H2A is closed. These two proteins have further downstream affects in regulating the RAS/ERK and JAK/STAT pathway via EGRF signalling. By closing this loop, the FGF signalling pathway is upregulated by direct and indirect interactions of VPA which promote the MAPK1 expression and activity. This is a gateway control for initiating the MAPK pathway, which is involved in several neural differentiation lineages. VPA also has an activity in oxidative stress which also acts as a dualistic interaction hub for MAPK pathway promotion.

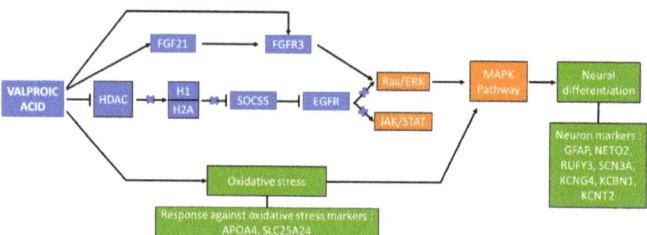

Figure 6. Reductive schematic of the proposed VPA induction pathway in the treatment of ADSCs toward neural differentiation.

Table 2. The gene ontology of proteins associated in the neural-related ClueGO interaction and signalling network map.

GO Term	GO:ID	Number of Proteins	Associated Proteins Found	Percentage of Associated Proteins in GO	Term P-Value
organelle transport along microtubule	GO:0072384	5	[CDC42, LAMP1, SUN1, SYNE2, UCHL1]	4.72	9.03×10^{-3}
regulation of NMDA receptor activity	GO:2000310	3	[DLG1, HSPA8, MAPK1]	5.56	2.70×10^{-2}
response to fibroblast growth factor	GO:0071774	9	[CCN2, FGF21, FGF3, FGFR3, MAPK1, POSTN, PTPN11, TFAP2C, THBS1]	4.95	3.59×10^{-4}
membrane assembly	GO:0071709	6	[ANXA2, CAV1, FLOT1, MAPK1, PDCD6IP, SPTBN1]	11.54	3.57×10^{-5}
cell-substrate junction assembly	GO:0007044	14	[BMX, CTTN, FN1, FYN, LAMB2, LRP1, PLEC, PPM1F, PTPRK, RAC1, RHOA, ROCK1, THBS1, THY1]	10.22	1.08×10^{-9}
transforming growth factor beta production	GO:0071604	3	[ITGAV, MTCO2P12, THBS1]	5.88	2.32×10^{-2}
regulation of myelination	GO:0031641	3	[DLG1, SOS1, TYMP]	6.12	2.09×10^{-2}
positive regulation of cell projection organization	GO:0031346	24	[AP2A1, ARPC2, BMX, CDC42, DDX21, FN1, FSCN1, FYN, HSPA5, HSPA8, ITGA3, KDM1A, LAP3, LRP1, NME2, PDCD6IP, PICALM, PSEN1, RAB21, RAC1, RHOA, SCARB2, SOS1, TMEM30A]	4.60	1.90×10^{-8}
cellular response to nerve growth factor stimulus	GO:1990090	3	[ARF6, HSPA5, PDCD6IP]	4.05	5.94×10^{-2}
cellular response to epidermal growth factor stimulus	GO:0071364	5	[EGFR, GSTP1, PDCD6IP, PTPN11, TFAP2C]	6.33	2.60×10^{-3}
neuron projection regeneration	GO:0031102	5	[GFAP, LAMB2, LRP1, SOS1, THY1]	6.94	1.73×10^{-3}
action potential	GO:0001508	8	[CACNB3, CAMK2D, CAV1, DLG1, KCNB1, MYH14, SCN2A, SCN3A]	4.68	1.09×10^{-3}
regulation of receptor signalling pathway via STAT	GO:1904892	8	[CAV1, FGFR3, FYN, HGS, IL3, JAK3, KLK3, TFRC]	4.26	1.99×10^{-3}
neurotransmitter uptake	GO:0001504	3	[FLOT1, GFAP, PSEN1]	4.92	3.69×10^{-2}

Table 2. Cont.

GO Term	GO:ID	Number of Proteins	Associated Proteins Found	Percentage of Associated Proteins in GO	Term P-Value
cellular response to fibroblast growth factor stimulus	GO:0044344	9	[CCN2, FGF21, FGF3, FGFR3, MAPK1, POSTN, PTPN11, TFAP2C, THBS1]	5.26	2.26×10^{-4}
cellular response to amyloid-beta	GO:1904646	5	[FYN, ICAM1, LRP1, PARP1, PSEN1]	8.77	5.98×10^{-4}
midbrain development	GO:0030901	8	[ACTB, CALM2, CDC42, HSPA5, PICALM, POTEF, RHOA, SOS1]	6.15	1.75×10^{-4}
response to epidermal growth factor	GO:0070849	6	[EGFR, GSTP1, MAPK1, PDCD6IP, PTPN11, TFAP2C]	7.14	5.19×10^{-4}
regulation of neuron projection regeneration	GO:0070570	3	[LRP1, SOS1, THY1]	7.14	1.39×10^{-2}
regulation of axon extension	GO:0030516	5	[CTTN, FN1, LRP1, RAB21, RTN4]	4.46	1.13×10^{-2}
negative regulation of ERK1 and ERK2 cascade	GO:0070373	6	[DLG1, EIF3A, GSTP1, MAPK1, PDCD6IP, TIMP3]	6.19	1.11×10^{-3}
negative regulation of neuron apoptotic process	GO:0043524	8	[BAX, FYN, LRP1, MSH2, PSEN1, RHOA, ROCK1, TFRC]	4.04	2.74×10^{-3}
regulation of ERK1 and ERK2 cascade	GO:0070372	18	[CCN2, DLG1, EGFR, EIF3A, FGF21, FGFR3, FN1, GNAI2, GSTP1, ICAM1, LRP1, MAPK1, MIF, PDCD6IP, PPP3CA, PTPN11, TFRC, TIMP3]	4.46	1.94×10^{-6}
regulation of neuron apoptotic process	GO:0043523	11	[BAX, FYN, KCNB1, LRP1, MSH2, PARP1, PCSK9, PSEN1, RHOA, ROCK1, TFRC]	4.03	4.76×10^{-4}
ERK1 and ERK2 cascade	GO:0070371	20	[CCN2, DLG1, EGFR, EIF3A, FGF21, FGFR3, FN1, GNAI2, GSTP1, ICAM1, ITGAV, LRP1, MAPK1, MIF, PDCD6IP, PPP3CA, PTPN11, TFAP2C, TFRC, TIMP3]	4.56	3.60×10^{-7}
glial cell activation	GO:0061900	3	[EGFR, LRP1, PSEN1]	4.62	4.32×10^{-2}
telencephalon glial cell migration	GO:0022030	4	[PDCD6IP, RTN4, SUN1, SYNE2]	9.30	1.72×10^{-3}
telencephalon cell migration	GO:0022029	7	[EGFR, PDCD6IP, PSEN1, RHOA, RTN4, SUN1, SYNE2]	7.69	1.12×10^{-4}

Table 2. Cont.

GO Term	GO:ID	Number of Proteins	Associated Proteins Found	Percentage of Associated Proteins in GO	Term P-Value
cerebral cortex development	GO:0021987	11	[ATIC, BAX, EGFR, KDM1A, LRP1, PDCD6IP, PSEN1, RHOA, RTN4, SUN1, SYNE2]	6.63	5.33×10^{-6}
cerebral cortex neuron differentiation	GO:0021895	3	[HPRT1, NCOA3, PSEN1]	7.89	1.05×10^{-2}
forebrain cell migration	GO:0021885	7	[EGFR, PDCD6IP, PSEN1, RHOA, RTN4, SUN1, SYNE2]	7.45	1.37×10^{-4}
cell morphogenesis involved in differentiation	GO:0000904	37	[ARPC2, BMX, CALM2, CAMK2A, CDC42, CTTN, FAM129B, FLOT1, FN1, FYN, GRB7, HPRT1, HSP90AA1, ITGAV, KRT7, LAMB2, LRP1, MAPK1, MYH9, NCOA3, PICALM, POSTN, PPP3CA, PSEN1, PTPN11, RAB21, RAC1, RB1, RHOA, ROCK1, RTN4, SOS1, SPTBN1, THY1, TUBB3, UCHL1, VAMP3]	4.03	7.39×10^{-11}
cell motility involved in cerebral cortex radial glia guided migration	GO:0021814	3	[PDCD6IP, SUN1, SYNE2]	18.75	8.49×10^{-4}
cerebral cortex radial glia guided migration	GO:0021801	4	[PDCD6IP, RTN4, SUN1, SYNE2]	9.30	1.72×10^{-3}
cerebral cortex radially oriented cell migration	GO:0021799	4	[PDCD6IP, RTN4, SUN1, SYNE2]	7.84	3.24×10^{-3}
cerebral cortex cell migration	GO:0021795	7	[EGFR, PDCD6IP, PSEN1, RHOA, RTN4, SUN1, SYNE2]	9.46	2.95×10^{-5}
glial cell development	GO:0021782	7	[EGFR, GFAP, GSTP1, LAMB2, LRP1, PSEN1, VTA1]	4.67	2.25×10^{-3}
dendritic spine development	GO:0060996	6	[ARF4, ARF6, CAMK2A, CDC42, MAPK1, PSEN1]	4.58	5.02×10^{-3}
substantia nigra development	GO:0021762	7	[ACTB, CALM2, CDC42, HSPA5, PICALM, POTEF, RHOA]	10.45	1.53×10^{-5}
pallium development	GO:0021543	13	[ALK, ATIC, ATP2B4, BAX, EGFR, KDM1A, LRP1, PDCD6IP, PSEN1, RHOA, RTN4, SUN1, SYNE2]	5.31	8.59×10^{-6}
telencephalon development	GO:0021537	15	[ALK, ATIC, ATP2B4, BAX, EGFR, HPRT1, KDM1A, LRP1, MAPK1, PDCD6IP, PSEN1, RHOA, RTN4, SUN1, SYNE2]	4.34	1.97×10^{-5}

Table 2. Cont.

GO Term	GO:ID	Number of Proteins	Associated Proteins Found	Percentage of Associated Proteins in GO	Term P-Value
epidermal growth factor-activated receptor activity	GO:0005006	4	[EFEMP1, EGFR, PSEN1, SOCS5]	9.76	1.44×10^{-3}
NMDA glutamate receptor activity	GO:0004972	3	[DLG1, HSPA8, MAPK1]	5.26	3.10×10^{-2}
neuron maturation	GO:0042551	3	[KDM1A, NCOA3, RB1]	4.41	4.83×10^{-2}
ionotropic glutamate receptor activity	GO:0004970	4	[DLG1, HSPA8, MAPK1, NETO2]	4.44	2.31×10^{-2}
activation of MAPKK activity	GO:0000186	5	[EGFR, MAPK1, PDCD6IP, PSEN1, TFRC]	4.63	9.75×10^{-3}
MAP kinase kinase activity	GO:0004708	5	[EGFR, MAPK1, PDCD6IP, PSEN1, TFRC]	4.03	1.69×10^{-2}
Wnt signalling pathway, planar cell polarity pathway	GO:0060071	11	[AP2A1, AP2A2, AP2B1, CDC42, PDCD6IP, PSMA1, PSMA3, PSMB9, PSMD4, RAC1, RHOA]	8.09	7.54×10^{-7}
Bergmann glial cell differentiation	GO:0060020	3	[GFAP, MAPK1, PTPN11]	33.33	1.36×10^{-4}
dendrite development	GO:0016358	14	[ARF4, ARF6, CALM2, CAMK2A, CDC42, FYN, HPRT1, MAPK1, PDCD6IP, PICALM, PPP3CA, PSEN1, RAB21, RHOA]	4.52	2.39×10^{-5}
neural retina development	GO:0003407	3	[ATP2B4, PSEN1, THY1]	4.05	5.94×10^{-2}
neurotransmitter biosynthetic process	GO:0042136	6	[ATP2B4, CAV1, HSP90AA1, ICAM1, MTCO2P12, RAC1]	4.84	3.84×10^{-3}
Wnt signalling pathway	GO:0016055	25	[AP2A1, AP2A2, AP2B1, CALM2, CAMK2A, CAV1, CDC42, CHD8, CTNND1, EGFR, G3BP1, ITGA3, LRP1, PDCD6IP, PICALM, PLCB3, PPP3CA, PRKAA1, PSEN1, PSMA1, PSMA3, PSMB9, PSMD4, RAC1, RHOA]	4.05	1.10×10^{-7}
gliogenesis	GO:0042063	18	[ANXA1, EGFR, GFAP, GSTP1, KRT7, LAMB2, LRP1, MAPK1, PDCD6IP, PSEN1, PSMD4, PTPN11, RELA, RHOA, RTN4, SUN1, SYNE2, VTA1]	4.81	6.45×10^{-7}

Table 2. Cont.

GO Term	GO:ID	Number of Proteins	Associated Proteins Found	Percentage of Associated Proteins in GO	Term P-Value
regulation of epidermal growth factor receptor signalling pathway	GO:0042058	9	[CDC42, EGFR, EPN1, HGS, PDCD6IP, PSEN1, RAB7A, SOCS5, SOS1]	7.63	1.26×10^{-5}
neurotrophin signalling pathway	GO:0038179	4	[CTNND1, PDCD6IP, PTPN11, SOS1]	6.45	6.53×10^{-3}
ERBB2 signalling pathway	GO:0038128	4	[EGFR, GRB7, HSP90AA1, SOS1]	9.52	1.58×10^{-3}
regulation of neurotransmitter uptake	GO:0051580	3	[FLOT1, GFAP, PSEN1]	12.50	2.86×10^{-3}
p38MAPK cascade	GO:0038066	4	[DLG1, PDCD6IP, SOS1, TFAP2C]	6.56	6.16×10^{-3}
neuron apoptotic process	GO:0051402	14	[BAX, FYN, HSPA5, KCNB1, LRP1, MSH2, PARP1, PCSK9, PSEN1, RB1, RHOA, ROCK1, SCN2A, TFRC]	4.50	2.47×10^{-5}
positive regulation of neuron death	GO:1901216	7	[BAX, CALM2, FYN, PARP1, PCSK9, PICALM, RHOA]	5.98	5.27×10^{-4}
Schwann cell differentiation	GO:0014037	3	[LAMB2, RELA, VTA1]	6.00	2.21×10^{-2}
astrocyte development	GO:0014002	5	[EGFR, GFAP, LAMB2, LRP1, PSEN1]	8.33	7.58×10^{-4}
regulation of ERBB signalling pathway	GO:1901184	10	[CDC42, EGFR, EPN1, HGS, PDCD6IP, PSEN1, RAB7A, RTN4, SOCS5, SOS1]	7.87	3.09×10^{-6}
negative regulation of neuron projection development	GO:0010977	9	[ARF6, GFAP, LRP1, MAPK1, PPP3CA, PSEN1, RHOA, RTN4, THY1]	4.59	6.15×10^{-4}
positive regulation of neuron projection development	GO:0010976	18	[AP2A1, BMX, DDX21, FN1, FYN, HSPA5, HSPA8, ITGA3, KDM1A, LRP1, NME2, PDCD6IP, PSEN1, RAB21, RHOA, SCARB2, SOS1, TMEM30A]	4.75	7.81×10^{-7}
regulation of p38MAPK cascade	GO:1900744	3	[DLG1, PDCD6IP, SOS1]	6.00	2.21×10^{-2}
regulation of glutamate receptor signalling pathway	GO:1900449	5	[DLG1, FYN, HSPA8, MAPK1, NETO2]	5.49	4.79×10^{-3}

Table 2. Cont.

GO Term	GO:ID	Number of Proteins	Associated Proteins Found	Percentage of Associated Proteins in GO	Term P-Value
non-canonical Wnt signalling pathway	GO:0035567	16	[AP2A1, AP2A2, AP2B1, CALM2, CAMK2A, CDC42, PDCD6IP, PICALM, PLCB3, PPP3CA, PSMA1, PSMA3, PSMB9, PSMD4, RAC1, RHOA]	8.56	9.57×10^{-10}
negative regulation of cell morphogenesis involved in differentiation	GO:0010771	7	[MAPK1, POSTN, PPP3CA, PSEN1, RHOA, RTN4, THY1]	5.69	7.11×10^{-4}
positive regulation of cell morphogenesis involved in differentiation	GO:0010770	8	[ARPC2, CDC42, FN1, LRP1, NCOA3, RAB21, RAC1, RHOA]	4.12	2.41×10^{-3}
negative regulation of axonogenesis	GO:0050771	5	[MAPK1, PSEN1, RHOA, RTN4, THY1]	5.32	5.49×10^{-3}
positive regulation of plasma membrane bounded cell projection assembly	GO:0120034	7	[ARPC2, CDC42, FN1, FSCN1, LAP3, PICALM, RAC1]	4.64	2.33×10^{-3}
neuron projection fasciculation	GO:0106030	3	[BMX, MAPK1, RTN4]	8.57	8.40×10^{-3}
neuron projection organization	GO:0106027	6	[CDC42, CTTN, FYN, ITGA3, MAPK1, PSEN1]	4.62	4.84×10^{-3}
neural nucleus development	GO:0048857	7	[ACTB, CALM2, CDC42, HSPA5, PICALM, POTEF, RHOA]	7.69	1.12×10^{-4}
regulation of neurotransmitter receptor activity	GO:0099601	5	[ATXN2, DLG1, HSPA8, MAPK1, NETO2]	4.72	9.03×10^{-3}
dendrite morphogenesis	GO:0048813	9	[CALM2, CAMK2A, CDC42, FYN, HPRT1, MAPK1, PICALM, PPP3CA, RAB21]	4.48	7.36×10^{-4}
postsynapse organization	GO:0099173	12	[ACTB, ARF4, ARF6, CDC42, CTTN, DLG1, FYN, ITGA3, MAPK1, PDCD6IP, POTEF, VTA1]	5.22	2.26×10^{-5}
astrocyte differentiation	GO:0048708	8	[EGFR, GFAP, KRT7, LAMB2, LRP1, MAPK1, PSEN1, PTPN11]	7.27	5.41×10^{-5}

Table 2. Cont.

GO Term	GO:ID	Number of Proteins	Associated Proteins Found	Percentage of Associated Proteins in GO	Term P-Value
regulation of postsynaptic membrane neurotransmitter receptor levels	GO:0099072	5	[AP2B1, CTNND1, DLG1, HSP90AA1, HSPA8]	5.56	4.57×10^{-3}
response to axon injury	GO:0048678	5	[ARF4, BAX, GNAI2, LAMB2, LRP1]	5.15	9.03×10^{-3}
axon extension	GO:0048675	7	[CTTN, FN1, HSP90AA1, LAMB2, LRP1, RAB21, RTN4]	4.70	2.70×10^{-2}
regulation of action potential	GO:0098900	5	[CACNB3, CAMK2D, CAV1, DLG1, KCNB1]	7.04	3.59×10^{-4}
thymus development	GO:0048538	3	[MAPK1, PRKDC, PSEN1]	4.92	3.57×10^{-5}
synaptic vesicle endocytosis	GO:0048488	6	[ACTB, ARF6, CALM2, PICALM, POTEF, ROCK1]	8.33	1.08×10^{-9}
glial cell differentiation	GO:0010001	13	[EGFR, GFAP, GSTP1, KRT7, LAMB2, LRP1, MAPK1, PSEN1, PSMD4, PTPN11, RELA, RHOA, VTA1]	4.74	2.32×10^{-2}
regulation of fibroblast proliferation	GO:0048145	10	[ANXA2, BAX, EGFR, FN1, GSTP1, MIF, PDCD6IP, PML, PPP3CA, PRKDC]	8.06	2.09×10^{-2}
receptor signalling pathway via STAT	GO:0097696	10	[CAV1, FGFR3, FYN, HGS, IL3, JAK3, KLK3, SOCS5, STAT1, TFRC]	4.67	1.90×10^{-8}
astrocyte activation	GO:0048143	3	[EGFR, LRP1, PSEN1]	9.38	5.94×10^{-2}
calcium ion transmembrane import into cytosol	GO:0097553	9	[ATP2B4, BAX, CALM2, CAMK2D, FYN, PICALM, PLCB3, TFRC, THY1]	4.46	2.60×10^{-3}
neurotrophin TRK receptor signalling pathway	GO:0048011	3	[CTNND1, PTPN11, SOS1]	6.38	1.73×10^{-3}
dendritic spine organization	GO:0097061	5	[CDC42, CTTN, FYN, ITGA3, MAPK1]	4.39	1.09×10^{-3}
fibroblast growth factor receptor signalling pathway	GO:0008543	8	[CCN2, FGF21, FGF3, FGFR3, MAPK1, POSTN, PTPN11, THBS1]	6.15	1.99×10^{-3}
glial cell migration	GO:0008347	5	[LRP1, PDCD6IP, RTN4, SUN1, SYNE2]	6.58	3.69×10^{-2}
regulation of receptor signalling pathway via JAK-STAT	GO:0046425	8	[CAV1, FGFR3, FYN, HGS, IL3, JAK3, KLK3, TFRC]	4.37	2.26×10^{-4}
neuron recognition	GO:0008038	3	[BMX, MAPK1, RTN4]	4.55	5.98×10^{-4}

Table 2. Cont.

GO Term	GO:ID	Number of Proteins	Associated Proteins Found	Percentage of Associated Proteins in GO	Term P-Value
neuron migration	GO:0001764	9	[BAX, CAMK2A, ELP3, FYN, ITGA3, NAV1, PDCD6IP, PSEN1, RAC1]	4.39	1.75×10^{-4}
endoderm development	GO:0007492	5	[BPTF, FN1, ITGAV, LAMB2, TFAP2C]	5.62	5.19×10^{-4}
axonal fasciculation	GO:0007413	3	[BMX, MAPK1, RTN4]	8.57	1.39×10^{-2}
axonogenesis	GO:0007409	24	[BMX, CALM2, CTTN, FAM129B, FLOT1, FN1, FYN, GRB7, HSP90AA1, LAMB2, LRP1, MAPK1, PICALM, PSEN1, PTPN11, RAB21, RAC1, RHOA, RTN4, SOS1, SPTBN1, THY1, TUBB3, UCHL1]	4.05	1.13×10^{-2}
tyrosine phosphorylation of STAT protein	GO:0007260	5	[CAV1, FGFR3, FYN, IL3, JAK3]	4.72	1.11×10^{-3}
receptor signalling pathway via JAK-STAT	GO:0007259	10	[CAV1, FGFR3, FYN, HGS, IL3, JAK3, KLK3, SOCS5, STAT1, TFRC]	4.81	2.74×10^{-3}
Wnt signalling pathway, calcium modulating pathway	GO:0007223	5	[CALM2, CAMK2A, PICALM, PLCB3, PPP3CA]	9.80	1.94×10^{-6}
glutamate receptor signalling pathway	GO:0007215	6	[DLG1, FYN, HSPA8, KCNB1, MAPK1, NETO2]	4.62	4.76×10^{-4}
epidermal growth factor receptor signalling pathway	GO:0007173	15	[ARF4, CDC42, CTNND1, EFEMP1, EGFR, EPN1, GRB7, HGS, HSP90AA1, PDCD6IP, PSEN1, PTPN11, RAB7A, SOCS5, SOS1]	9.20	3.60×10^{-7}

Table 3. Proteins involved in the proposed VPA induction pathway of neural differentiation of ADSCs.

Protein Name	Gene	Accession Numbers	Molecular Weight (Da)	Identification Probability	Gene Ontology
Signal transducer and activator of transcription 1-alpha/beta	STAT1	P42224	87,336.90	100%	GO:0007259
Calcium-binding mitochondrial carrier protein SCaMC-1	SLC25A24	Q6NUK1-2	53,356.60	92.60%	GO:0034599
Fibroblast growth factor 21	FGF21	Q9NSA1	22,300.60	92.50%	GO:0090080
Advillin	AVIL	O75366-2	92,029.10	92.20%	GO:0007399
Potassium channel subfamily T member 2	KCNT2	Q6UVM3-2, Q6UVM3-3	130,506.30	89.50%	GO:0005249
Mitogen-activated protein kinase 1	MAPK1	P28482-2	41,391.90	86.90%	GO:0000165
Neuropilin and tolloid-like protein 2	NETO2	Q8NC67-3	59,393.90	85.80%	GO:2000312
Tyrosine-protein kinase JAK3	JAK3	P52333-2	125,101.70	81.90%	GO:0046425
Sodium/calcium exchanger 3	SLC8A3	P57103-2, P57103-6, P57103-7	103,011.70	77.90%	GO:0060291
Signal transducer and activator of transcription 6	STAT6	P42226	94,136.90	59.90%	GO:0019221
Glial fibrillary acidic protein	GFAP	P14136-2, P14136-3	49,881.40	35.40%	GO:0031102
Potassium voltage-gated channel subfamily B member 1	KCNB1	Q14721	95,881.40	14.40%	GO:1900454
Potassium voltage-gated channel subfamily G member 4	KCNG4	Q8TDN1	58,981.00	11.80%	GO:0005251
Fibroblast growth factor receptor 3	FGFR3	P22607-2	877,100.00	6.20%	GO:0043410

4. Discussion

The variety of neural related applications of Valproic acid, including its use as an anticonvulsant to use in treating disorders, such as epilepsy, bipolar, Schizophrenia, Parkinson's, and stroke, holds significant value in its role in directing in vivo neural cell modulation and repair. In vitro studies have observed a VPA effect on several factors in molecular responses of stem cells treated with the chemical, indicating shifts toward neural-like outgrowth with the expression of specific markers and morphological ques associated with differentiation. In this study we aimed to observe and measure the effect of VPA on the wide changes over chosen time points of the proteome of adult stem cells to gain a global understanding of the early mechanisms that are involved in the VPA induction of stem cells.

4.1. Cellular Morphology

The microscopy analysis exhibits the first evidence of differentiation. VPA induces morphological changes on the ADSCs within 3 h, and the cells show long cytoplasmic extensions and become thicker relative to the untreated cells. This indicates that VPA may influence cytoskeletal modifications. Dendrite-like structures appear from 6 h provides further evidence that ADSCs are taking on a neuronal differentiation path. At the final time point, examined at 24 h, the treated cells have a vastly changed appearance from the original form. Much of the population appears slender and has a directed polar outward growth pattern. Furthermore, the dendrite extensions are present in most cells. VPA does not have an influence on the death rate, the cell population has had minimal variation over the treatment time points as opposed to studies with other small chemicals, such as BME and DMSO [2,3,23]. The cell counts and subsequent ALP and Reazurin assays support the stability of the cell culture population with nominal changes over time.

4.2. Secreted Molecules Role in Signalling Pathways Controlling Neural Differentiation

The pleiotropic nature of secreted cytokines assists in the molecular signalling and pathway modulation across various systems in almost all cell types. They are particularly interesting due to the multifunctional roles within cellular responses and differentiation, by primarily promoting or closing pathways as well as regulating the expression of specific cascades leading to the release of neurotrophic factors in the case of neural differentiation. Tracking their expression patterns from treated cells utilizing the Bioplex system, allows for a relative quantification and group clustering to identify trends between multiple molecules.

In the Bioplex results, it is noticeable that for almost all cytokines, post VPA treatment, the quantified amounts are reduced from that time point. The levels seem to increase by the final time point with variable expression patterns that are cytokine specific.

We found that VPA has effects on every cytokine measured within this study, thus it has a large action spectrum of modulating cytokine expression, however, is very specific for targets such as IP-10 and MIP-1b. For these two cytokines, IP-10 and MIP-1b, VPA definitively stops their expression upon treatment. IP-10 is not detected after the first control time point across all replicates. This may indicate that VPA has an irreversible action on these particular cytokines. Whereas, the other cytokine trends indicate possible reversible action as variable expression patterns are viewed across time points. IP-10 and MIP-1b have known interactions and roles with the JAK/STAT protein pathway [24,25]. The JAK/STAT canonical pathway is a system of linked interactions involved in the phosphorylation of tyrosine residues in receptors creating active binding sites for proteins with Src-Homology (SH2) domains.

In this receptor—SH2 activation the ligand proteins are translocated to the cell nucleus to initiate the transcription of genes that are vital in development, immunity and oncogenesis [26]. MIP-1b and STAT-1 protein interaction were previously implicated in the development of human glial cells and astrocytes [27]. IP-10 has also been shown to play a critical role in the maintenance of maturing astrocytes in vitro [28]. The limitation of these two molecules expression and subsequent interactions could limit the astroglial lineage commitment and instead promote neuronal development via the MAPK pathway. Supporting this, astrogliogenesis has been noted to require a high expression of neuroinflammatory cytokines IL-1β, IL-6, and TNF-α during the development process [29].

These molecules were detected within the VPA treatments at levels substantially below the non-treated ADSC controls. Higher expression levels of IL-1β [30,31], IL-6 [32] and TNF-α [33] are known to be inhibitory or to limit to neurogenesis as well as promote cellular proliferation. Chen et al., found that increased IL-1β limited neurogenesis by co-stimulation of STAT in the JAK/STAT pathway [34]. Jian et al., noted that the repression of the STAT occurs by activating the MAPK pathway [35], thus supporting the dualistic nature of JAK/STAT versus MAPK. The reduced expression of the abovementioned cytokines by modulation of VPA treatment favours neurogenesis induction over astrogliogenesis.

The expression changes in cytokines involved in one or several pathways like the ERK/MAPK or JAK/STAT pathways affect, even if it is temporally, the pathways and inductive effects on the cellular cycle and the induction of differentiation.

4.3. Protein Expression and Interaction Pathways Affected by VPA Treatment

The proteomics and network analysis show that VPA induces the expression of a variety of neural developmental and differentiation related proteins. An interesting protein expressed due to VPA influence is SOCS5. It is found in the 3 h samples, so the VPA effect on its expression is short; however, its functional role is considerable. SOCS5 is categorised in the protein family group of suppressors of cytokine signalling. SOCS5 gene expression is repressed by histone deacetylation [36], and we know that VPA inhibits class I HDAC [11]. Thus, VPA treatment assists in increasing the expression of SOCS5 by inhibiting the HDAC. Studies proved that SOCS5 inhibits the JAK/STAT pathway [37] by decreasing STATs activation [38]. SOCS5 is also involved in the negative regulation of IL4 and IL7 signalling [38]; this is seen in this studies Bioplex results. The expression of SOCS5 could be one of the responsible elements in decreasing IL4 and IL7 expression and possibly other cytokines. Its effect may only be temporary for most of the cytokines expressions and definitive for IP-10 and MIP-1b.

SOCS5 has also been previously annotated to interact with epidermal growth factor receptor (EGFR). EGFR primary binding partner is epidermal growth factor (EGF) which activates several signal transduction pathways including PI3K/AKT, RAS/ERK and JAK/STAT pathways [39]. The role of EGFR is particularly important for maintaining proliferative capacities in cells which is directly promotes JAK/STAT family proteins and dysregulates mTOR pathways useful in downstream neurogenesis. Furthermore, EGFR role in JAK/STAT promotes gliogenesis in direct competitive opposition to the activation of the Ras/ERK-MAPK signalling pathway [40]. The interaction of SOCS5 and EGFR is a SH-2 domain associated inhibition of EGFR, thereby the SOCS5 again has another multifunctional influence on limiting the JAK/STAT pathway [41]. SOCS5 could indirectly activate the MAPK pathway through this pathway alternation. Furthermore, the appearance of JAK3 protein in the last time points could prove that the JAK/STAT is downregulated and an intermediary protein of the cascade of reaction as JAK3 accumulates. The events conducting to this result require further investigation. By this protein interactivity the expression of SOCS5 downregulates the activation of the RAS/ERK and JAK/STAT pathways.

4.4. The Oxidative Stress Role in Neural Differentiation Activation

Oxidative stress is another effect of VPA treatment, by increasing the formation of reactive oxygen species [42]. In several case studies, it was noted that increasing levels of oxidative stress can be counterproductive to cellular function; however, there is now a growing body of evidence that indicates that oxidative stress is necessary in neurogenesis [43]. A recent study by Okubo et al. [44] supports VPAs role in modulating oxidative stress by through NO-signalling. The expression of apolipoprotein A-4 (APOA4) is a marker of cellular response against oxidative stress [45]. Similarly, the calcium binding mitochondrial carrier proteins (SLC25A24) is also expressed by the cells to protect themselves from oxidative stress [46]. Within the biological process GO graph (Figure 4), these proteins were found to be database annotated [47] in cell differentiation and neuron specific ontologies, namely; generation of neurons, neurogenesis, neuron development and neuron projection development. These ontologies were found to have several subsidiary groupings, examined through the ClueGo interaction map (Figure 5), to specific neuronal developmental checkpoints supported by pathway signalling. The presence of p38 MAPKs allows for the activation of the MAPK cascade and mitotic arrest under a low level of oxidative stress, which has also been reported by Kurata et al. [48]. VPA's role in p38 MAPK expression and the subsequent activation of the MAPK cascade is a supplementary route over the Ras/ERK signalling forbearer activation of MAPK and neurogenesis pathways. VPA creates an environment with low oxidative stress triggering the ADSCs to activating the MAPK cascade.

4.5. Functional Roles of Identified Neural Proteins in VPA Treated MSCs

Studies show that VPA promotes the production of Fibroblast growth factor 21 (FGF21) while suppressing HDAC [49]. FGF21 expression in this study was noted onward from the 6 h time point FGF21 is a regulator of metabolic processes and has strong links to neurogenesis and neuron maturation and myelination [50]. Its receptor FGFR3 is expressed at 3 h, 6 h, and 24 h. Studies proved that following the FGF21 activation of FGFR, the MAPK pathway is initiated, involving phosphorylation of ERK 1 and 2 [51]. In the ClueGo analysis, the FGFR signalling pathway is proximal to several downstream processes, particularly in cerebral cortex development and neuron maturation. In a recent study by Shahror et al. [52] it was shown that MSCs over expressing FGF21 transplanted to a mouse model enhanced neurogenesis and recovery. Furthermore, their results also show the FGF21 promoted maturation of the hippocampal neurons. The expression of the FGF21 and FGFR3 post VPA treatment of the stem cells is useful indicator of the neurogenic potential of VPA and MSCs.

A pertinent dataset, supportive of neuronal induction and differentiation, is the presence of neuronal markers, which appear from the first treatment time point. Table 2 presents a list of identified proteins and their correlative biological process in neurodevelopment according to gene ontology. Exploring several key markers and their interaction partners allows for a greater view of the molecular changes occurring during treatment and differentiation. The early expression of glial fibril associated protein (GFAP), neuropilin and tolloid like 2 (NETO2), and RUN and FYVE Domain Containing 3 (RUFY3) are particularly interesting. GFAP is known to be expressed in developing central nervous systems, and is particularly expressed in glia, astrocytes, neural stem cells, and neuron progenitor cells, with its expression declining in mature neurons [53].

It plays a vital role in neuron development, and is classed in the GO category of neuron projections along with its GO category and interaction partner, Thy1-membrane glycoprotein (THY1). The interaction of these two proteins are thought to guide cell-to-cell extension in the early phases of synapse formation. The expression of NETO2 and RUFY3 were of great interest as these proteins were annotated as specifically expressed in neurons [54,55]. NETO2 interacts with several other proteins and falls in with certain ontologies related to neurotransmitter update and glutamate receptor regulation. NETO2 is also known to assist in the development of neurite outgrowth [55].

RUFY3 is also involved in the growth of neurons, specifically associated with the guidance of axon growth [54], fittingly, the ontologies analysis and graphs correlate its role in neuron development, the positive regulation of cell morphogenesis involved in differentiation, and the regulation of neuron projection development. Their presence in this study of treated stem cell samples eludes to the early stages of differentiation and commitment toward neuronal lineage. Some markers appear in later time points like advillin (AVIL) and proteins involved in voltage-gated channel and that are specific in generating the neuronal action potential, such as SCN3A, KCNG4, KCBN1 and KCNT2. AVIL is involved in neuron development by cytoskeletal organization in neuron projection and morphogenesis through its interaction with intermediary filaments and is a downstream partner in the MAPK pathway. These proteins are evidentiary developing neuron markers. Their presence in the VPA treated ADSCs shows that the cells are following a neuronal differentiation pathway.

5. Conclusions

In this study we presented the temporal treatment of VPA on ADSCs and the proteomic, Bioplex, interaction network and pathway analysis. We found that VPA induces a cascade of reactions using its different properties. Inhibiting HDACs, it promotes the expression of SOCS5, which downregulates the JAK/STAT pathway. In this way, the glial differentiation is silenced, and the neuronal differentiation can be promoted.

We demonstrated that VPA activates the MAPK cascade by creating a low oxidative stress and by upregulating the expression of FGF21. However, the ERK pathway is downregulated by SOCS5 as well; however, this can operate as a regulator of the activation of the ERK/MAPK cascade. Specific neuronal markers are found in the induced ADSCs and their expressions confirm that VPA induced a neuronal differentiation pathway on the ADSCs.

This study opens a new opportunity to further differentiate ADSCs into neurons using a chemical that is already used clinically. VPA can be a key to finding new neuro-regenerative methods.

Author Contributions: J.S. conceived and designed the experiments. T.H. performed cell culture, differentiation cell preparation for mass spectrometry. J.S. performed Bioplex and assays. J.S., T.H. and B.K.M. analyzed data and wrote paper. B.K.M. contributed reagents/materials, edited paper and supervised J.S. and T.H. All authors have read and agreed to the published version of the manuscript.

Funding: This research was partially funded by the Schwartz Foundation philanthropic donation to support research.

Acknowledgments: We would like to thank the UTS Proteomics Core Facility, Matt Padula for technical support and running samples on the Mass spectrometer.

Conflicts of Interest: The authors declare no conflict of interest.

Abbreviations

ADSCs	Adipose Derived Stem Cells
ALP	Alkaline phosphatase
AVIL	Advillin
BHA	butylated hydroxyanisole
BME	beta-mercaptoethanol
DMEM	Dulbecco's Modified Eagle's Medium: Nutrient Mixture F-12
DMSO	dimethylsulfoxide
ERK	Extracellular Receptor Kinase
FGF21	Fibroblast growth factor 21
FGFR3	Fibroblast growth factor receptor 3
GFAP	Glial fibrillary acidic protein
hADSCs	human Adipose Derived Stem Cells
HDAC	histone deacetylase
JAK	Janus kinase
JAK3	Tyrosine-protein kinase JAK3
KCNB1	Potassium voltage-gated channel subfamily B member 1
KCNG4	Potassium voltage-gated channel subfamily G member 4
KCNT2	Potassium channel subfamily T member 2
LC-MS/MS	Liquid chromatography tandem mass spectrometry
MAPK1	Mitogen-activated protein kinase
NETO2	Neuropilin and tolloid-like protein 2
PBS	Phosphate-buffered saline
RA	Retinoic acid
SLC25A24	Calcium-binding mitochondrial carrier protein SCaMC-1
SLC8A3	Sodium/calcium exchanger 3
STAT1	Signal transducer and activator of transcription 1-alpha/beta
STAT6	Signal transducer and activator of transcription 6
VPA	Valproic Acid

References

1. Franco Lambert, A.P.; Fraga Zandonai, A.; Bonatto, D.; Cantarelli Machado, D.; Pegas Henriques, J.A. Differentiation of human adipose-derived adult stem cells into neuronal tissue: Does it work? *Differ. Res. Biol. Divers.* **2009**, *77*, 221–228. [CrossRef]
2. Woodbury, D.; Schwarz, E.J.; Prockop, D.J.; Black, I.B. Adult rat and human bone marrow stromal cells differentiate into neurons. *J. Neurosci. Res.* **2000**, *61*, 364–370. [CrossRef]
3. Santos, J.; Milthorpe, B.K.; Herbert, B.R.; Padula, M.P. Proteomic Analysis of Human Adipose Derived Stem Cells during Small Molecule Chemical Stimulated Pre-neuronal Differentiation. *Int. J. Stem Cells* **2017**. [CrossRef]
4. Kondo, T.; Johnson, S.A.; Yoder, M.C.; Romand, R.; Hashino, E. Sonic hedgehog and retinoic acid synergistically promote sensory fate specification from bone marrow-derived pluripotent stem cells. *Proc. Natl. Acad. Sci. USA* **2005**, *102*, 4789–4794. [CrossRef]
5. Yu, J.M.; Bunnell, B.A.; Kang, S.K. Neural differentiation of human adipose tissue-derived stem cells. *Methods Mol. Biol. (Clifton, N.J.)* **2011**, *702*, 219–231. [CrossRef]
6. Mu, M.W.; Zhao, Z.Y.; Li, C.G. Comparative study of neural differentiation of bone marrow mesenchymal stem cells by different induction methods. *Genet. Mol. Res. GMR* **2015**, *14*, 14169–14176. [CrossRef] [PubMed]
7. Santos, J.; Milthorpe, B.K.; Padula, M.P. Proteomic Analysis of Cyclic Ketamine Compounds Ability to Induce Neural Differentiation in Human Adult Mesenchymal Stem Cells. *Int. J. Mol. Sci.* **2019**, *20*, 523. [CrossRef] [PubMed]
8. Talwadekar, M.; Fernandes, S.; Kale, V.; Limaye, L. Valproic acid enhances the neural differentiation of human placenta derived-mesenchymal stem cells in vitro. *J. Tissue Eng. Regen. Med.* **2017**, *11*, 3111–3123. [CrossRef] [PubMed]
9. Vukicevic, V.; Qin, N.; Balyura, M.; Eisenhofer, G.; Wong, M.L.; Licinio, J.; Bornstein, S.R.; Ehrhart-Bornstein, M. Valproic acid enhances neuronal differentiation of sympathoadrenal progenitor cells. *Mol. Psychiatry* **2015**, *20*, 941–950. [CrossRef]
10. Eckschlager, T.; Plch, J.; Stiborova, M.; Hrabeta, J. Histone Deacetylase Inhibitors as Anticancer Drugs. *Int. J. Mol. Sci.* **2017**, *18*, 1414. [CrossRef]
11. Gottlicher, M.; Minucci, S.; Zhu, P.; Kramer, O.H.; Schimpf, A.; Giavara, S.; Sleeman, J.P.; Lo Coco, F.; Nervi, C.; Pelicci, P.G.; et al. Valproic acid defines a novel class of HDAC inhibitors inducing differentiation of transformed cells. *EMBO J.* **2001**, *20*, 6969–6978. [CrossRef] [PubMed]
12. Yu, I.T.; Park, J.-Y.; Kim, S.H.; Lee, J.-S.; Kim, Y.-S.; Son, H. Valproic acid promotes neuronal differentiation by induction of proneural factors in association with H4 acetylation. *Neuropharmacology* **2009**, *56*, 473–480. [CrossRef]
13. Hsieh, J.; Nakashima, K.; Kuwabara, T.; Mejia, E.; Gage, F.H. Histone deacetylase inhibition-mediated neuronal differentiation of multipotent adult neural progenitor cells. *Proc. Natl. Acad. Sci. USA* **2004**, *101*, 16659–16664. [CrossRef] [PubMed]
14. Liu, X.S.; Chopp, M.; Kassis, H.; Jia, L.F.; Hozeska-Solgot, A.; Zhang, R.L.; Chen, C.; Cui, Y.S.; Zhang, Z.G. Valproic acid increases white matter repair and neurogenesis after stroke. *Neuroscience* **2012**, *220*, 313–321. [CrossRef] [PubMed]
15. Rezaei, F.; Tiraihi, T.; Abdanipour, A.; Hassoun, H.K.; Taheri, T. Immunocytochemical analysis of valproic acid induced histone H3 and H4 acetylation during differentiation of rat adipose derived stem cells into neuron-like cells. *Biotech. Histochem.* **2018**, *93*, 589–600. [CrossRef] [PubMed]
16. Long, X.; Olszewski, M.; Huang, W.; Kletzel, M. Neural cell differentiation in vitro from adult human bone marrow mesenchymal stem cells. *Stem Cells Dev.* **2005**, *14*, 65–69. [CrossRef] [PubMed]
17. Tomita, M.; Mori, T.; Maruyama, K.; Zahir, T.; Ward, M.; Umezawa, A.; Young, M.J. A comparison of neural differentiation and retinal transplantation with bone marrow-derived cells and retinal progenitor cells. *Stem Cells (Dayton, Ohio)* **2006**, *24*, 2270–2278. [CrossRef]
18. Galindo, L.T.; Filippo, T.R.M.; Semedo, P.; Ariza, C.B.; Moreira, C.M.; Camara, N.O.S.; Porcionatto, M.A. Mesenchymal Stem Cell Therapy Modulates the Inflammatory Response in Experimental Traumatic Brain Injury. *Neurol. Res. Int.* **2011**, *2011*, 564089. [CrossRef]
19. Štefková, K.; Procházková, J.; Pacherník, J. Alkaline phosphatase in stem cells. *Stem Int.* **2015**, *2015*, 628368. [CrossRef]

20. Hanna, H.; Mir, L.M.; Andre, F.M. In vitro osteoblastic differentiation of mesenchymal stem cells generates cell layers with distinct properties. *Stem Cell Res. Ther.* **2018**, *9*, 203. [CrossRef]
21. Taverner, T.; Karpievitch, Y.V.; Polpitiya, A.D.; Brown, J.N.; Dabney, A.R.; Anderson, G.A.; Smith, R.D. DanteR: An extensible R-based tool for quantitative analysis of -omics data. *Bioinformatics* **2012**, *28*, 2402–2406. [CrossRef] [PubMed]
22. Shannon, P.; Markiel, A.; Ozier, O.; Baliga, N.S.; Wang, J.T.; Ramage, D.; Amin, N.; Schwikowski, B.; Ideker, T. Cytoscape: A software environment for integrated models of biomolecular interaction networks. *Genome Res.* **2003**, *13*, 2498–2504. [CrossRef]
23. Lu, P.; Blesch, A.; Tuszynski, M.H. Induction of bone marrow stromal cells to neurons: Differentiation, transdifferentiation, or artifact? *J. Neurosci. Res.* **2004**, *77*, 174–191. [CrossRef] [PubMed]
24. Wang, W.; Tan, J.; Xing, Y.; Kan, N.; Ling, J.; Dong, G.; Liu, G.; Chen, H. p43 induces IP-10 expression through the JAK-STAT signaling pathway in HMEC-1 cells. *Int. J. Mol. Med.* **2016**, *38*, 1217–1224. [CrossRef] [PubMed]
25. Moshapa, F.T.; Riches-Suman, K.; Palmer, T.M. Therapeutic Targeting of the Proinflammatory IL-6-JAK/STAT Signalling Pathways Responsible for Vascular Restenosis in Type 2 Diabetes Mellitus. *Cardiol. Res. Pract.* **2019**, *2019*, 9846312. [CrossRef]
26. Jatiani, S.S.; Baker, S.J.; Silverman, L.R.; Reddy, E.P. JAK/STAT Pathways in Cytokine Signaling and Myeloproliferative Disorders: Approaches for Targeted Therapies. *Genes Cancer* **2010**, *1*, 979–993. [CrossRef]
27. Rezaie, P.; Trillo-Pazos, G.; Everall, I.P.; Male, D.K. Expression of beta-chemokines and chemokine receptors in human fetal astrocyte and microglial co-cultures: Potential role of chemokines in the developing CNS. *Glia* **2002**, *37*, 64–75. [CrossRef]
28. Choi, S.S.; Lee, H.J.; Lim, I.; Satoh, J.-I.; Kim, S.U. Human Astrocytes: Secretome Profiles of Cytokines and Chemokines. *PLoS ONE* **2014**, *9*, e92325. [CrossRef]
29. Wang, T.; Yuan, W.; Liu, Y.; Zhang, Y.; Wang, Z.; Zhou, X.; Ning, G.; Zhang, L.; Yao, L.; Feng, S.; et al. The role of the JAK-STAT pathway in neural stem cells, neural progenitor cells and reactive astrocytes after spinal cord injury. *Biomed. Rep.* **2015**, *3*, 141–146. [CrossRef]
30. Boehme, M.; Guenther, M.; Stahr, A.; Liebmann, M.; Jaenisch, N.; Witte, O.W.; Frahm, C. Impact of indomethacin on neuroinflammation and hippocampal neurogenesis in aged mice. *Neurosci. Lett.* **2014**, *572*, 7–12. [CrossRef]
31. Koo, J.W.; Duman, R.S. IL-1β is an essential mediator of the antineurogenic and anhedonic effects of stress. *Proc. Natl. Acad. Sci. USA* **2008**, *105*, 751–756. [CrossRef] [PubMed]
32. Monje, M.L.; Toda, H.; Palmer, T.D. Inflammatory blockade restores adult hippocampal neurogenesis. *Science* **2003**, *302*, 1760–1765. [CrossRef] [PubMed]
33. Johansson, S.; Price, J.; Modo, M. Effect of Inflammatory Cytokines on Major Histocompatibility Complex Expression and Differentiation of Human Neural Stem/Progenitor Cells. *Stem Cells (Dayton, Ohio)* **2008**, *26*, 2444–2454. [CrossRef] [PubMed]
34. Chen, E.; Xu, D.; Lan, X.; Jia, B.; Sun, L.; Zheng, J.C.; Peng, H. A Novel Role of the STAT3 Pathway in Brain Inflammation-induced Human Neural Progenitor Cell Differentiation. *Curr. Mol. Med.* **2013**, *13*, 1474–1484. [CrossRef]
35. Jain, N.; Zhang, T.; Fong, S.L.; Lim, C.P.; Cao, X. Repression of Stat3 activity by activation of mitogen-activated protein kinase (MAPK). *Oncogene* **1998**, *17*, 3157–3167. [CrossRef]
36. Kim, M.-H.; Kim, M.-S.; Kim, W.; Kang, M.A.; Cacalano, N.A.; Kang, S.-B.; Shin, Y.-J.; Jeong, J.-H. Suppressor of Cytokine Signaling (SOCS) Genes Are Silenced by DNA Hypermethylation and Histone Deacetylation and Regulate Response to Radiotherapy in Cervical Cancer Cells. *PLoS ONE* **2015**, *10*, e0123133. [CrossRef]
37. Cooney, R.N. Suppressors of cytokine signaling (SOCS): Inhibitors of the JAK/STAT pathway. *Shock (Augusta, Ga.)* **2002**, *17*, 83–90. [CrossRef]
38. Sharma, N.; Nickl, C.; Kang, H.; Winter, S.S.; Cannon, J.; Matlawska-Wasowska, K. SOCS5 Regulates JAK-STAT Signaling and T-ALL Development. *Blood* **2017**, *130*, 370.
39. Henson, E.S.; Gibson, S.B. Surviving cell death through epidermal growth factor (EGF) signal transduction pathways: Implications for cancer therapy. *Cell. Signal.* **2006**, *18*, 2089–2097. [CrossRef]
40. Bonni, A.; Sun, Y.; Nadal-Vicens, M.; Bhatt, A.; Frank, D.A.; Rozovsky, I.; Stahl, N.; Yancopoulos, G.D.; Greenberg, M.E. Regulation of gliogenesis in the central nervous system by the JAK-STAT signaling pathway. *Science* **1997**, *278*, 477–483. [CrossRef]

41. Kario, E.; Marmor, M.D.; Adamsky, K.; Citri, A.; Amit, I.; Amariglio, N.; Rechavi, G.; Yarden, Y. Suppressors of cytokine signaling 4 and 5 regulate epidermal growth factor receptor signaling. *J. Biol. Chem.* **2005**, *280*, 7038–7048. [CrossRef] [PubMed]
42. Tung, E.W.; Winn, L.M. Valproic acid increases formation of reactive oxygen species and induces apoptosis in postimplantation embryos: A role for oxidative stress in valproic acid-induced neural tube defects. *Mol. Pharmacol.* **2011**, *80*, 979–987. [CrossRef] [PubMed]
43. Yuan, T.-F.; Gu, S.; Shan, C.; Marchado, S.; Arias-Carrión, O. Oxidative Stress and Adult Neurogenesis. *Stem Cell Rev. Rep.* **2015**, *11*, 706–709. [CrossRef] [PubMed]
44. Okubo, T.; Fujimoto, S.; Hayashi, D.; Suzuki, T.; Sakaue, M.; Miyazaki, Y.; Tanaka, K.; Usami, M.; Takizawa, T. Valproic acid promotes mature neuronal differentiation of adipose tissue-derived stem cells through iNOS–NO–sGC signaling pathway. *Nitric Oxide* **2019**, *93*, 1–5. [CrossRef] [PubMed]
45. Han, E.-S.; Muller, F.L.; Pérez, V.I.; Qi, W.; Liang, H.; Xi, L.; Fu, C.; Doyle, E.; Hickey, M.; Cornell, J.; et al. The in vivo gene expression signature of oxidative stress. *Physiol. Genom.* **2008**, *34*, 112–126. [CrossRef] [PubMed]
46. Traba, J.; Del Arco, A.; Duchen, M.R.; Szabadkai, G.; Satrustegui, J. SCaMC-1 promotes cancer cell survival by desensitizing mitochondrial permeability transition via ATP/ADP-mediated matrix Ca(2+) buffering. *Cell Death Differ.* **2012**, *19*, 650–660. [CrossRef]
47. Mi, H.; Muruganujan, A.; Ebert, D.; Huang, X.; Thomas, P.D. PANTHER version 14: More genomes, a new PANTHER GO-slim and improvements in enrichment analysis tools. *Nucleic Acids Res.* **2018**, *47*, D419–D426. [CrossRef]
48. Kurata, S.-I. Selective Activation of p38 MAPK Cascade and Mitotic Arrest Caused by Low Level Oxidative Stress. *J. Biol. Chem.* **2000**, *275*, 23413–23416. [CrossRef]
49. Leng, Y.; Wang, J.; Wang, Z.; Liao, H.M.; Wei, M.; Leeds, P.; Chuang, D.M. Valproic Acid and Other HDAC Inhibitors Upregulate FGF21 Gene Expression and Promote Process Elongation in Glia by Inhibiting HDAC2 and 3. *Int. J. Neuropsychopharmacol.* **2016**, *19*. [CrossRef]
50. Kuroda, M.; Muramatsu, R.; Maedera, N.; Koyama, Y.; Hamaguchi, M.; Fujimura, H.; Yoshida, M.; Konishi, M.; Itoh, N.; Mochizuki, H.; et al. Peripherally derived FGF21 promotes remyelination in the central nervous system. *J. Clin. Investig.* **2017**, *127*, 3496–3509. [CrossRef]
51. Iwata, T.; Hevner, R.F. Fibroblast growth factor signaling in development of the cerebral cortex. *Dev. Growth Differ.* **2009**, *51*, 299–323. [CrossRef] [PubMed]
52. Shahror, R.A.; Linares, G.R.; Wang, Y.; Hsueh, S.C.; Wu, C.C.; Chuang, D.M.; Chiang, Y.H.; Chen, K.Y. Transplantation of Mesenchymal Stem Cells Overexpressing Fibroblast Growth Factor 21 Facilitates Cognitive Recovery and Enhances Neurogenesis in a Mouse Model of Traumatic Brain Injury. *J. Neurotrauma* **2019**. [CrossRef] [PubMed]
53. Miller, F.D.; Gauthier, A.S. Timing Is Everything: Making Neurons versus Glia in the Developing Cortex. *Neuron* **2007**, *54*, 357–369. [CrossRef] [PubMed]
54. Wei, Z.; Sun, M.; Liu, X.; Zhang, J.; Jin, Y. Rufy3, a protein specifically expressed in neurons, interacts with actin-bundling protein Fascin to control the growth of axons. *J. Neurochem.* **2014**, *130*, 678–692. [CrossRef] [PubMed]
55. Vernon, C.G.; Swanson, G.T. Neto2 Assembles with Kainate Receptors in DRG Neurons during Development and Modulates Neurite Outgrowth in Adult Sensory Neurons. *J. Neurosci. Off. J. Soc. Neurosci.* **2017**, *37*, 3352–3363. [CrossRef]

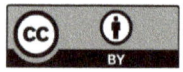

© 2020 by the authors. Licensee MDPI, Basel, Switzerland. This article is an open access article distributed under the terms and conditions of the Creative Commons Attribution (CC BY) license (http://creativecommons.org/licenses/by/4.0/).

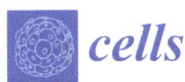

Article

The Phenotype and Secretory Activity of Adipose-Derived Mesenchymal Stem Cells (ASCs) of Patients with Rheumatic Diseases

Ewa Kuca-Warnawin [1,*], Urszula Skalska [1], Iwona Janicka [1], Urszula Musiałowicz [1], Krzysztof Bonek [2], Piotr Głuszko [2], Piotr Szczęsny [3], Marzena Olesińska [3] and Ewa Kontny [1]

1. Department of Pathophysiology and Immunology, National Institute of Geriatrics, Rheumatology and Rehabilitation, 02-637 Warsaw, Poland; ula.skalska@gmail.com (U.S.); zaklad.patofizjologii@spartanska.pl (I.J.); zbiu@op.pl (U.M.); ewa.kontny@spartanska.pl (E.K.)
2. Department of Rheumatology, National Institute of Geriatrics, Rheumatology and Rehabilitation, 02-637 Warsaw, Poland; krzysztof.bonek@gmail.com (K.B.); piotr.gluszko@spartanska.pl (P.G.)
3. Clinic of Connective Tissue Diseases, National Institute of Geriatrics, Rheumatology and Rehabilitation, 02-637 Warsaw, Poland; piotr_szczesny@live.com (P.S.); marzena.olesinska@vp.pl (M.O.)
* Correspondence: ewa.kuca-warnawin@spartanska.pl; Tel.: +48-(22)-6709260

Received: 7 November 2019; Accepted: 14 December 2019; Published: 17 December 2019

Abstract: Mesenchymal stem/stromal cells (MSCs) have immunosuppressive and regenerative properties. Adipose tissue is an alternative source of MSCs, named adipose-derived mesenchymal stem cells (ASCs). Because the biology of ASCs in rheumatic diseases (RD) is poorly understood, we performed a basic characterization of RD/ASCs. The phenotype and expression of adhesion molecules (intracellular adhesion molecule (ICAM)-1 and vascular cell adhesion molecule (VCAM)-1) on commercially available healthy donors (HD), ASC lines (n = 5) and on ASCs isolated from patients with systemic lupus erythematosus (SLE, n = 16), systemic sclerosis (SSc, n = 17) and ankylosing spondylitis (AS, n = 16) were analyzed by flow cytometry. The secretion of immunomodulatory factors by untreated and cytokine-treated ASCs was measured by ELISA. RD/ASCs have reduced basal levels of CD90 and ICAM-1 expression, correlated with interleukin (IL)-6 and transforming growth factor (TGF)-β1 release, respectively. Compared with HD/ASCs, untreated and tumour necrosis factor (TNF) + interferon (IFN)-γ (TI)-treated RD/ASCs produced similar amounts of prostaglandin E2 (PGE$_2$), IL-6, leukemia inhibiting factor (LIF), and TGF-β1, more IL-1Ra, soluble human leukocyte antigen G (sHLA-G) and tumor necrosis factor-inducible gene (TSG)-6, but less kynurenines and galectin-3. Basal secretion of galectin-3 was inversely correlated with the patient's erythrocyte sedimentation rate (ESR) value. IFN-α and IL-23 slightly raised galectin-3 release from SLE/ASCs and AS/ASCs, respectively. TGF-β1 up-regulated PGE$_2$ secretion by SSc/ASCs. In conclusion, RD/ASCs are characterized by low basal levels of CD90 and ICAM-1 expression, upregulated secretion of IL-1Ra, TSG-6 and sHLA-G, but impaired release of kynurenines and galectin-3. These abnormalities may modify biological activities of RD/ASCs.

Keywords: adipose-derived mesenchymal stem cells; phenotype; secretory potential; ankylosing spondylitis; systemic lupus erythematosus; systemic sclerosis

1. Introduction

Rheumatic diseases (RD), triggered by a complex interplay of genetic and environmental factors and mediated by autoimmune and/or autoinflammatory mechanisms, are characterized by chronic inflammation, progressive damage and functional impairment of affected tissues and organs [1]. Systemic lupus erythematosus (SLE) is a multisystemic disease of autoimmune background.

Overactivation of B cells, production of numerous autoantibodies, and defective immunoregulation are pivotal in SLE pathogenesis [2]. Systemic sclerosis (SSc), a rare autoimmune disease, is characterized by vascular derangement, abnormal fibroblast activation and progressive multi-organ fibrosis [3]. In SSc and SLE, serious life-threatening manifestations are common. Patients require long-term conventional immunosuppression but, despite an improvement in treatment opportunities, both diseases are still incurable [2,3]. Ankylosing spondylitis (AS) is accompanied by inflammatory back pain, damage to joint structures, and pathological bone formation, leading to spine ankylosis. Early long-lasting anti-inflammatory therapy may slow the progression of this irreversible structural damage [4]. This disease has certain autoinflammatory features and is mediated by interactions between innate and adaptive immune cells and cytokines [4,5].

Mesenchymal stromal/stem cells (MSCs), present in many embryonic and adult tissues, are endowed with regenerative potential and exert immunomodulatory effects on different components of the immune system, acting through cell-to-cell contact and/or secreted factors [6,7]. For these reasons, MSCs are thought to represent a promising therapeutic tool in autoimmune and inflammatory diseases [8]. However, depending on local conditions, tissue-resident MSCs can exhibit either anti- or pro-inflammatory capabilities, and thus may exert either protective effects or contribute to disease development [9]. In SLE and SSc, a growing body of data indicates numerous abnormalities of bone marrow derived MSCs (BM-MSCs), suggesting their possible contribution to disease pathology and raising questions about their autologous therapeutic application [10–13]. The knowledge about BM-MSC biology in AS is much less; limited data show aberrant function of these cells, and therefore several ongoing clinical trials apply allogenic MSCs [14–16]. Because of low expression of class II major histocompatibility complex (MHC) molecules, MSCs are claimed to be immune privileged and allogenic MSC therapy is generally regarded as harmless [17]. However, animal studies question this dogma by showing recipient immune responses and rejection of transplanted allogenic MSCs [18,19]. In humans, the clinical consequences of the therapeutic application of MHC-mismatched MSCs are unknown and, if possible, administration of autologous MSCs is recommended [19]. Human adipose tissue is a rich source of MSCs that possess stronger immunomodulatory capability than BM-MSCs [20,21]. Little is known about the biological properties of adipose tissue-derived MSCs (ASCs) from SLE, SSc and AS patients. These cells have been assessed in several SLE and SSc animal models with promising results [10]. At present, several clinical trials for curing SLE and SSc patients with allogeneic or autologous stromal vascular fraction (SVF), obtained from adipose tissue, are in progress (National Clinical Trials: NCT 02975960, NCT 02866552, NCT 02741362, clinicaltrials.gov) [22]. Unfortunately, SVF preparations contain variable proportions of ASCs and other cells, which may lead to unpredictable effects, makes standardization difficult and limits SVF therapeutic application [10]. By contrast, ASCs represent a more homogeneous population of cells and early phase clinical trials reported beneficial effects of autologous ASC transplantation in the alleviation of cutaneous symptoms in SSc patients [23–25]. However, there is still controversy over the use of autologous or allogeneic ASCs in the clinic because there are studies suggesting functional alterations of these cells in SSc [26,27]. Therefore, with the view of the potential therapeutic application of autologous ASCs in mind, we have performed a basic characterization of these cells and compared the phenotype and secretory potential of RD patients' ASCs (RD/ASCs) with the corresponding features of ASC lines originating from healthy donors (HDs).

2. Materials and Methods

2.1. Patients and Sample Collection

Three groups of patients who fulfilled the criteria for SLE (n = 16), SSc (n = 17) or AS (n = 16), were included in the study [28–30]. This study meets all criteria contained in the Declaration of Helsinki and was approved by the Ethics Committee of the National Institute of Geriatrics, Rheumatology, and Rehabilitation, Warsaw, Poland (approval protocol number: KBT-8/4/20016). All patients gave their written informed consent prior to enrolment.

2.2. ASC Isolation and Culture

Specimens of subcutaneous abdominal fat (approximately 300 mg) were taken from the patients by 18 G needle biopsy. Tissue processing, ASC isolation and culture were performed as described previously [31]. Five human adipose-derived mesenchymal cell lines (Lonza Group, Lonza Walkershille Inc., MD, USA, donor numbers: 0000440549, 0000410252, 0000535975, 0000605220, 0000550179) were used as a control. All experiments were performed using ASCs at 3–5 passages. The medium used for ASC culture was composed of DMEM/F12 (PAN Biotech UK Ltd., Wimborn, UK), 10% fetal calf serum (FCS) (Biochrom, Berlin, Germany), 200 U/mL penicillin, 200 µg/mL streptomycin (Polfa Tarchomin S.A., Warsaw, Poland) and 5 µg/mL plasmocin (InvivoGen, San Diego, CA, USA). For some experiments, ASCs were stimulated for 24 h with recombinant human tumor necrosis factor (TNF)-α and interferon (IFN)-γ (both from R & D Systems, Minneapolis, MN, USA; each used at 10 ng/mL), 2000 U/mL of IFN-α, (R&D Systems), 5 ng/mL of transforming growth factor (TGF-β1) or 20 ng/mL of interleukin (IL)-23 (both from PeproTech Inc. Rocky Hill, NY, USA). Then, culture supernatants (SNs) and cells were harvested for further analysis by enzyme-linked immunosorbent assays (ELISAs) or flow cytometry, respectively.

2.3. Flow Cytometry Analysis

For ASC phenotype analysis, cells were treated with non-enzymatic cell dissociation solution (ATCC Manassas, VA, USA) and washed with FACS buffer (phosphate-buffered saline, 0.1% NaN3, 1% FCS). Then, 5×10^4 cells were resuspended in 50 µL of FACS buffer and stained for 30 min on ice with fluorochrome conjugated murine anti-human monoclonal antibodies against the following surface markers: CD90-FITC, CD105-PE, CD73-APC (eBioscience, San Diego, CA, USA), CD34-PE-Cy7, CD45-PE, CD19-PE and CD14-APC (BD Pharmingen, San Diego, CA, USA). For evaluation of intracellular adhesion molecule 1 (ICAM-1) and vascular cell adhesion molecule 1 (VCAM-1) expression, ASCs were detached as described above, then stained with anti-ICAM-1-PE and anti-VCAM-1-APC antibodies (both from Biolegend, San Diego, CA, USA). After the washing step, cells were acquired and analyzed using a FACSCanto cell sorter/cytometer and Diva software. The gating strategy and applied isotype controls are shown in Figure S1 in the Supplementary Materials.

2.4. ELISAs

The concentrations of cytokines were measured in culture SNs in duplicate using specific ELISAs. The IL-6 ELISA was performed according to our own procedure using a goat polyclonal neutralizing antibody specific for human IL-6 (R & D Systems, Minneapolis, MN, USA), and an IL-6 specific rabbit polyclonal antibody (Sigma-Aldrich, St. Louis, MO, USA) as the capture and detection antibodies, respectively, followed by horseradish peroxidase-conjugated goat anti-rabbit immunoglobulins and o-phenylenediamine dihydrochloride (OPD) (both from Sigma) as a substrate. Human recombinant IL-6 (R & D Systems) was used a standard. The concentrations of TGF-β1, galectin-3, leukemia inhibiting factor (LIF) and IL-1 receptor antagonist (IL-1Ra) were measured using ELISA DuoSet kits, while PGE$_2$ was measured using the Parameter kit (all from R & D Systems). The soluble form of human leukocyte antigen G (sHLA-G) concentration was measured using a specific ELISA kit from Biovendor, Brno, Czech Republic. Tumor necrosis factor-inducible gene 6 protein (TSG-6) concentration was assessed using a specific ELISA from RayBiotech, Norcross, GA, USA. Kynurenine concentration was measured spectrophotometrically as described elsewhere [32]. Briefly, SNs were mixed with 30% trichloroacetic acid at a 2:1 ratio and incubated for 30 min at 5 °C, then centrifuged at 10,000× g for 5 min and finally diluted at a 1:1 ratio in Ehrlich's reagent (100 mg p-dimethyl benzaldehyde and 5 mL glacial acetic acid; Sigma-Aldrich). The optical density of the samples was measured at wavelength of 490 nm. L-kynurenine (Sigma-Aldrich) diluted in culture medium was used to prepare the standard curve.

2.5. Data Analysis

Data were analyzed using GraphPad Prism software version 7. The Shapiro–Wilk test was used as a normality test. The results are shown as median ± interquartile range (IQR) or range. One-way analysis of variance (ANOVA) with repeated measures and post-hoc Tukey test was used to compare untreated and cytokine-treated ASCs. The differences between ASC lines from healthy donors (HD/ASCs) and ASCs from SLE (SLE/ASCs), SSc (SSc/ASCs) and AS (AS/ASCs) patients were analyzed using the Kruskal–Wallis and Dunn's multiple comparison tests. For comparison of two groups (e.g., HD/ASCs vs. SLE/ASCs for IFN-α-treated cells), the Mann–Whitney U test was applied. Parametric (Pearson's linear) and non-parametric (Spearman's rank) correlation tests were used to assess an association between tested parameters. Probability values less than 0.05 were considered significant.

3. Results

3.1. Patients

The patient cohort was heterogeneous with respect to demographic and clinical data (Table 1). There were no significant differences between patient groups in body mass index (BMI), disease duration, and erythrocyte sedimentation rate (ESR) values, but SLE patients were younger than SSc patients, and AS patients had a slightly higher concentrations of C-reactive protein (CRP) than other patients. All AS patients were HLA-B27 positive and they were mostly treated with non-steroid anti-inflammatory drugs (NSAIDs). The majority of SLE and SSc patients had disease-specific autoantibodies (anti-dsDNA or Scl70, respectively) and received immunosuppressive drugs, usually with (SLE) or without (SSc) glucocorticosteroids. A similar proportion of SSc patients had localized (52.9%) or diffused (47%) disease form. A minority of patients received non-biologic disease-modifying anti-rheumatic drugs (DMARDs).

Table 1. Demographic and clinical characteristics of the patients.

Parameters	Systemic Lupus Erythematosus (SLE) (n = 16)	Systemic Sclerosis (SSc) (n = 17)	Ankylosing Spondylitis (AS) (n = 16)
Demographics			
Age, years	41 (20–54) [#]	52 (20–77)	43 (25–70)
Sex, female (F)/male (M), n	15 F/1 M	12 F/7 M	8 F/8 M
BMI	24.3 (16.4–39.1)	25.8 (16.5–38.7)	26.9 (21.4–35.8)
Disease duration, years	8 (0–47)	3 (1–23) [a]/5 (1–40) [b]	6 (1.5–17)
Clinical data			
Disease activity *, score	7 (0–32)	1 (0–8)	6.3 (1.0–8.2)
Laboratory values			
CRP, mg/L	5 (1–23)	5 (3–18)	8 (5–59) [##]
ESR, mm/h	16.5 (3–73)	16 (4–59)	15 (1–59)
Proteinuria, mg/24 h	185 (0–7550)	0 (0–0.2)	n/a
C3, mg/dL	73.5 (23.2–133)	98.1 (65.8–141)	n/a
C4, mg/dL	15.45 (5.38–20.6)	17.35 (13–27.1)	n/a
ANA, titre (1:x)	960 (160–10,240)	2560 (320–20,480)	n/a
anti-dsDNA antibody, %	75	n/a	n/a
anti-dsDNA antibody, IU/mL	68.85 (0–666.9)	n/a	n/a
Scl-70 antibody, %	n/a	88.9	n/a
Autoantibody specificities, no.	3 (1–7)	3 (2–4)	n/a
Medications, %			
NSAIDs			81.25
Immunosuppressive drugs	92.8	55	0
Non-biologic DMARDs	28.6	27.3	37.5
Glucocorticosteroids	75	23.5	21.25

Except where indicated otherwise, values are the median (range). BMI, body mass index; * SLEDAI, SLE Disease Activity Index, * EUSTAR, the European League Against Rheumatism Scleroderma Trials and Research revised index, or * BASDAI, Bath Ankylosing Spondylitis Disease Activity Index; CRP, C-reactive protein; ESR, erythrocyte sedimentation rate; C, complement components; ANA, antinuclear antibody; Scl-70, anti-topoisomerase I antibody; NSAIDs, non-steroid anti-inflammatory drugs; DMARDs, disease-modifying anti-rheumatic drugs; n/a, not applicable. [#] $p = 0.03$ for SLE vs. SSc patient comparison; [##] $p = 0.03$ for AS vs. SLE and SSc comparisons.

3.2. Phenotype of ASCs

Almost all HD/ASCs and RD/ASCs possessed MSC specific surface markers (CD105, CD90, CD73) and the percentage of triple positive cells was similar in every group (Figure 1A). There was also no significant difference in the level of CD105 and CD73 marker expression, shown as the median fluorescence intensity (MFI). However, RD/ASCs expressed less CD90 molecules than HD/ASCs, both on triple (CD105+/CD90+/CD73+) (Figure 1B) and single (CD90+) (data not shown) positive cells. The proportion of ASCs expressing hematological markers was low and similar in every group, i.e., less than 4% of HD/ASCs and RD/ASCs were positive for CD14, CD19, CD45, or CD34 (Figure 1C,D). However, four RD/ASC lines contained ≥10% CD34+ cells. The median percentage of HLA-DR$^+$ cells was below 10, and the majority of HD/ASCs and RD/ASCs lines contained less than 1–2% of HLA-DR+ cells. Nevertheless, some of them (one HD/ASC and seven RD/ASCs) contained ≥20% of these cells (Figure 1D). There was a strong inverse correlation between CD90 MFI on HD/ASCs and basal secretion of PGE$_2$ by these cells (Figure 1E), while in the RD group, CD90 MFI correlated positively but moderately with IL-6 secretion (Figure 1F). Both HD/ASCs and RD/ASCs differentiated in vitro into osteoblastic, chondrogenic and adipogenic lineages (data not shown; manuscript in preparation).

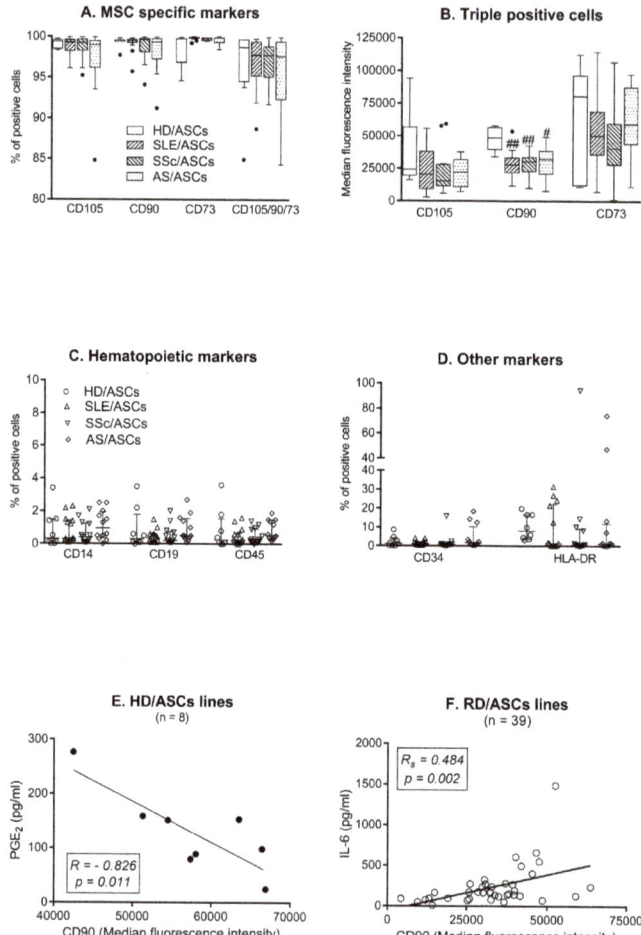

Figure 1. The phenotype of ASCs from healthy donors (HD) and patients with rheumatic diseases (RD). Expression of MSC specific (**A,B**) and non-specific (**C,D**) markers was assessed quantitatively (**B**) and/or qualitatively (**A,C,D**) using ASCs from healthy donors (HD/ASCs; n = 5), systemic lupus erythematosus (SLE/ASCs; n = 14), systemic sclerosis (SSc/ASCs; n = 13) and ankylosing spondylitis (AS/ASCs; n = 12) patients. Data are expressed as the median (horizontal line) with interquartile range (IQR, box), lower and upper whiskers (data within 3/2xIQR) and outliers (points) (Tukey's box) (**A,B**) or as the median with IQR (**C,D**). # p = 0.05–0.01; ## p = 0.01–0.001 for HD/ASCs versus RD/ASCs comparison. Pearson's (R) and Spearman's rank (R_s) correlation coefficients. Solid cirle—HD/ASC samples, hollow circles RD/ASC samples (**E,F**).

3.3. Expression of Adhesion Molecules by ASCs

A similar proportion of untreated and cytokine (TNFα + IFNγ; TI) treated HD/ASCs and RD/ASCs expressed the surface adhesion molecules ICAM-1 and VCAM-1 (Figure 2A,B). VCAM-1 was co-expressed by a small fraction of ICAM-1+ cells and no single VCAM-1+ cells were found. By contrast, the frequency of single ICAM-1+ cells predominated over the proportion of double ICAM-1+/VCAM-1+ cells. Amongst untreated cells, a slightly higher proportion of SSc/ASCs co-expressed ICAM-1 and VCAM-1 compared to other RD/ASCs (Figure 2A). Upon TI treatment, the percentage of single positive, double positive, and consequently all ICAM-1+ cells increased significantly (Figure 2B). Basal levels

(MFI) of VCAM-1 expression on HD/ASCs and RD/ASCs were similar (Figure 2C), and TI treatment did not modify it (Figure 2D). However, basal levels of ICAM-1 expression on single and double positive cells were significantly lower in SSc/ASCs and AS/ASCs than in HD/ASCs, and in the case of SLE/ASCs, a similar tendency was also noted (Figure 2C). Upon TI treatment, these differences disappeared (Figure 2D). In the RD group, the ICAM-1 MFI on ASCs positively correlated with TGF-β secretion by these cells (Figure S2, Supplementary Materials).

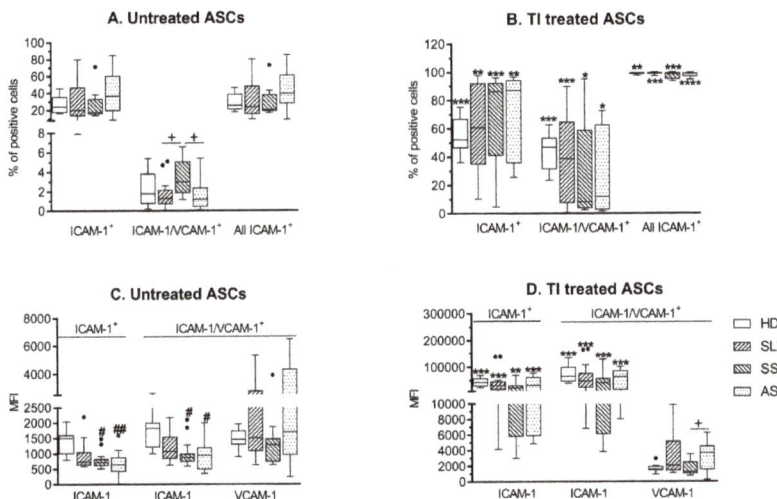

Figure 2. Expression of adhesion molecules on untreated and cytokine-treated ASCs. Healthy donors (HD; n = 5), systemic lupus erythematosus (SLE; n = 16), systemic sclerosis (SSc; n = 16) and ankylosing spondylitis (AS; n = 15) ASCs were cultured in medium alone (untreated ASCs) or in the presence of tumor necrosis factor (TNF)-α and interferon (IFN)-γ (TI treated ASCs) for 24 h. The qualitative (**A,B**) and quantitative (**C,D**) assessments of intracellular adhesion molecule (ICAM)-1 and vascular cell adhesion molecule (VCAM)-1 expression were performed. Results are expressed as the Tukey's boxes (see Figure 1). # p = 0.05–0.01, ## p = 0.01–0.001 for HD/ASCs versus patients' ASCs, while * p = 0.05–0.01, ** p = 0.01–0.001, *** p = 0.001–0.0001 for untreated versus TI treated ASC comparisons, + p = 0.05–0.01 for patients' versus patients' ASCs. Solid circles (points) represents outliers.

3.4. Basal and Cytokine-Triggered Secretory Activity of ASCs

As shown in Figure 3A,B, both untreated and cytokine-stimulated RD/ASCs secreted significantly smaller amounts of kynurenines and galectin-3 than HD/ASCs. Treatment with TI, but not other cytokines, significantly increased kynurenine secretion in HD/ASCs and, to a lesser extent, in RD/ASC cultures (Figure 3A), but failed to change the release of galectin-3 by both HD/ASCs and RD/ASCs (Figure 3B). However, the slight elevation of galectin-3 secretion by RD/ASCs was observed when disease-specific cytokines (IFN-α for SLE/ASCs and IL-23 for AS/ASCs) were used as the stimuli (Figure 3B). In addition, basal release of galectin-3 by RD/ASCs correlated weakly and inversely with patient ESR value, especially in the SSc group in which the correlation was much stronger (Figure 3C,D). On the other hand, RD/ASCs released more IL-1Ra, sHLA-G and TSG-6 than HD/ASCs, and cytokine treatment had a significant effect on their secretion (Figure 4). By contrast, both untreated and cytokine-stimulated HD/ASCs and RD/ASCs released similar amounts of the other tested factors (PGE$_2$, IL-6, TGF-β and LIF) (Figure 5). Upon TI treatment, HD/ASCs and RD/ASCs upregulated their secretion of IL-6; there was also increased release of LIF from HD/ASCs and PGE$_2$ from RD/ASCs while no changes were observed in the case of TGF-β, with the only exception of a smaller secretion of this cytokine by TI treated compared to untreated SSc/ASCs.

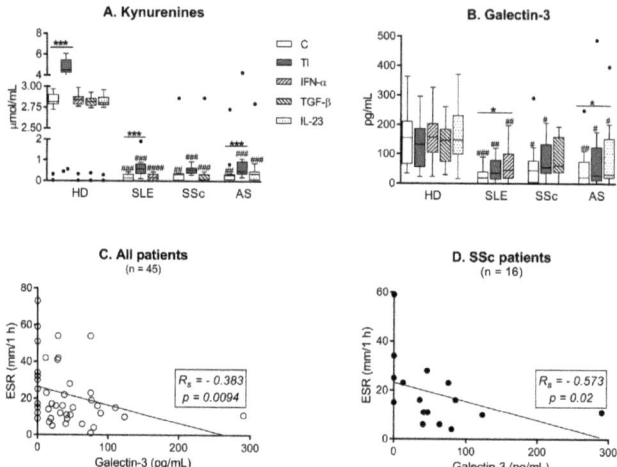

Figure 3. Impaired secretion of galectin-3 and kynurenines by ASCs of patients with rheumatic diseases (RD). Five healthy donor (HD) ASCs lines from two different passages (n = 10), systemic lupus erythematosus (SLE; n = 16), systemic sclerosis (SSc; n = 16–17) and ankylosing spondylitis (AS; n = 15) patients' ASCs were cultured in medium alone (C, control), or in the presence of the indicated cytokines (TI, TNF-α + IFN-γ). Galectin-3 and kynurenine concentrations were measured in culture supernatants. (**A**,**B**) Data are expressed as Tukey's boxes (see Figure 1); * p = 0.05–0.01, *** p = 0.001–0.0001 for control versus cytokine-treated cells; # p = 0.05–0.01, ## p = 0.01–0.001, ### p = 0.001–0.0001, #### p < 0.0001 for HD/ASCs versus RD/ASCs comparisons. (**C**,**D**) R_s, Spearman's rank correlation coefficient. Hollow circles represents RD/ASC samples, solid circle represents SSc/ASC samples. ESR - erythrocyte sedimentation rate.

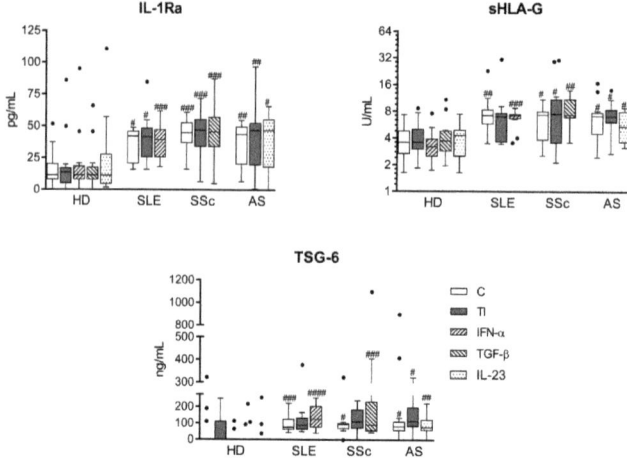

Figure 4. Enhanced secretion of IL-1Ra, soluble human leukocyte antigen G (sHLA-G) and tumor necrosis factor-inducible gene (TSG)-6 by ASCs of patients with rheumatic diseases (RD). Culture conditions of ASC lines from healthy donors (HD; n = 10), systemic lupus erythematosus (SLE; n = 12–16), systemic sclerosis (SSc; n = 10–17) and ankylosing spondylitis (AS; n = 9–15) patients were the same as described in Figure 3. Concentrations of indicated factors were measured in culture supernatants. Data are expressed as the Tukey's boxes (see Figure 1). No differences between untreated (C) and cytokine-stimulated cells were found. # p = 0.05–0.01; ## p = 0.01–0.001; ### p = 0.001–0.0001; #### p < 0.0001 for HD/ASCs versus RD/ASCs comparison.

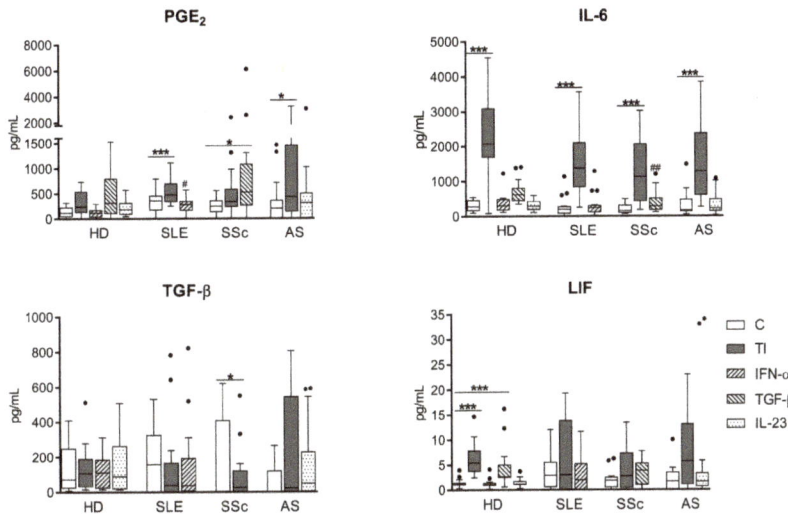

Figure 5. Similar secretion of other factors by ASCs of healthy donors and patients with rheumatic diseases. Culture conditions of ASC lines from healthy donors (HD; n = 10) and from patients with rheumatic diseases (RD), i.e., systemic lupus erythematosus (SLE; n = 16), systemic sclerosis (SSc; n = 16–17) and ankylosing spondylitis (AS; n = 15), were the same as described in Figure 3. Concentrations of indicated factors were measured in culture supernatants. Data are expressed as the Tukey's boxes (see Figure 1). * p = 0.05–0.01, *** p = 0.001–0.0001 for untreated (C) versus cytokine-treated cells; # p = 0.05–0.01, ## p = 0.01–0.001 for HD/ASCs versus RD/ASCs.

4. Discussion

MSCs are not constitutively immunosuppressive but acquired such capabilities upon exposure to appropriate local environments, and control immune responses through cell–cell contact and paracrine secretion of numerous soluble factors [9]. To assess the basic biological features of RD/ASCs, the cells exposed in vivo to chronic inflammatory milieu, we first analyzed the phenotype of these cells. According to a revised statement of the International Fat Applied Technology Society (IFATS), there are three minimal criteria for the definition of ASCs: plastic adherence, differentiation potential into adipocytes, chondrocytes and osteoblasts, as well as characteristic surface phenotype. More than 80% of these cells should express primary stable positive markers (CD105, CD90, CD73), while the expression of primary negative markers (CD45 and others) should be below 2% [33]. Other authors observed expression of positive and negative markers on more than 90% and less than 5% of ASCs, respectively [34]. The present results show that ASCs isolated from subcutaneous abdominal adipose tissue of RD patients fulfill the above phenotypic criteria of MSCs (Figure 1A,C,D). Observed individual variation in the proportion of CD34+ cells in ASC lines of both HD and RD patients (Figure 1D) may be explained by unique features of this molecule, which is a primary unstable ASC positive marker, present at variable levels and lost gradually during cell culture [33]. Although MSCs are thought to be devoid of surface HLA-DR, expression of these molecules on ASCs has been reported [35]. Thus, presence of HLA-DR molecules on some HD/ASC and RD/ASC lines, observed in our study (Figure 1D), is unsurprising. Altogether, our results show that in terms of surface marker expression, RD/ASCs resemble ASCs obtained from healthy volunteers, which is consistent with other reports [36–38].

In comparison with HD/ASCs, we found significantly reduced levels of CD90 expression on RD/ASCs (Figure 1B). CD90 is a glycoprotein endowed with numerous immunological and non-immunological functions, including cell–cell and cell–matrix interactions, cell motility, inflammation, and fibrosis [39]. It was reported that CD90 expressed on MSCs promotes osteogenic differentiation, but inhibits adipogenic differentiation of these cells, while MSCs with reduced expression of CD90 lose their immunosuppressive activity [40,41]. Therefore, it is likely that impaired CD90 expression on RD/ASCs contributes to the abnormal regenerative and immunoregulatory function of these cells. Consistent with this supposition, our results suggest that the level of CD90 expression may affect the secretory potential of ASCs (Figure 1E,F). According to our observation, high CD90 expression may restrict PGE_2 release in HD/ASCs, while it may promote IL-6 secretion in RD/ASCs. The reason for CD90 downregulation on RD/ASCs is unknown, but prolonged in vivo exposure of these cells to inflammatory milieu is the probable cause. Unfortunately, we failed to notice any significant changes in CD90 expression after three days exposure of HD/ASCs and RD/ASCs to TI stimulation (data not shown). Although this observation does not rule out the likelihood of CD90 loss due to the action of other factors contributing to chronic inflammation, alternative explanations, e.g., intrinsic defects, also exist [12].

The adhesion molecules ICAM-1 and VCAM-1 regulate the migration of MSCs and provide their interaction with co-operating immune cells, making them indispensable for MSC-mediated immunosuppression [42,43]. Similar to other reports [18], we failed to observe single VCAM-1 bearing ASCs, found mostly single positive ICAM-1 cells and, less frequently, cells co-expressing both of these molecules (Figure 2A). Importantly, compared with HD/ASCs, both single and double positive RD/ASCs had lower basal ICAM-1 expression (Figure 1C), which, in addition, correlated moderately with TGF-β1 release by these cells (Figure S2, Supplementary Materials), suggesting that ICAM-1 may also have an impact on RD/ASC secretory function. Upon TI treatment, there was a similar upregulation of ICAM-1, but not VCAM-1, expression on HD/ASCs and RD/ASCs (Figure 1B,D). Therefore, the reason for impaired basal ICAM-1 expression on RD/ASCs is not related to pro-inflammatory cytokine exposure in vivo. Based on the present findings, we conclude that reduced basal expression levels of CD90 and ICAM-1 are characteristic for RD/ASCs. Neither the reason nor the consequences of these abnormalities are known yet. We did not find any association between basal CD90 and ICAM-1 expression and patient demographic and clinical data, including age, BMI, disease duration, ESR/CRP values, disease activity, etc. (data not shown). Nevertheless, our results suggest that both defects may affect RD/ASC secretory activity.

MSCs regulate immune responses by the release of various immunomodulatory factors and indoleamine 2,3-dioxogenase (IDO)-1-mediated catabolism of tryptophan into kynurenines [6,35,44]. Our results show significant differences between RD/ASCs and HD/ASCs in the secretion of these factors. Firstly, both untreated and cytokine-treated RD/ASCs produced less kynurenines and galectin-3 (Figure 3A,B). Activation of the kynurenine pathway, triggered mostly by IFN-γ, mediates the immunosuppressive action of MSCs in vitro and in vivo and exerts strong inhibitory effects mostly on the proliferation and cytotoxicity of T cells and natural killer (NK) cells [44]. Galectin-3, a member of the β-galactoside binding protein family, is a multifunctional protein with immunomodulatory effects on cell apoptosis, activation, differentiation and migration [45]. This protein is a critical mediator of MSC suppression of T cell proliferation and its secretion is considered as a biomarker for the immunomodulatory potential of MSCs [46]. We observed that TI treatment upregulated kynurenine release by HD/ASCs and RD/ASCs, but the latter cells responded poorly, suggesting that they are rather refractory to kynurenine pathway activation. In addition, we found that disease-specific cytokines were unable to trigger the kynurenine pathway in ASCs, while IFN-α and IL-23 activated, to a small extent, the galectin-3 pathway in SLE/ASCs and AS/ASCs, respectively. In contrast, secretion of galectin-3 by HD/ASCs was stable, which is consistent with its reported constitutive expression in BM-MSCs [47]. Since we found an inverse correlation between basal secretion of galectin-3 by RD/ASCs and ESR value (Figure 3C,D), it is likely that impairment of galectin-3 production by ASCs may contribute to inefficient control of systemic inflammation in these patients.

Secondly, compared with HD/ASCs, we found significant elevation of IL-1Ra, sHLA-G, and TSG-6 secretion by RD/ASCs (Figure 4). Applied stimuli did not alter the release of these factors. IL-1Ra counteracts the inflammatory effects of IL-1; its role in mediating the immunosuppressive effect of MSCs lies mostly in the polarization of macrophages toward the anti-inflammatory M2 phenotype and inhibition of B cell differentiation [48]. In collagen-induced arthritis in mice, inhibition of T-helper (Th)17 cells generation by IL-1Ra producing MSCs was also shown [49]. HLA-G, a non-classical HLA class I molecule, inhibits functions of innate and adaptive immune cells. Both surface-expressed and soluble forms (present in body fluids) of HLA-G are involved in the suppression of the cytotoxic function of T cells and NK cells, the maturation and function of dendritic cells (DC), and the generation of regulatory T cells (Tregs) [50]. TSG-6 mediates many of the immunomodulatory and reparative activities of MSCs and exerts therapeutic effects in various animal disease models [50]. This protein acts by binding to numerous ligands, e.g., extracellular matrix components and chemokines, where it inhibits neutrophil migration and macrophage activation and promotes M2 macrophage switching and Treg generation [51].

Independently of activation status, HD/ASCs and RD/ASCs secreted similar amounts of the other tested factors (PGE$_2$, IL-6, TGF-β1, and LIF; Figure 5). In general, RD/ASCs and HD/ASCs responded in similar way to applied stimuli, and a significant increase of secretion, if any, was triggered by TI treatment. The only exception was an elevation of PGE$_2$ release by TGF-β1 treated SSc/ASCs (Figure 5). All these ASC-derived factors were reported to mediate the immunomodulatory effects of MSCs in several ways, including inhibition of T cell proliferation. In addition, IL-6 and PGE$_2$ were shown to inhibit maturation of DCs and mediate switching of M1 inflammatory macrophages to an M2-like phenotype, while LIF and TGF-β1 were suggested to contribute to Treg generation [52–54].

As discussed above, there is a redundancy in the biological activities of MSC secreted factors. In addition, to achieve therapeutic immunosuppressive effects, a combination of these factors is usually required. For example, in SLE patients, the therapeutic effect of allogeneic MSC application was accompanied by an upregulation of Tregs and downregulation of Th17 cells, which was dependent on sHLA-G and TGF-β1, or PGE$_2$ action, respectively [55,56]. Therefore, it is hard to predict how the presently found abnormalities in the secretory activity of RD/ASCs may affect the immunoregulatory function of these cells. Nevertheless, observed upregulation of IL-1Ra, sHLA-G and TSG-6 secretion and normal release of IL-6, PGE$_2$, TGF-β1 and LIF suggest that RD/ASCs, exposed in vivo to a chronic inflammatory microenvironment, may preferentially use these factors to control excessive immune responses. However, impaired kynurenine and galectin-3 secretion may contribute to inefficiency of ASC control. It is likely that galectin-3 deficiency is more critical, as low production of this protein by RD/ASCs is associated with higher-grade systemic inflammation. Interestingly, disease-specific cytokines seem to trigger a compensatory mechanism by upregulating the release of galectin-3 from ASCs in SLE and AS and PGE$_2$ secretion in SSc patients.

Our study has some limitations. Firstly, it is well known that the type of harvesting procedure used may affect viability, yield or the biology of ASCs [57]. Because of ethical reasons, we had to apply the needle-aspiration technique, which is not commonly used. However, for ASC isolation, we utilized the enzymatic digestion-based method [31], intended mainly for experimental purposes [57]. In addition, to perform these analyses, isolated ASCs had to be expanded in vitro. Fortunately, the applied ASC isolation method turned out to be good enough to obtain a homogeneous population of cells with the MSC phenotype (Figure 1), even from scanty specimens of adipose tissue. Secondly, our RD patient cohort was heterogeneous in terms of some demographic data (age), clinical symptoms and treatment (Table 1). Obviously, these differences may also influence the phenotype and secretory activity of ASCs. Surprisingly, despite all the differences between SLE, SSc and AS patients, their ASCs show similar alterations in CD90 and ICAM-1 expression and immunoregulatory factor release. Because the aforementioned RDs are inflammatory disorders, chronic in vivo exposure of ASCs to the inflammatory environment of adipose tissue is a more likely explanation for the observed abnormalities.

5. Conclusions

In summary, we report that RD/ASCs are characterized by a low basal level of CD90 and ICAM-1 expression, elevated spontaneous secretion of IL-1Ra, TSG-6 and sHLA-G, but impaired release of kynurenines and galectin-3, and there are only small differences between ASCs obtained from SLE,

SSc, and AS patients. Exposure of RD/ASCs to a pro-inflammatory cytokine cocktail (TI) normalizes ICAM-1 expression, but not the secretion of immunoregulatory factors. We suggest that the observed alterations are caused by in vivo exposure of ASCs to an inflammatory milieu and may contribute to the inadequate immunoregulatory function of these cells.

Supplementary Materials: The following are available online at http://www.mdpi.com/2073-4409/8/12/1659/s1, Figure S1: Representative gating strategy and representative dot plots/histograms for assessing ASC phenotype, Figure S2: Correlation of basal ICAM-1 expression and TGF-β release by ASCs of patients with rheumatic diseases. The quantitative assessment of basal ICAM-1 expression (MFI, median fluorescence intensity) on ASCs obtained from patients with rheumatic diseases (RD/ASC lines) and basal secretion of TGF-β by these cells were done as described in the Materials and Methods. The correlation was assessed using Spearman's rank test; Rs and p values are shown. Note that the regression lines were used for graphic purposes only.

Author Contributions: E.K.-W. and U.S. designed experiments, performed flow cytometry experiments and data analysis. U.M. performed ELISA tests. I.J. was responsible for cell isolation and culture. K.B., P.G., P.S. and M.O. helped with recruited patients, acquired and analysed clinical data. E.K. wrote the manuscript.

Funding: This research was funded by the National Science Centre, Poland, grant number UMO-2016/21/B/NZ5/00500.

Acknowledgments: We are grateful to all patients who donated their adipose tissue for our research.

Conflicts of Interest: The authors declare that they have no competing interests. The funder (National Science Centre) had no role in the design of the study; in the collection, analyses, or interpretation of data; in the writing of the manuscript, or in the decision to publish the results.

Abbreviations

ANA	antinuclear antibody
APC	allophycocyanin
AS	ankylosing spondylitis
ASCs	adipose-derived mesenchymal stem cells
BASDAI	Bath Ankylosing Spondylitis Disease Activity Index;
BM-MSCs	bone marrow derived mesenchymal stem/stromal cells MSCs
C	complement components
CD	cluster of differentiation
CRP	C-reactive protein
DMARDs	disease-modifying anti-rheumatic drugs
ELISA	enzyme-linked immunosorbent assay
ESR	erythrocyte sedimentation rate
EUSTAR	European League Against Rheumatism Scleroderma Trials and Research revised index
FACS	fluorescence-activated cell sorting
FITC	fluorescein isothiocyanate
HD	healthy donors
HLA-B27	human leukocyte antigen B27
ICAM-1	intracellular adhesion molecule 1
IDO-1	indoleamine 2,3-dioxogenase 1
IFN-α	interferon-α
IFN-γ	interferon-γ
IL	interleukin
IL-1Ra	IL-1 receptor antagonist
IQR	interquartile range
LIF	leukemia inhibiting factor
MFI	median fluorescence intensity
MHC	major histocompatibility complex
MSCs	mesenchymal stem/stromal cells
NCT	National Clinical Trial
NSAIDs	non-steroid anti-inflammatory drugs
OPD	o-phenylenediamine dihydrochloride
PE	phycoerythrin

PE-Cy7	tandem fluorochrome of phycoerythrin coupled to the cyanine dye Cy7
PGE$_2$	prostaglandin E2
RD	rheumatic diseases
Scl-70	anti-topoisomerase I antibody
sHLA-G	soluble human leukocyte antigen G
SLE	systemic lupus erythematosus
SLEDAI	SLE Disease Activity Index
SN	supernatants
SSc	systemic sclerosis
SVF	stromal vascular fraction
TGF-β1	transforming growth factor β1
TI	TNF-α + IFN-γ
TNF-α	tumor necrosis factor α
TSG-6	tumor necrosis factor-inducible gene 6 protein
VCAM-1	vascular cell adhesion molecule-1

References

1. McGonagle, D.; McDermott, M.F. A proposed classification of the immunological diseases. *PLoS Med.* **2006**, *3*, e297. [CrossRef]
2. Pan, L.; Lu, M.P.; Wang, J.H. Immunological pathogenesis and treatment of systemic lupus erythematosus. *World J. Pediatrics* **2019**, *22*, 1–22. [CrossRef] [PubMed]
3. Denton, C.P.; Khanna, D. Systemic sclerosis. *Lancet* **2017**, *390*, 1685–1699. [CrossRef]
4. López-Medina, C.; Moltó, A. Update on the epidemiology, risk factors, and disease outcomes of axial spondyloarthritis. *Best Pract. Res. Clin. Rheumatol.* **2018**, *32*, 241–253. [CrossRef] [PubMed]
5. Generali, E.; Bose, T. Nature versus nurture in the spectrum of rheumatic diseases: Classification of spondyloarthritis as autoimmune or autoinflammatory. *Autoimm. Rev.* **2018**, *7*, 95–941. [CrossRef] [PubMed]
6. Cagliani, J.; Grande, D. Immunomodulation by mesenchymal stromal cells and their clinical application. *J Stem Cell Regen. Biol.* **2017**, *3*. [CrossRef]
7. Maumus, M.; Jorgensen, C. Mesenchymal stem cells in regenerative medicine applied to rheumatic diseases: Role of secretome and exosomes. *Biochimie* **2013**, *95*, 2229–2234. [CrossRef]
8. Klinker, M.W.; Wei, C.-H. Mesenchymal stem cells in the treatment of inflammatory and autoimmune diseases in experimental animal models. *World J. Stem Cells* **2015**, *7*, 556–567. [CrossRef]
9. Cao, W.; Cao, K.; Cao, J.; Wang, Y.; Shi, Y. Mesenchymal stem cells and adaptive immune response. *Immunol. Lett.* **2015**, *168*, 147–153. [CrossRef]
10. Marie, A.T.J.; Maumus, M. Adipose-derived mesenchymal stem cells in autoimmune disorders: State of art and perspectives for systemic sclerosis. *Clin. Rev. Allergy Immunol.* **2017**, *52*, 234–259. [CrossRef]
11. Gao, L.; Slack, M. Cell senescence in lupus. *Curr. Rheumatol. Rep.* **2019**, *21*. [CrossRef] [PubMed]
12. Zhu, Y.; Feng, X. Genetic contribution to mesenchymal stem cell dysfunction in systemic lupus erythematosus. *Stem Cell Res.* **2018**, *9*, 149. [CrossRef] [PubMed]
13. Cipriani, P.; Marrelli, A. Scleroderma mesenchymal stem cells display a different phenotype from healthy controls; implication for regenerative medicine. *Angiogenesis* **2013**, *16*, 595–607. [CrossRef] [PubMed]
14. Krajewska-Włodarczyk, M.; Owczarczyk-Saczonek, A. Role of stem cells in pathophysiology and therapy of spondyloarthropathies – new therapeutic possibilities? *Int. J. Mol. Sci.* **2018**, *19*, 80. [CrossRef]
15. Wu, Y.; Ren, M. Reduced immunomodulation potential of bone marrow-derived mesenchymal stem cells induced CCR4+CCR6+ Th/Treg cell subset imbalance in ankylosing spondylitis. *Arthritis Res.* **2011**, *13*, R29. [CrossRef]
16. Xie, Z.; Wang, P. Imbalance between bone morphogenic protein 2 and noggin induces abnormal osteogenic differentiation of mesenchymal stem cells in ankylosing spondylitis. *Arthritis Rheum* **2016**, *68*, 430–440. [CrossRef]
17. Le Blanc, K.; Tammik, C. HLA expression and immunologic properties of differentiated and undifferentiated mesenchymal stem cells. *Exp. Hematol.* **2003**, *31*, 890–896. [CrossRef]
18. Schu, S.; Nosov, M. Immunogenicity of allogeneic mesenchymal stem cells. *J. Cell. Mol. Med.* **2012**, *16*, 2094–2103. [CrossRef]

19. Berglund, A.K.; Fortier, L.A. Immunoprivileged no more: Measuring the immunogenicity of allogenic adult mesenchymal stem cells. *Stem Cell Res.* **2017**, *8*, 288. [CrossRef]
20. Hass, R.; Kasper, C. Different populations and sources of human mesenchymal stem cells (MSC): A comparison of adult and neonatal tissue-derived MSC. *Cell Commun. Sign* **2011**, *9*, 12. [CrossRef]
21. Li, C.; Wu, X. Comparative analysis of human mesenchymal stem cells from bone marrow and adipose tissue under xeno-free conditions for cell therapy. *Stem Cell Res Ther.* **2015**, *6*, 55. [CrossRef] [PubMed]
22. U.S. National Library of Medicine. Available online: https://clinicaltrials.gov/ (accessed on 14 December 2019).
23. Scuderi, N.; Ceccarelli, S.; Onest, M.G.; Fioramonti, P.; Guidi, C.; Romano, F.; Frati, L.; Angeloni, A.; Marchese, C. Human adipose-derived stromal cells for cell-based therapies in the treatment of systemic sclerosis. *Cell Transpl.* **2013**, *22*, 779–795. [CrossRef] [PubMed]
24. Onest, M.G.; Fioramonti, P.; Carella, S.; Fino, P.; Marchese, C.; Scuderi, N. Improvement of mouth functional disability in systemic sclerosis patients over one year in a trial of fat transplantation versus adipose-derived stromal cells. *Stem Cells Int.* **2016**, *2016*, 2416192. [CrossRef] [PubMed]
25. Rozier, P.; Maria, A.; Goulabchand, R.; Jorgensen, C.; Guilpain, P.; Noël, D. Mesenchymal stem cells in systemic sclerosis: Allogenic or autologous approaches for therapeutic use? *Front. Immunol.* **2018**, *9*, 2938. [CrossRef]
26. Manetti, M.; Romano, E.; Rosa, I.; Fioretto, B.S.; Praino, E.; Guiducci, S.; Iannone, F.; Ibba-Manneschi, L.; Matucci-Cerinic, M. Systemic sclerosis serum steers the differentiation of adipose-derived stem cells toward profibrotic myofibroblasts: Pathophysiologic implications. *J. Clin. Med.* **2019**, *8*, 1256. [CrossRef]
27. Lee, R.; Del Papa, N.; Introna, M.; Reese, C.F.; Zemskova, M.; Bonner, M.; Carmen-Lopez, G.; Helke, K.; Hoffman, S.; Tourkina, E. Adipose-derived mesenchymal stromal/stem cells in systemic sclerosis: Alterations in function and beneficial effect on lung fibrosis are regulated by caveolin-1. *J. Scleroderma Relat. Disord.* **2019**, *4*, 127–136. [CrossRef]
28. Perti, M.; Orbai, A.M. Derivation and validation of the Systemic Lupus International Collaborating Clinics classification criteria for systemic lupus erythematosus. *Arthritis Rheum.* **2012**, *64*, 2677–2686.
29. Van den Hoogen, F.; Khanna, D. 2013 classification criteria for systemic sclerosis: An American College of Rheumatology/European League against Rheumatism collaborative initiative. *Arthritis Rheum.* **2013**, *65*, 2737–2747. [CrossRef]
30. Rudwaleit, M.; van der Heijde, D. The development of ASSessment of SpondyloArthritis international Society classification criteria for axial spoandyloarthritis (part II): Validation and final selection. *Ann. Rheum. Dis.* **2009**, *68*, 777–783. [CrossRef]
31. Skalska, U.; Kontny, E. Intra-articular adipose-derived mesenchymal stem cells from rheumatoid arthritis patients maintain the function of chondrogenic differentiation. *Rheumatology* **2012**, *51*, 1757–1764. [CrossRef]
32. Van Buul, G.M.; Villafuertes, E. Mesenchymal stem cells secrete factors that inhibit inflammatory processes in short-term osteoarthritic synovium and cartilage explants culture. *Osteoartrhritis Cartil.* **2012**, *20*, 1186–1196. [CrossRef] [PubMed]
33. Bourin, P.; Bunnell, B.A. Stromal cells from the adipose tissue-derived stromal vascular fraction and culture expanded adipose tissue-derived stromal/stem cells: A joint statement of the International Federation for Adipose Therapeutics (IFATS) and Science and the International Society for Cellular Therapy (ISCT). *Cytotherapy* **2013**, *15*, 641–648. [PubMed]
34. Baer, P.C.; Kuçi, S.; Krause, M.; Kuçi, Z.; Zielen, S.; Geiger, H.; Bader, P.; Schubert, R. Comprehensive phenotypic characterization of human adipose-derived stromal/stem cells and their subsets by a high throughput technology. *Stem Cells Dev.* **2013**, *22*, 330–339. [CrossRef] [PubMed]
35. Dubey, N.K.; Mishra, V.K. Revisiting the advances in isolation, characterization and secretome of adipose-derived stromal/stem cells. *Int. J. Mol. Sci.* **2018**, *19*, 2200. [CrossRef] [PubMed]
36. Nie, Y.; Lau, G.S. Defective phenotype of mesenchymal stem cells in patients with systemic lupus erythematosus. *Lupus* **2010**, *19*, 850–859. [CrossRef]
37. Capelli, C.; Zaccara, E. Phenotypical and functional characteristics of in vitro-expanded adipose-derived mesenchymal stromal cells from patients with systemic sclerosis. *Cell Transpl.* **2017**, *26*, 841–854. [CrossRef]
38. Liu, Z.; Gao, Z. TNF-α induced the enhanced apoptosis of mesenchymal stem cells in ankylosing spondylitis by overexpressing TRAIL-R2. *Stem Cells Int.* **2017**, 4521324. [CrossRef]
39. Rege, T.A.; Hagood, J.S. Thy-1, a versatile modulator of signalling affecting cellular adhesion, proliferation, survival, and cytokine/growth factor responses. *Biochim. Biophys. Acta* **2006**, *1763*, 991–999. [CrossRef]

40. Saalbach, A.; Anderegg, U. Thy-1: More than a marker for mesenchymal stromal cells. *FASEB J.* **2019**, *33*, 6689–6696. [CrossRef]
41. Campioni, D.; Rizzo, R. A decreased positivity for CD90 on human mesenchymal stromal cells (MSCs) is associated with a loss of immunosuppressive activity by MSCs. *Cytom. B Clin. Cytom.* **2009**, *76*, 225–230. [CrossRef]
42. Ren, G.; Roberts, A.I. Adhesion molecules. Key players in mesenchymal stem cell-mediated immunosuppression. *Cell Adhes. Migr.* **2011**, *50*, 20–22. [CrossRef] [PubMed]
43. Rubtsov, Y.; Goryunov, K. Molecular mechanisms of immunomodulation properties of mesenchymal stromal cells: A new insight into the role of ICAM-1. *Stem Cells Int.* **2017**, 6516854. [CrossRef] [PubMed]
44. Jones, S.P.; Guillemin, G.J. The kynurenine pathway in stem cell biology. *Int. J. Tryptophan Res.* **2013**, *6*, 57–66. [CrossRef] [PubMed]
45. De Oliveira, F.L.; Gatto, M. Galectin-3 in autoimmunity and autoimmune diseases. *Exp. Biol. Med.* **2015**, *240*, 1019–1028. [CrossRef] [PubMed]
46. Liu, G.Y.; Xu, Y.; Li, Y. Secreted galectin-3 as a possible biomarker for the immunomodulatory potential of human umbilical cord mesenchymal stromal cells. *Cytotherapy* **2013**, *15*, 1208–1217. [CrossRef] [PubMed]
47. Sioud, M. New insights into mesenchymal stromal cell-mediated T-cell suppression through galectins. *Scand. J. Immunol.* **2011**, *73*, 79–84. [CrossRef]
48. Luz-Crawford, P.; Djouad, F. Mesenchymal stem cell-derived interleukin 1 receptor antagonist promotes macrophage polarization and inhibits B cell differentiation. *Stem Cells* **2016**, *34*, 483–492. [CrossRef]
49. Lee, K.; Park, N. Mesenchymal stem cells ameliorate experimental arthritis via expression of interleukin-1 receptor antagonist. *PLoS ONE* **2018**, *13*, e0193086. [CrossRef]
50. Rebmann, V.; König, L. The potential of HLA-G-bearing extracellular vesicles as a future element in HLA-G immune biology. *Front. Immunol.* **2016**, *7*, 173. [CrossRef]
51. Day, A.J.; Milner, C.M. TSG-6: A multifunctional protein with anti-inflammatory and tissue-protective properties. *Matrix Biol.* **2019**, *78*, 60–83. [CrossRef]
52. Fontaine, M.J.; Shih, H. Unraveling the mesenchymal stromal cells' paracrine immunomodulatory effects. *Transfus. Med. Rev.* **2016**, *30*, 37–43. [CrossRef] [PubMed]
53. Manferdini, C.; Paolella, F. Adipose stromal cells mediated switching of the pro-inflammatory profile of M1-like macrophages is facilitated by PGE_2: In vitro evaluation. *Osteoarthr. Cartil.* **2017**, *25*, 1161–1171. [CrossRef] [PubMed]
54. Philipp, D.; Shur, L. Preconditioning of bone marrow-derived mesenchymal stem cells highly strengthens their potential to promote IL-6-dependent M2b polarization. *Stem Cell Res. Ther.* **2018**, *9*, 286. [CrossRef] [PubMed]
55. Chen, C.; Liang, J. Mesenchymal stem cells upregulate Treg cells via sHLA-G in SLE patients. *Int. Immunopharmacol.* **2017**, *44*, 234–241. [CrossRef] [PubMed]
56. Wang, D.; Huang, S. The regulation of the Treg/Th17 balance by mesenchymal stem cells in human systemic lupus erythematosus. *Cell Mol. Immunol.* **2017**, *14*, 423–431. [CrossRef]
57. Palumbo, P.; Lombardi, F.; Siragusa, G.; Cifone, M.G.; Cinque, B.; Giuliani, M. Methods of isolation, characterization and expansion of human adipose-derived stem cells (ASCs): An overview. *Int. J. Mol. Sci.* **2018**, *19*, 1897. [CrossRef]

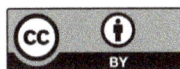

© 2019 by the authors. Licensee MDPI, Basel, Switzerland. This article is an open access article distributed under the terms and conditions of the Creative Commons Attribution (CC BY) license (http://creativecommons.org/licenses/by/4.0/).

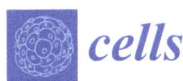

Article

Natural Histogel-Based Bio-Scaffolds for Sustaining Angiogenesis in Beige Adipose Tissue

Margherita Di Somma [1,†], Wandert Schaafsma [2,†], Elisabetta Grillo [1], Maria Vliora [1,3], Eleni Dakou [4], Michela Corsini [1], Cosetta Ravelli [1], Roberto Ronca [1], Paraskevi Sakellariou [3], Jef Vanparijs [5], Begona Castro [2] and Stefania Mitola [1,*]

1. Department of Molecular and Translational Medicine, University of Brescia, 25121 Brescia, Italy; m.disomma88@gmail.com (M.D.S.); elisabetta.grillo@unibs.it (E.G.); mvliora@gmail.com (M.V.); michela.corsini@unibs.it (M.C.); cosetta.ravelli@unibs.it (C.R.); roberto.ronca@unibs.it (R.R.)
2. Histocell, S.L.Parque Tecnológico 801A, 2o 48160 Derio—BIZKAIA, Spain; wandertschaafsma@gmail.com (W.S.); bcastro@histocell.com (B.C.)
3. FAME Laboratory, Department of Exercise Science, University of Thessaly, 38221 Trikala, Greece; sakellariou.elvina@gmail.com
4. Laboratory of Cell Genetics, Department of Biology, Faculty of Science and Bioengineering Sciences, Vrije Universiteit Brussel, 1050 Brussels, Belgium; Eleni.Dakou@vub.be
5. Department of Human Physiology, Faculty of Physical Education and Physical Therapy, Vrije Universiteit Brussel, 1050 Brussels, Belgium; Jef.Vanparijs@vub.be
* Correspondence: stefania.mitola@unibs.it
† Equally contributed.

Received: 28 October 2019; Accepted: 13 November 2019; Published: 18 November 2019

Abstract: In the treatment of obesity and its related disorders, one of the measures adopted is weight reduction by controlling nutrition and increasing physical activity. A valid alternative to restore the physiological function of the human body could be the increase of energy consumption by inducing the browning of adipose tissue. To this purpose, we tested the ability of Histogel, a natural mixture of glycosaminoglycans isolated from animal Wharton jelly, to sustain the differentiation of adipose derived mesenchymal cells (ADSCs) into brown-like cells expressing UCP-1. Differentiated cells show a higher energy metabolism compared to undifferentiated mesenchymal cells. Furthermore, Histogel acts as a pro-angiogenic matrix, induces endothelial cell proliferation and sprouting in a three-dimensional gel in vitro, and stimulates neovascularization when applied in vivo on top of the chicken embryo chorioallantoic membrane or injected subcutaneously in mice. In addition to the pro-angiogenic activity of Histogel, also the ADSC derived beige cells contribute to activating endothelial cells. These data led us to propose Histogel as a promising scaffold for the modulation of the thermogenic behavior of adipose tissue. Indeed, Histogel simultaneously supports the acquisition of brown tissue markers and activates the vasculature process necessary for the correct function of the thermogenic tissue. Thus, Histogel represents a valid candidate for the development of bioscaffolds to increase the amount of brown adipose tissue in patients with metabolic disorders.

Keywords: angiogenesis; adipose derived mesenchymal cells; Histogel

1. Introduction

Obesity represents a major health problem associated with increased mortality and co-morbidities, including many metabolic diseases [1]. Obesity is characterized by an increase in adipose mass due to increased energy intake, decreased energy expenditure, or both. Several elements including lifestyle, environmental, neuro-psychological, genetic, and epigenetic factors contribute to increase the energy intake (calories) and to reduce the energy expenditure (metabolic and physical activity). The treatment options for patients with severe obesity are the modification of lifestyle, limiting the intake of total fats and sugars, increasing consumption of fruits, vegetables, and whole grains and practicing regular physical activity or pharmacological treatments currently available in the market, which are commonly associated with severe side effects. Indeed, increased risk of psychiatric disorders and non-fatal myocardial infarction or stroke have been described in pharmacologically treated patients [2–4]. In the treatment of obesity, only 1% of patients receive bariatric surgery despite its safety and the better outcomes achieved [5]. Therefore, several groups are working on the development of different and new therapeutic approaches [3]. The increase of energy consumption through the increase of metabolism and thermogenesis of the adipose tissue may be a valid alternative [6].

Adipose tissue (AT) contains adipocytes and pre-adipocytes surrounded by stromal cells (fibroblasts, endothelial cells, macrophages), which make the adipose tissue the most plastic organ in the human body. AT is the major organ that controls the overall energy homeostasis in a living organism, storing the superabundant nutrients in the form of triglycerides, and suppling the nutrients to other tissues through lipolysis [7]. Two different types of adipose tissue have been described in mammalians. White adipose tissue (WAT) stores energy, while brown adipose tissue (BAT) is specialized for energy expenditure. The cellular structure of these tissues well reflects their biological functions: WAT contains adipocytes with a single large lipid droplet and few mitochondria, while BAT cells are characterized by the presence of several small lipid droplets and many mitochondria expressing uncoupling proteins (UCPs). UCP-1 contributes to energy loss as heat; in particular, it controls the dissipation as heat of the proton gradient produced by the mitochondria respiration chain. In humans, BAT mass declines with age, and it is less active in obese patients. The adipose tissue (AT) can be considered an endocrine organ, as both WAT and BAT secrete many cytokines, hormones, and adipokines. Recently, an additional/intermediate AT cell type termed "beige" has been described. Beige adipocytes sporadically reside with white adipocytes and emerge in response to certain environmental cues [8]. Under specific stimuli, beige adipocytes can exert BAT-like or WAT-like functions. Although beige adipocytes express a low level of UCP-1, they retain a remarkable ability to activate the expression of this gene powerfully and to turn on a robust program of respiration and energy expenditure that is equivalent to that of classical brown fat cells [8,9]. These cells represent a cellular mechanism to provide flexibility in adaptive thermogenesis and metabolism. Thus, the possibility to generate and control the amount of beige adipocytes may represent an alternative therapy for obese patients.

Blood vessels play a key role in the regulation of AT behavior. AT is the most plastic organ in the human body, subjected to continuous expansion and regression. This plasticity requires constant growth, regression, and remodeling of blood vessels, under the control of several metabolites secreted by AT itself. The adipose vasculature supports AT in multiple manners. The vascular network provides nutrients and oxygen, which are essential for tissue maintenance, and removes metabolic products of AT. Moreover, it exports the AT derived growth factors, adipokines, and cytokines from AT to body tissues, regulating physiological functions via an endocrine mechanism [10]. Furthermore, similar to mesenchymal cells [11], the adipocyte precursor cells within WAT and BAT express VEGF-A, promoting the angiogenic process and endotheliogenesis through VEGFR2 signaling [12].

Tissue engineering represents an interdisciplinary approach to regenerate damaged tissues, instead of replacing them, by developing biological substitutes that improve or restore tissue functions. Tissue engineering can help to boost human metabolism through the integration of cell biology and biomaterial sciences [13]. With particular attention to adipose tissue, tissue engineering is a promising approach to improve energy balance and metabolic homeostasis controlling the amount of beige cells [14,15]. Several biological or synthetic scaffolds have been developed to support and/or promote tissue regeneration or organ repair [16–20]. All the scaffolds share some characteristics including biocompatibility, neglectable immunoreactivity, and suitability for cell growth. Furthermore, scaffolds should be biodegradable, and their derivates should not be toxic to the body.

Here, we tested the ability of a novel bioscaffold able to promote both the differentiation of mesenchymal cells into beige adipose tissue and to sustain the angiogenic process. The Histogel-alginate scaffold promotes adipose tissue derived stem cell (ADSC) differentiation into adipocytes expressing PPARγ, PdK4, and UCP1 proteins supporting vessel recruitment and growth. Our results suggest that Histogel based scaffolds may represent good candidates for the development of scaffolds aimed at regulating energy expenditure in obese patients.

2. Materials and Methods

2.1. Hyaluronan Analysis

Commercial low, high molecular weight HA was electrophoretically analyzed on 1% agarose gel and stained with Stains-All solution HA (25 mg in 500 mL ethanol:water 50:50) overnight in the dark. Then, agarose gels were de-stained with water. The same protocol was used to explore the amount and the molecular weight of HA in Histogel preparations.

2.2. Cell Cultures and Differentiation

ADSCs were isolated from lipoaspirate (Histocell, Spain, in compliance with Certification of Laboratory 4269-E for the manufacture of research drugs (cell therapy products), Spanish Agency of Drugs and Medical Devices (Agencia Española de Medicamentos y Productos Sanitarios, AEMPS) and were cultured in DMEM, complemented with Glutamax, penicillin/streptomycin, 10% FBS, and gentamicin sulfate (identified as basal medium). ADSCs were differentiated for 15 days in basal medium in the presence of 20 nM insulin (Sigma, St. Louis, MO, USA), 5 μM dexamethasone (Sigma), 125 μM indomethacin (Sigma), 1 nM triiodothyronine (T3) and 0.5 mM 3-isobutyl-1-methylxanthine (IBMX). Lipid vesicles formed starting from Day 6 of differentiation [21]. Human umbilical vein endothelial cells (HUVECs) were isolated from umbilical cords from healthy informed volunteers and used at early passages (I–IV). Cells were grown on culture plates coated with Porcine Gelatin Type I, in M199 medium supplemented with 20% FCS, endothelial cell growth factor (10 μg/mL), and porcine heparin (100 μg/mL) [22].

2.3. Identification of Angiogenic Factors

Pro- and anti-angiogenic molecules released by ADSCs and ADSC derived beige cells were analyzed using the Human Angiogenesis Antibody Array (R&D System) according to the manufacturer's instructions.

2.4. Quantitative RT-PCR

The expression of brown adipocyte markers was analyzed by RT-PCR. Briefly, total RNA was isolated using TRIzol reagent (Invitrogen, Carlsbad, CA, USA) according to the manufacturer's instructions from 3 independent differentiation experiments. Two micrograms of total RNA were retro-transcribed with M-MLV reverse transcriptase (Invitrogen, Carlsbad, CA, USA) using random hexaprimers in a final 20 μL volume. Quantitative RT-PCR was performed using the iTaq™ Universal SYBR® Green Supermix (Bio-Rad, Hercules, CA, USA). Each PCR reaction was performed in triplicate on one plate, and fluorescence data were recorded using a Viia7 Real Time PCR System (Thermo Fisher Scientific, Waltham, MA, USA). Relative expression ratios were calculated by the Relative Expression Software Tool. The mRNA expression levels of target genes were normalized to the level of GAPDH transcript.

The following specific primers were used: Hs UCP1_Fw CGCAGGGAAAGAAACAGCAC; Hs UCP1_Rv TTCACGACCTCTGTGGGTTG; HsPdk4_FwATTTAAGAATGCAATGCGGGC; HsPdk 4_RvACACCACCTCCTCTGTCTGA; Hs PPARγ_Fw CCGTGGCCGCAGAAATGA; Hs PPARγ_Rv TGATCCCAAAGTTGGTGGGC; MmCD31 FwAAGCCAAGGCCAAACAGA; Mm_CD31_Rv GGGTT TTACTGCATCATTTCC; Mm_CD45_Fw TATCGCGGTGTAAAACTCGTCAA; Mm_CD45

_Rv GCTCAGGCCAAGAGACTAACGTT; Hs GAPDH_Fw GAAGGTCGGAGTCAACGGATT; Hs_ GAPDH_Rv TGACGGTGCCATGGAATTTG.

2.5. Mitochondrial Activity

Mitochondrial activity was monitored with Seahorse XFe24 instrument technology analysis. Oxygen consumption rate (OCR) (pmol/minute) was monitored over time before and after sequential injection of oligomycin (100 μM), carbonyl cyanide p-trifluoromethoxy-phenylhydrazone (FCCP, 100 μM), and rotenone/antimycin A (50 μM) inhibitors (which inhibit ATPase, the proton gradient, and complex I/III, respectively). Thus, ATP-linked respiration and maximal respiration were measured. Extracellular acidification rate (ECAR; mpH/minute) was also measured to observe glycolytic capability. The colorimetric 3-(4,5-dimethylthiazol-2-yl)-2,5-diphenyltetrazolium bromide (MTT) test was used to analyze the effect of isoproterenol and norepinephrine on the metabolic activity of cells, using the reducing ability of ubiquinone and CyrC and B of the mitochondrial electron transport system. For this, differentiated ADSCs were treated with 10 μM isoproterenol or 1 mM norepinephrine for 24 h. Then, cells were incubated in the presence of 0.2 mg/mL of MTT substrate for 1 h. The amount of metabolized formazan was measured by recording absorbance at 570 nm using a plate reader spectrophotometer (ELx-800 Bio-Tec Instrument).

2.6. EC Sprouting Assay

The collagen gel invasion assay was performed on HUVEC spheroids [23]. Briefly, spheroids were prepared in 20% methylcellulose medium, embedded in collagen gel or collagen gel:Histogel (1:5) in the absence or in the presence of ADSCs or differentiated cells. The formation of radially growing cell sprouts was observed during the next 24 h. Sprouts were counted and photographed using an Axiovert 200M microscope equipped with an LD A PLAN 20X/0,30PH1 objective (Carl Zeiss, Oberkochen, Germany).

2.7. In Vitro Angiogenesis Assay

Wells of μ-Slide Angiogenesis chambers (Ibidi, Martine Marne, Germany) were coated with a 0.8 mm thick layer of gel matrix by adding 10 μL of Cultrex Reduced Growth Factor Basement Membrane Matrix. After gel polymerization, 5000 HUVECs were seeded in M199 added with 5% FCS and treated with conditioned medium of undifferentiated or differentiated ADSCs. Cell viability was confirmed using calcein-AM. In live cells, the non-fluorescent calcein-AM is converted into green-fluorescent calcein. Calcein-AM is a permeant dye. After 5 h, samples were photographed using an inverted Axiovert 200 M epifluorescence microscope equipped with an LD A PLAN 20X/0,30PH1 objective (Carl Zeiss, Oberkochen, Germany). Images were analyzed using ImageJ software with the Angiogenesis plugin to detect total closed structures [24].

2.8. Immunofluorescence Analysis

Cells were seeded on glass coverslips and fixed in 4.0% paraformaldehyde (PFA)/2.0% sucrose in PBS, permeabilized with 0.5% Triton-X100, and saturated with goat serum in PBS. Then, cells were incubated with UCP-1 (sc-6529, SantaCruz, CA, USA), PPARγ (sc-7273, SantaCruz), and ACRP30 (sc-26497, SantaCruz) antibodies. Cells were analyzed using a Zeiss Axiovert 200M epifluorescence microscope equipped with a Plan-Apochromat 63X/1.4 NA oil objective.

2.9. CAM Assay

Alginate beads containing PBS, or 100 ng of recombinant human VEGF-A, or 5% of Histogel, or 30,000 cells were placed on the chicken chorioallantoic membrane (CAM) of fertilized white Leghorn chicken eggs at Day 11 of incubation [25]. After 72 h, newly formed blood vessels converging toward the implant were counted at 5× magnification using an STEMI SR stereo-microscope equipped with an objective f of 100 mm with adapter ring 475,070 (Zeiss, Oberkochen, Germany).

2.10. Murine Angiogenic Assay

All the procedures involving mice and their care conformed to institutional guidelines that complied with national and international laws and policies (EEC Council Directive 86/609, OJ L 358, 12 December 1987). Seven-week-old C57BL/6 mice (Charles River Laboratories International, Inc., Wilmington, MA, USA) were injected subcutaneously with 400 µL of 5% alginic acid (Sigma) containing PBS or 500 ng of VEGF-A, in the absence or in the presence of 5% Histogel solution. One week after injection, mice were sacrificed, and plugs were harvested and processed for RT-qPCR as previously described [26]. The mRNA expression levels of murine CD31 and CD45 were normalized to the levels of human GAPDH. Data are expressed as relative expression ratios ($\Delta\Delta Ct$—fold increase) using one PBS plug as the reference.

2.11. Data Representation and Statistical Analyses

Data are expressed as the mean ± SEM. Statistical analyses were performed using one-way ANOVA followed by Bonferroni's test or Student's *t*-test. The indicated *p*-value was set as statistically significant.

3. Results

3.1. Histogel Is a Pro-Angiogenic Bio-Scaffold

Histogel is a natural mixture of glycosaminoglycans including, among others, high grade hyaluronic acid (HA) and chondroitin sulfate obtained from the Wharton jelly found in umbilical cords of animal origin [20]. Histogel modulates inflammation, induces the release of extracellular matrices (ECM), and supports cell recruitment and growth [20]. On these bases, Histogel represents a suitable scaffold to drive cell differentiation. Since hyaluronan is a mix of molecules with different masses and the molecular weight confers different biological properties to hyaluronan preparations, a first set of experiments was performed to compare the amount and the molecular weight of hyaluronan contained in different Histogel preparations. Two different Histogel preparations were analyzed, pre-autoclaved (p.a.) or not, on agarose gel, and stained with Stains-All reagent. The amount of HA was similar in both analyzed batches, and it was around 76–80%. Moreover, the ratio between high and low molecular weight molecules remained approximately constant. Of note, this ratio is not affected by the autoclave sterilization cycles used for the preparation of 5% Histogel working dilutions (Figure 1a). Next, we tested the proangiogenic activity of Histogel preparation in several in vitro angiogenesis assays. Angiogenesis is a multistep process starting with the activation of endothelial cells (ECs) and the degradation of ECM of the basal membrane. Then, ECs invade the surrounding tissue, proliferate, and reorganize themselves in capillary-like structures. Among the variety of in vitro, ex vivo, and in vivo assays that mimic the individual aspects of the angiogenic cascade, in vitro models of angiogenesis represent cost effective and rapid tools for testing angiogenic compounds. In particular, the use of 3D culture techniques able to recapitulate all steps of endothelial capillary sprout formation may serve as an effective strategy for these purposes. 3D endothelial cell spheroids were embedded in collagen or collagen:5% Histogel (1:1 ratio) gels. VEGF-A was used as the positive control and as the reference for the angiogenic activity. Figure 1b shows that, in keeping with the pro-angiogenic activity of commercial high molecular weight HA (Figure A1a,b), Histogel stimulates the formation of endothelial cell sprouts from aggregates of HUVEC cells embedded in a 3D gel. To assess the in vivo pro-angiogenic activity, Histogel loaded alginate beads were implanted onto the chicken embryo CAMs at 11 days of development. After 72 h, a robust angiogenic response was observed around the Histogel implants when compared to alginate or VEGF engrafted embryos (Figure 1c). The number of vessels converging towards the pellets was equal to 7.4 ± 0.6, 33.1 ± 1.0, and 58.3 ± 9.1 for alginate, VEGF, and Histogel implants, respectively. In keeping with these observations, Histogel modulates the recruitment of CD45$^+$ cells and the consequent pro-angiogenic response when injected subcutaneously in mice (Figure 1d). All these data suggest that Histogel is endowed with stronger pro-angiogenic activity if compared to VEGF-A. The pro-angiogenic ability of Histogel makes it a suitable candidate for the development of a bioscaffold for BAT differentiation.

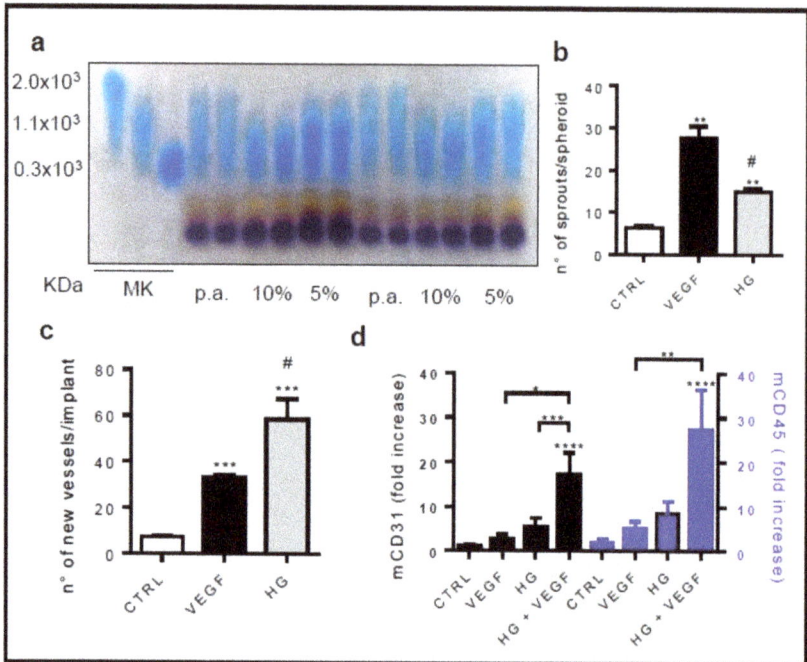

Figure 1. Histogel modulates the angiogenic response. (**a**) Five percent and 10% of two different Histogel preparations were electrophoretically analyzed on agarose gel and stained with Stains-All solution. p.a., pre-autoclaved. Three different standard molecules (2×10^3, 1.1×10^3, 300 kDa) were used as markers of molecular weight (MK). (**b**) HUVEC spheroids were embedded in collagen or in collagen:5% Histogel 1:1 (HG) gels. Fifty nanograms per milliliter of VEGFA$_{165}$ were used as the positive control. The formation of radially growing sprouts was evaluated after 24 h of incubation. Data are the mean ± SEM of three independent experiments (** $p < 0.001$ vs. CTRL; # $p < 0.001$ vs. VEGF, one-way ANOVA followed by Bonferroni's test versus the control). (**c**) Alginate beads containing vehicle, or 100 ng of VEGFA$_{165}$, or 5% Histogel (v/v 1:1) were implanted on the top of chick embryo chorioallantoic membrane (CAM) at Day 11 of development. After 72 h, newly formed blood vessels converging toward the implant were counted in ovo at 5× magnification using an STEMI SR stereomicroscope equipped with an objective f equal to 100 mm with adapter ring 475,070 (Carl Zeiss). Data are the mean ± SEM (n = 6–8) (*** $p < 0.0001$ vs. control; # $p < 0.0001$ vs. VEGF, one-way ANOVA followed by Bonferroni's test versus the control). (**d**) Five percent of liquid alginic acid was mixed with 1.0 μg/mL VEGFA$_{165}$ in the absence or in the presence of v/v 1:1 of 5% Histogel and injected subcutaneously into the flank of C57BL/6 mice. Plugs with vehicle alone were used as negative controls (CTRL). One week after injection, plugs were harvested. CD31 and CD45 mRNA expression levels were measured by RT-qPCR. Data are the mean ± SEM (n = 10) and are expressed as relative expression ratios (ΔΔCt – fold increase) using one vehicle plug as the reference. * $p < 0.05$; ** $p < 0.01$; *** $p < 0.005$; **** $p < 0.001$, one-way ANOVA followed by Bonferroni's test versus the control.

3.2. ADSCs Differentiate in Beige Adipocytes

Several protocols for ADSCs' differentiation were tested. ADSCs were maintained for 15 days in commercial specific media (such as StemMACS AdipoDiff Media from Milteny Biotec), or in DMEM supplemented with hBMP7, or supplemented with adipo-growth factors and analyzed for the expression of adipocyte markers including PPARγ, AdipoR, Prdm16, UCP-1, and Pdk4 (Figure A2). Among all the tested conditions, the custom medium was found to be the most promising in terms of expression of brown tissue markers. Thus, in all the experiments listed below, confluent ADSCs were cultured for 15 days in basal medium complemented with insulin and dexamethasone to stimulate adipogenic differentiation, indomethacin, and 3-isobutyl-1-methylxanthine (IBMX) to modulate the expression of the PPARγ receptor and with triiodothyronine (T3) to increase UCP-1 expression. Figure 2a shows the morphological changes occurring in ADSCs upon differentiation. A clear sign of differentiation was the presence of small lipid droplets in differentiated ADSCs' cytoplasm. Immunofluorescence and RT-PCR analyses for the expression of PPARγ, ACRP30, UCP-1, and PdK4 confirmed that ADSCs acquired brown cell molecular markers during the differentiation protocol (Figure 2b–d). Finally, we tested the metabolic activity of differentiated ADSCs using the Seahorse Cell Mito Stress Test. Although the basal oxygen consumption (OCR) of undifferentiated and differentiated ADSC seemed to be very similar, the maximal mitochondrial activity was significantly increased in differentiated ADSCs as demonstrated by the higher oxygen consumption measured by treating cells with the uncoupling agent FCCP. Furthermore, extracellular acidification increased in differentiated ADSCs compared to control ADSCs (Figure 2e,f). These data were confirmed by the ability of norepinephrine and isoproterenol to positively modulate the mitochondrial activity (Figure 2g) of differentiated ADSCs. Taken together, our results confirm that our protocol was suitable to drive ADSCs differentiation into ADSC derived beige cells.

3.3. ADSCs-Derived Beige Cells Show Pro-Angiogenic Properties

It is well known that mesenchymal stem cells support vessel recruitment and growth by producing and releasing several growth factors and chemokines. To assess whether ADSC derived beige cells maintain this pro-angiogenic activity, we evaluated their capacity to activate HUVECs in different angiogenic assays. To this, conditioned mediums were collected from ADSCs or ADSC derived beige cells cultured in basal medium for 48 h and tested in the tube formation assay. The conditioned medium of ADSC derived beige cells accelerated the morphogenesis of HUVE cells as demonstrated by the higher number of closed structures formed in 18 h compared to that induced by the conditioned medium of undifferentiated ADSCs (Figure 3a). Of note, VEGF-A, used as a positive control, exerted a pro-angiogenic effect, comparable to the one of the conditioned medium of undifferentiated ADSCs. The presence of pro-angiogenic factors in the conditioned medium of ADSC derived beige cells was confirmed by the human angiogenesis antibody array. For this, all proteins of conditioned medium were labelled with biotinylated antibodies and incubated on a spotted specific capture antibody membrane. The antibody array showed that ADSC derived beige cells continued to express and release in the extracellular environment high levels of several pro-angiogenic molecules including VEGF, FGF, PlGF, and PDGF (Figure 3b). To overcome the possible partial or total degradation of the soluble factors contained in the conditioned medium and to ensure a continuous release of soluble molecules, we set up an in vitro endothelial–ADSC co-culture system in which ADSCs were plated and differentiated for 15 days in the same well used for the co-culture. Then, 3D Cultrex gel was stratified in the well, and HUVECs were plated on it. Again, the ADSC derived beige cells accelerated the morphogenesis of HUVEC cells in terms of the number of closed structures. Of note, HUVECs cultured with undifferentiated ADSCs remained non-organized (Figure 4a,b). ADSC derived beige cells induced more sprouts from HUVEC-formed spheroids when embedded in 3D collagen gel in the co-culture system (Figure 4c,d). Importantly, in both co-culture systems, no physical interaction occurred between HUVEC and ADSCs. Furthermore, to mimic the co-culture system in an in vivo assay, ADSCs and ADSC derived beige cells were delivered on the top of the chick embryo chorioallantoic membrane

(CAM) at Day 11 of development. In agreement with the in vitro results, ADSC derived beige cells supported the recruitment of host vessels from the surrounding tissues into the cell-enriched-3D scaffold on chick embryo CAM (Figure 4e,f).

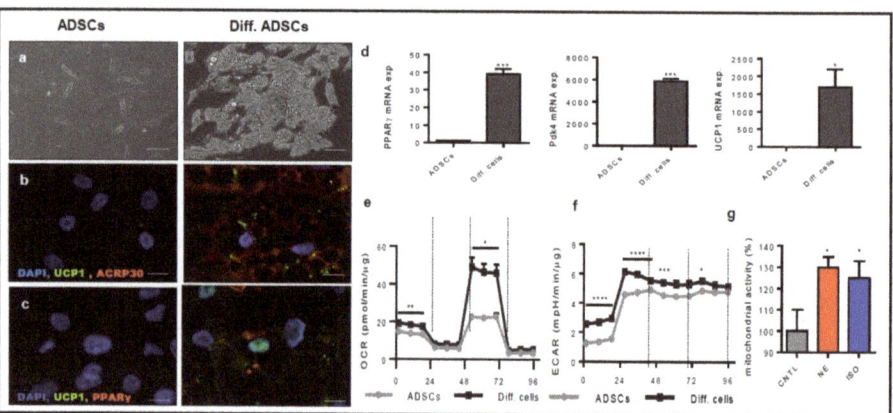

Figure 2. ADSCs differentiate into beige-like adipocytes. (**a**) The morphology of ADSCs and ADSC derived beige cells (Diff.) was analyzed at Day 15 of differentiation (Scale bar 100 μm). (**b,c**) Immunofluorescent detection of expression levels of UCP-1 (green) and ACRP30 (red) (**b**) and PPARγ (red) (**c**). Nuclei were counterstained with DAPI. (Scale bar 10 μm). (**d**) PPARγ, Pdk4, and UCP1 mRNA expression levels were measured by RT-qPCR analysis. Data are the mean ± SEM (n = 6) and are expressed as relative expression ratios (ΔΔCt – fold increase). (**e,f**) Mitochondrial energy metabolism was measured using the Agilent Seahorse Cell Mito Stress Test. The oxygen consumption rate (OCR) (**e**) and extracellular acidification rate (ECAR) (**f**) of ADSCs and ADSC derived beige cells was recorded before and after treatment with 10 μM oligomycin, 10 μM carbonyl cyanide p-trifluoromethoxy-phenylhydrazone (FCCP), and 5 μM rotenone/antimycin A. Data were analyzed according to the Agilent Seahorse XF Cell Mito Stress Test Report Generator. (**g**) Mitochondrial activity of ADSC derived beige cells was measured by the MTT test in the absence or in the presence of norepinephrine and isoproterenol. * $p < 0.05$; ** $p < 0.01$; *** $p < 0.005$; **** $p < 0.001$, one-way ANOVA followed by Bonferroni's test versus the control.

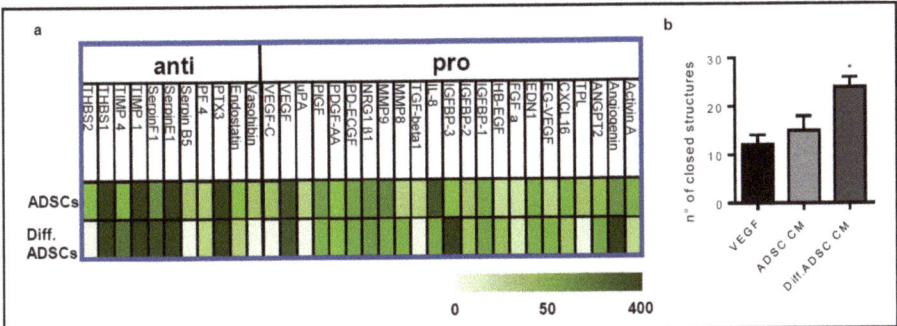

Figure 3. Conditioned medium of ADSC derived beige cells contains pro-angiogenic factors. Conditioned media were collected from confluent ADSCs and ADSC derived beige cells (Diff. ADSCs) cultured in basal medium for 48 h. (**a**) HUVEC cells (40,000 cells/cm^2) were plated on reduced growth factor Cultrex and stimulated with conditioned medium obtained from ADSCs or ADSC derived beige cells. After 5 h, endothelial cell morphogenesis in terms of the formation of closed structures was examined using ImageJ software. Data are the mean ± SEM of three measurements per sample. * $p < 0.05$, Student's t-test. (**b**) The Proteome Profiler Human Angiogenesis Antibody Array was used to detect angiogenesis related proteins in the conditioned medium of ADSCs and ADSC derived beige cells. Densitometry analysis of positive spot signals was normalized to positive and negative antibody array controls. Data are the mean of duplicate spots and expressed by color code (n = 2). Negative spots in both ADSCs and ADSC derived beige cell conditioned medium were not included in the analysis.

3.4. Histogel Supports the Pro-Angiogenic Activity of ADSC-Derived Beige Cells

Finally, we tested whether the pro-angiogenic ability of Histogel supports beige adipocyte potentiality. ADSC or ADSC derived beige cells were embedded in a co-culture system in a 3D bioscaffold containing a 1:1 ratio of Histogel/collagen on HUVEC sprout growth. Of note, the Histogel/collagen scaffold did not affect cell viability of either ADSCs or ADSC derived beige cells as demonstrated by the ability of their intracellular esterase to hydrolyze calcein-AM also for a long time (Figure 5a). ADSCs and ADSC derived beige cells were seeded and covered by HUVEC spheroids incorporated in the Histogel/collagen bioscaffold prototype. Results demonstrated that brown-like cells, also in the presence of the Histogel based bioscaffold, increased by 33% the angiogenic capacity of HUVEC cells as demonstrated by the higher number of newly formed sprouts (Figure 5b,c). ADSC derived beige cells synergized with the Histogel-collagen scaffold to induce angiogenesis as demonstrated by the ratio between endothelial sprouts formed in the 3D Histogel/collagen gel with respect to the 3D collagen gel co-cultured respectively with ADSCs or ADSC derived beige cells (Figure 5c).

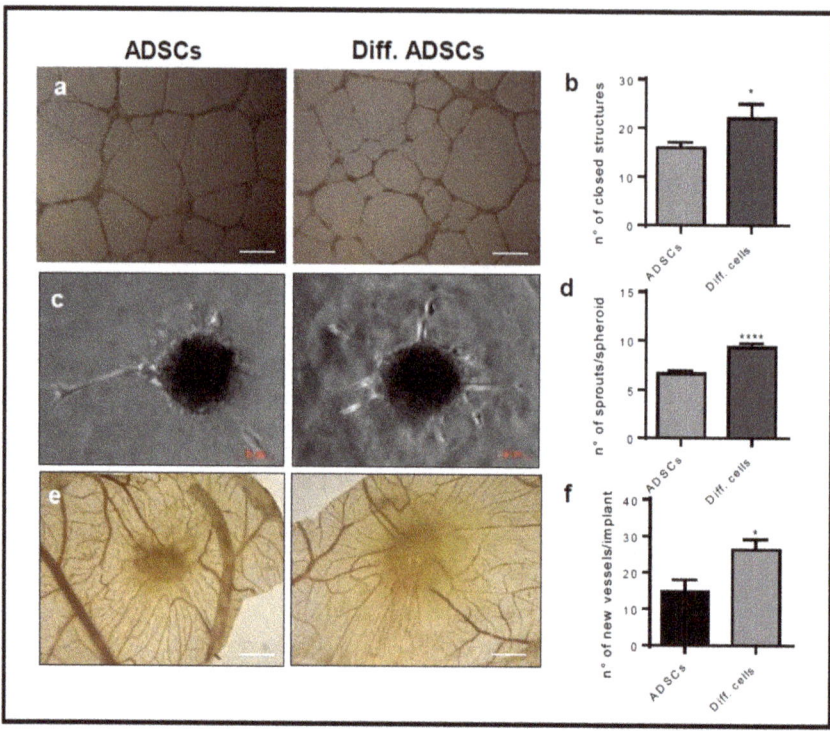

Figure 4. The differentiation into ADSC derived beige cells positively modulates the pro-angiogenic ability of ADSCs. (**a**) Confluent monolayers of ADSCs and ADSC derived beige cells (Diff.cells) were cultured in 24 wells. Two-hundred microliters of growth factor reduced Cultrex were added on the monolayers, and HUVEC cells were plated on gel. After 18 h, the formation of capillary-like structures was examined using a Zeiss Axiovert 200 M microscope (Scale bar 500 µm). Data are the mean ± SEM of three measurements per sample. * $p < 0.05$, Student's *t*-test. (**b**) The number of closed structures. (**c–d**) HUVEC spheroids embedded in collagen gel and plated on an ADSC monolayer. The formation of radially growing sprouts was evaluated after 24 h of incubation. Data are the mean ± SEM of three independent experiments (* $p < 0.05$, **** $p < 0.001$, one-way ANOVA followed by Bonferroni's test versus the control). (**e–f**) Alginate beads containing 3×10^4 ADSCs or ADSC derived beige cells were implanted on the top of chick embryo chorioallantoic membranes (CAMs) at Day 11 of development. After 72 h, newly formed blood vessels converging toward the implant were counted in ovo at 5× magnification using an STEMI SR stereomicroscope equipped with an objective f equal to 100 mm with adapter ring 475,070 (Carl Zeiss) (Scale bar 2 mm). Data are the mean ± SEM (n = 6–8) (* $p < 0.05$, one-way ANOVA followed by Bonferroni's test versus the control).

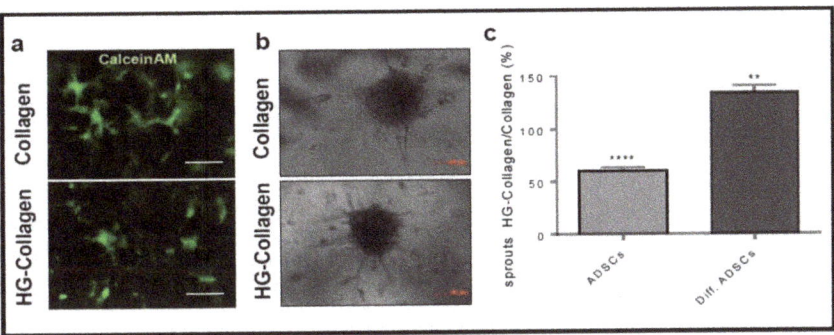

Figure 5. Histogel supports the angiogenic ability of ADSC derived beige cells. (**a**) ADSC derived beige cells were cultured in collagen or collagen:5% Histogel 1:1 for five days. Cells were photographed after 1 h of calcein-AM treatment (Scale bar 200 µm). (**b**,**c**) HUVEC spheroids were embedded in collagen gel or in collagen:5% Histogel 1:1 and plated on confluent monolayers of ADSCs and ADSC derived beige cells. The formation of radially growing sprouts was evaluated after 24 h of incubation. Representative figures (**b**). (**c**) describes the ratio of the number of sprouts formed from the endothelial cell spheroid co-cultured in 5% Histogel-collagen or in collagen gel with ADSCs or ADSC derived beige cells (ratio ± SEM of three independent experiments (**** $p < 0.0001$, ** $p < 0.01$, Student's t-test versus the control).

4. Discussion

Obesity and its related disorders are mostly preventable conditions, but their treatment has proven to be a complex endeavor that has been mostly unsuccessful. The countermeasure usually suggested against overweightness and obesity is an increase in physical activity and/or a reduction of energy intake. A valid alternative to restore the normal physiological function of the human body could be the increase of energy consumption. BAT regulates the thermoregulation and metabolism, generating heat via non-shivering thermogenesis. In addition, beige adipocytes located in WAT also have thermogenic properties characterized by the expression of UCP1 [14]. Thus, the increase of brown tissue mass may represent a healthy and practical way to increase energy consumption, thus helping the individuals to control the weight balance [27]. For this purpose, here, we proposed the use of Histogel based bioscaffolds to promote the browning of adipose tissue. Histogel is a natural bioscaffold derived from porcine Wharton jelly. It is non-cytotoxic and non-hemolytic, and it does not induce inflammation [20]. Wharton jelly is a porous connective tissue found in umbilical cords of animal origin, forming a 3D spongy structure of fibrillar collagen and highly hydrated mucopolysaccharides, including hyaluronic acid proteoglycans [28,29]. The physiological function of Wharton jelly is to prevent the compression of the umbilical cord vessels. Decellularized Wharton jelly is a biocompatible scaffold with mechanical properties suitable to support cell adhesion, proliferation, and reorganization in 3D structures [30], appropriate for tissue engineering [31]. Furthermore, the low cost to obtain it and the "zero waste" material should not be underestimated. Histogel was isolated from porcine farming systems and by transforming them into high-end products with high potentiality for regenerative medicine and cosmetic devices by means of an eco-friendly processing. Here, we showed that Histogel promoted an angiogenic response both in vitro and in vivo. Histogel induced the migration, invasion, and reorganization into a tube-like structure of HUVEC cells and supported the recruitment of new blood vessels when implanted on the chorioallantoic membrane of chick embryos. Of note, the angiogenic process is necessary in tissue regeneration; thus, the pro-angiogenic ability of Histogel makes it a good bioscaffold for tissue engineering.

Biodegradability and porosity are critical features to keep in mind when designing bioscaffolds for tissue engineering. A good bioscaffold must remain in the tissue for the time necessary to support the engraftment of implanted cells, the recruitment of cells from surrounding tissue, and to sustain the metabolism of cells. Thus, the bioscaffold must remain in the host for a long time and not be degraded too quickly. To delay Histogel degradation and to achieve a longer permanence of Histogel in the host, we combined it with alginate or type I collagen gels. Both matrices are currently used in the production of scaffolds for tissue engineering. Alginate is a polymer of mannuronic and glucuronic acid, extracted from brown algae [32]. Alginate has found numerous applications in biomedical sciences and engineering, such as controlled drug delivery for cartilage repair and regeneration [33]. Mammals lack alginase; thus, alginate results in being a non-degradable polymer. Therefore, in our protocol, alginate depolymerization was only dependent on the presence of monovalent ions in the microenvironment [34]. One critical drawback of alginate is its inherent lack of cell adhesivity [35]. In our system, this drawback was overcome by the high adhesivity of Histogel. Then, we tested Histogel-Type I collagen combinations. Type I collagen is a biodegradable material with remarkable water retention ability, low antigenicity, and cytocompatibility. Collagen is an efficient scaffold used for bone repair. It is also employed in regenerative medicine to promote regeneration of skin, cartilage, or ligaments [36]. The presented results supported that both Histogel based materials were biocompatible and provided good mechanical support, creating a scaffold suitable for cell adhesion and proliferation. Histogel based scaffolds allowed adhesion, migration, and endothelial cell reorganization and supported the adhesion and the survival of undifferentiated and differentiated ADSCs in vitro and in vivo.

Both histogel-alginate and Histogel-type I collagen gel scaffolds well supported on the one hand the differentiation of adipose tissue derived stem cells (ADSCs) into brown-like adipose cells expressing PPARγ, PdK4, and UCP-1 proteins and on the other hand the recruitment of blood vessels. The expression of specific adipose markers and the increase of OCR in differentiated ADSCs confirmed that our models well supported ADSCs differentiation. As expected, norepinephrine and isoproterenol increased the mitochondrial activity of ADSC derived beige cells [37,38].

Blood vessels are a necessary requirement to support BAT maintenance. In human adults, BAT consists of brown adipocytes, adipocyte progenitor cells, and blood vessels. BAT is a highly vascularized tissue located in the thorax in quantities inversely proportional to the size of the animal. Therefore, to increase brown adipose tissue or to promote the browning of WAT, it is essential to support the growth of new blood vessels. In our model, the ADSC derived beige cells produced and released in the microenvironment several pro-angiogenic factors, which, in association with the pro-angiogenic behavior of the Histogel based scaffolds, may contribute to supporting the vascularization of BAT.

The regeneration of BAT has been largely ignored in tissue engineering. Here, we proposed the use of biological scaffolds to support the proliferation and differentiation of the adipose tissue resident stem cells into a brown-like tissue and to allow the recruitment of vessels from the surrounding tissues. The employment of such devices will result in heavy BAT mass gain and efficient body weight loss. This would substantially improve the already existing applications in regenerative medicine and metabolic disease treatments.

Author Contributions: Conceptualization, M.D.S., W.S., E.G., and S.M.; Methodology, M.D.S., W.S., E.G., C.R., M.C., E.K., M.V., E.S., J.V., and R.R.; Formal analysis, M.D.S., W.S., E.G.; Investigation, M.D.S., W.S., E.G., C.R., M.C., E.K., M.V., E.D., E.S., J.V., P.S. and R.R.; Resources, B.C., R.R., J.V. and S.M.; Data curation, M.D.S., W.S.; Writing, original draft preparation, M.D.S., M.V., E.G., and S.M.; Writing, review and editing, M.D.S., E.G., and S.M.; Supervision, S.M.

Funding: This work was supported by H2020-MSCA-RISE-2014 (Grant No. 645640–SCAFFY) to S.M., V.M., B.C., E.D., W.S., J.V., C.R., E.S., M.D.S., and E.G.; by Associazione Italiana per la Ricerca sul Cancro (AIRC) IG 17276 grants to S.M.; and by MFAG-18459 to RR. EG was supported by Associazione Italiana per la Ricerca sul Cancro (AIRC) fellowships.

Conflicts of Interest: The authors declare no conflict of interest.

Appendix A

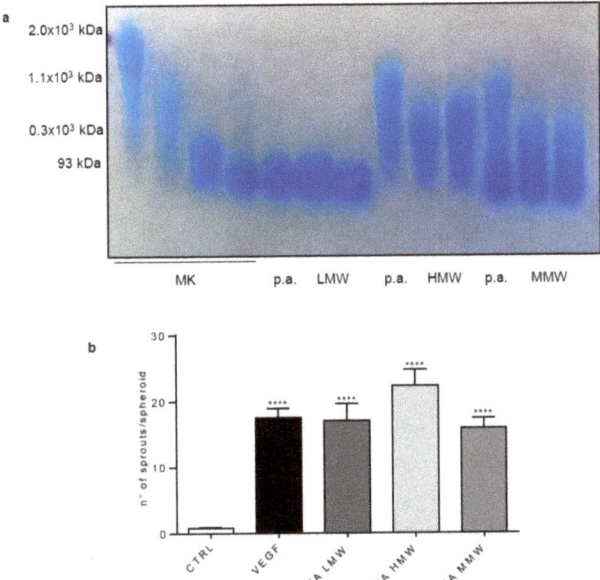

Figure A1. (**a**) Commercial low, high molecular weight HA was electrophoretically analyzed on agarose gel and stained with Stains-All solution. p.a. means pre-autoclaved. Three different standard molecules (2×10^3, 1.1×10^3, 300 kDa) were used as markers of molecular weight (MK). (**b**) HUVEC spheroids embedded in collagen gel were stimulated with commercial HA. The formation of radially growing sprouts was evaluated after 24 h of incubation. Data are the mean ± SEM of three independent experiments (** $p < 0.001$, one-way ANOVA followed by Bonferroni's test versus the control).

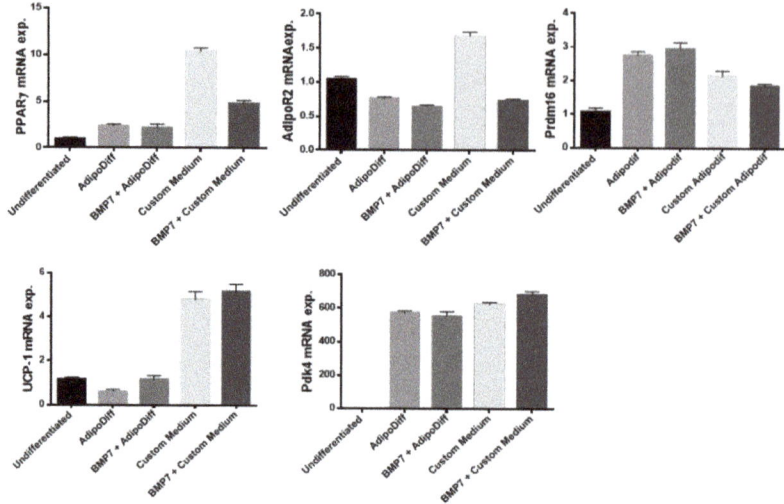

Figure A2. Confluent ADSCs were differentiated in different conditions, i.e., DMEM 10% FCS, AdipoDiff (Milteny Biotech), DMEM complemented with 10% FCS and 3.3 nM of BMP7, DMEM 10% complemented with 20 nM insulin (Sigma), 5 µM dexamethasone (Sigma), 125 µM indomethacin (Sigma), 1 nM triiodothyronine (T3), and 0.5 mM 3-isobutyl-1-methylxanthine (IBMX) in the absence or in the presence of 3.3 nM of hBMP7 for 15 days. Expression of adipose markers was analyzed by RT-PCR. ADSC derived beige cells were analyzed on Day 15 of differentiation. PPARγ, AdipoR, Prdm16, UCP-1, and Pdk4 mRNA expression levels were measured by RT-qPCR analysis. Data are the mean ± SEM (n = 5) and are expressed as relative expression ratios (ΔΔCt − fold increase).

References

1. James, P.T.; Leach, R.; Kalamara, E.; Shayeghi, M. The Worldwide Obesity Epidemic. *Obes. Res.* **2001**, *9*, 228S–233S. [CrossRef] [PubMed]
2. Kang, S.-I.; Shin, H.-S.; Kim, H.-M.; Hong, Y.-S.; Yoon, S.-A.; Kang, S.-W.; Kim, J.-H.; Ko, H.-C.; Kim, S.-J. Anti-Obesity Properties of a Sasa quelpaertensis Extract in High-Fat Diet-Induced Obese Mice. *Biosci. Biotechnol. Biochem.* **2012**, *76*, 755–761. [CrossRef] [PubMed]
3. Cristina Oliveira de Lima, V.; Piuvezam, G.; Leal Lima Maciel, B.; Heloneida de Araújo Morais, A. Trypsin inhibitors: Promising candidate satietogenic proteins as complementary treatment for obesity and metabolic disorders? *J. Enzym. Inhib. Med. Chem.* **2019**, *34*, 405–419. [CrossRef] [PubMed]
4. Komarnytsky, S.; Cook, A.; Raskin, I. Potato protease inhibitors inhibit food intake and increase circulating cholecystokinin levels by a trypsin-dependent mechanism. *Int. J. Obes.* **2011**, *35*, 236–243. [CrossRef] [PubMed]
5. Panteliou, E.; Miras, A.D. What is the role of bariatric surgery in the management of obesity? *Climacteric* **2017**, *20*, 97–102. [CrossRef] [PubMed]
6. Lee, J.H.; Park, A.; Oh, K.-J.; Lee, S.C.; Kim, W.K.; Bae, K.-H. The Role of Adipose Tissue Mitochondria: Regulation of Mitochondrial Function for the Treatment of Metabolic Diseases. *Int. J. Mol. Sci.* **2019**, *20*, 4924. [CrossRef]
7. Granneman, J.G.; Li, P.; Zhu, Z.; Lu, Y. Metabolic and cellular plasticity in white adipose tissue I: effects of β3-adrenergic receptor activation. *Am. J. Physiol. Metab.* **2005**, *289*, E608–E616. [CrossRef]
8. Wu, J.; Boström, P.; Sparks, L.M.; Ye, L.; Choi, J.H.; Giang, A.-H.; Khandekar, M.; A Virtanen, K.; Nuutila, P.; Schaart, G.; et al. Beige adipocytes are a distinct type of thermogenic fat cell in mouse and human. *Cell* **2012**, *150*, 366–376. [CrossRef]
9. Park, A.; Kim, W.K.; Bae, K.-H. Distinction of white, beige and brown adipocytes derived from mesenchymal stem cells. *World J. Stem Cells* **2014**, *6*, 33–42. [CrossRef]

10. Cao, Y. Angiogenesis modulates adipogenesis and obesity. *J. Clin. Investig.* **2007**, *117*, 2362–2368. [CrossRef]
11. Zhou, Y.; Cheng, Z.; Wu, Y.; Wu, Q.; Liao, X.; Zhao, Y.; Li, J.; Zhou, X.; Fu, X. Mesenchymal stem cell-derived conditioned medium attenuate angiotensin II-induced aortic aneurysm growth by modulating macrophage polarization. *J. Cell. Mol. Med.* **2019**, *23*, 8233–8245. [CrossRef] [PubMed]
12. Almalki, S.G.; Agrawal, D.K. ERK signaling is required for VEGF-A/VEGFR2-induced differentiation of porcine adipose-derived mesenchymal stem cells into endothelial cells. *Stem Cell Res. Ther.* **2017**, *8*, 113. [CrossRef] [PubMed]
13. Zambon, J.P.; Atala, A.; Yoo, J.J. Methods to Generate Tissue-Derived Constructs for Regenerative Medicine Applications. *Methods* **2019**. [CrossRef]
14. Srivastava, S.; Veech, R.L. Brown and Brite: The Fat Soldiers in the Anti-Obesity Fight. *Front. Physiol.* **2019**, *10*, 38. [CrossRef] [PubMed]
15. Brown, A.C. Brown adipocytes from induced pluripotent stem cells-how far have we come? *Ann. N. Y. Acad. Sci.* **2019**. [CrossRef]
16. Dave, K.; Gomes, V.G. Interactions at scaffold interfaces: Effect of surface chemistry, structural attributes and bioaffinity. *Mater. Sci. Eng. C* **2019**, *105*, 110078. [CrossRef]
17. Luo, H.; Cha, R.; Li, J.; Hao, W.; Zhang, Y.; Zhou, F. Advances in tissue engineering of nanocellulose-based scaffolds: A review. *Carbohydr. Polym.* **2019**, *224*, 115144. [CrossRef]
18. Pandit, A.H.; Mazumdar, N.; Ahmad, S. Periodate oxidized hyaluronic acid-based hydrogel scaffolds for tissue engineering applications. *Int. J. Boil. Macromol.* **2019**, *137*, 853–869. [CrossRef]
19. Son, Y.J.; Tse, J.W.; Zhou, Y.; Mao, W.; Yim, E.K.F.; Yoo, H.S. Biomaterials and controlled release strategy for epithelial wound healing. *Biomater. Sci.* **2019**, *7*, 4444–4471. [CrossRef]
20. Herrero-Mendez, A.; Palomares, T.; Castro, B.; Herrero, J.; Granado, M.H.; Bejar, J.M.; Alonso-Varona, A. HR007: A family of biomaterials based on glycosaminoglycans for tissue repair. *J. Tissue Eng. Regen. Med.* **2017**, *11*, 989–1001. [CrossRef]
21. Shinoda, K.; Ohyama, K.; Hasegawa, Y.; Chang, H.-Y.; Ogura, M.; Sato, A.; Hong, H.; Hosono, T.; Sharp, L.Z.; Scheel, D.W.; et al. Phosphoproteomics Identifies CK2 as a Negative Regulator of Beige Adipocyte Thermogenesis and Energy Expenditure. *Cell Metab.* **2015**, *22*, 997–1008. [CrossRef] [PubMed]
22. Grillo, E.; Ravelli, C.; Corsini, M.; Ballmer-Hofer, K.; Zammataro, L.; Oreste, P.; Zoppetti, G.; Tobia, C.; Ronca, R.; Presta, M.; et al. Monomeric gremlin is a novel vascular endothelial growth factor receptor-2 antagonist. *Oncotarget* **2016**, *7*, 35353–35368. [CrossRef] [PubMed]
23. Rezzola, S.; Di Somma, M.; Corsini, M.; Leali, D.; Ravelli, C.; Polli, V.A.B.; Grillo, E.; Presta, M.; Mitola, S. VEGFR2 activation mediates the pro-angiogenic activity of BMP4. *Angiogenesis* **2019**. [CrossRef] [PubMed]
24. Nowak-Sliwinska, P.; Alitalo, K.; Allen, E.; Anisimov, A.; Aplin, A.C.; Auerbach, R.; Augustin, H.G.; Bates, D.O.; Van Beijnum, J.R.; Bender, R.H.F.; et al. Consensus guidelines for the use and interpretation of angiogenesis assays. *Angiogenesis* **2018**, *21*, 425–532. [CrossRef] [PubMed]
25. Ravelli, C.; Mitola, S.; Corsini, M.; Presta, M. Involvement of alphavbeta3 integrin in gremlin-induced angiogenesis. *Angiogenesis* **2013**, *16*, 235–243. [CrossRef]
26. Corsini, M.; Moroni, E.; Ravelli, C.; Andrés, G.; Grillo, E.; Ali, I.H.; Brazil, D.P.; Presta, M.; Mitola, S.M.F. Cyclic Adenosine Monophosphate-Response Element–Binding Protein Mediates the Proangiogenic or Proinflammatory Activity of Gremlin. *Arter. Thromb. Vasc. Boil.* **2014**, *34*, 136–145. [CrossRef]
27. Ling, Y.; Carayol, J.; Galusca, B.; Canto, C.; Montaurier, C.; Matone, A.; Vassallo, I.; Minehira, K.; Alexandre, V.; Cominetti, O.; et al. Persistent low body weight in humans is associated with higher mitochondrial activity in white adipose tissue. *Am. J. Clin. Nutr.* **2019**, *110*, 605–616. [CrossRef]
28. Ferguson, V.L.; Dodson, R.B. Bioengineering aspects of the umbilical cord. *Eur. J. Obstet. Gynecol. Reprod. Boil.* **2009**, *144*, S108–S113. [CrossRef]
29. Jadalannagari, S.; Converse, G.; McFall, C.; Buse, E.; Filla, M.; Villar, M.T.; Artigues, A.; Mellot, A.J.; Wang, J.; Detamore, M.S.; et al. Decellularized Wharton's Jelly from human umbilical cord as a novel 3D scaffolding material for tissue engineering applications. *PLoS ONE* **2017**, *12*, e0172098. [CrossRef]
30. Kehtari, M.; Beiki, B.; Zeynali, B.; Hosseini, F.S.; Soleimanifar, F.; Kaabi, M.; Soleimani, M.; Enderami, S.E.; Kabiri, M.; Mahboudi, H. Decellularized Wharton's jelly extracellular matrix as a promising scaffold for promoting hepatic differentiation of human induced pluripotent stem cells. *J. Cell. Biochem.* **2019**, *120*, 6683–6697. [CrossRef]

31. Beiki, B.; Zeynali, B.; Seyedjafari, E. Fabrication of a three dimensional spongy scaffold using human Wharton's jelly derived extra cellular matrix for wound healing. *Mater. Sci. Eng. C* **2017**, *78*, 627–638. [CrossRef] [PubMed]
32. Augst, A.D.; Kong, H.J.; Mooney, D.J. Alginate Hydrogels as Biomaterials. *Macromol. Biosci.* **2006**, *6*, 623–633. [CrossRef] [PubMed]
33. Pelletier, S.; Hubert, P.; Payan, E.; Marchal, P.; Choplin, L.; Dellacherie, E. Amphiphilic derivatives of sodium alginate and hyaluronate for cartilage repair: rheological properties. *J. Biomed. Mater. Res.* **2001**, *54*, 102–108. [CrossRef]
34. Lee, K.Y.; Mooney, D.J. Alginate: properties and biomedical applications. *Prog. Polym. Sci.* **2012**, *37*, 106–126. [CrossRef]
35. Koo, L.Y.; Irvine, D.J.; Mayes, A.M.; A Lauffenburger, D.; Griffith, L.G. Co-regulation of cell adhesion by nanoscale RGD organization and mechanical stimulus. *J. Cell Sci.* **2002**, *115*.
36. Yang, C.; Hillas, P.J.; A B??ez, J.; Nokelainen, M.; Balan, J.; Tang, J.; Spiro, R.; Polarek, J.W.; Baez, J.A. The Application of Recombinant Human Collagen in Tissue Engineering. *BioDrugs* **2004**, *18*, 103–119. [CrossRef]
37. Braun, K.; Li, Y.; Westermeier, J.; Klingenspor, M. Opposing Actions of Adrenocorticotropic Hormone and Glucocorticoids on UCP1-Mediated Respiration in Brown Adipocytes. *Front. Physiol.* **2018**, *9*, 1931. [CrossRef]
38. Del Mar Gonzalez-Barroso, M.; Pecqueur, C.; Gelly, C.; Sanchis, D.; Alves-Guerra, M.C.; Bouillaud, F.; Ricquier, D.; Cassard-Doulcier, A.M. Transcriptional activation of the human ucp1 gene in a rodent cell line. Synergism of retinoids, isoproterenol, and thiazolidinedione is mediated by a multipartite response element. *J. Biol. Chem.* **2000**, *275*, 31722–31732. [CrossRef]

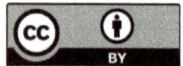

© 2019 by the authors. Licensee MDPI, Basel, Switzerland. This article is an open access article distributed under the terms and conditions of the Creative Commons Attribution (CC BY) license (http://creativecommons.org/licenses/by/4.0/).

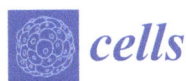

Article

Differences in the Emission of Volatile Organic Compounds (VOCs) between Non-Differentiating and Adipogenically Differentiating Mesenchymal Stromal/Stem Cells from Human Adipose Tissue

Ann-Christin Klemenz [1], Juliane Meyer [2], Katharina Ekat [2], Julia Bartels [1], Selina Traxler [1], Jochen K. Schubert [1], Günter Kamp [3], Wolfram Miekisch [1,†] and Kirsten Peters [2,*,†]

1. Department of Anesthesiology and Intensive Care Medicine, University Medical Centre Rostock, Schillingallee 35, 18057 Rostock, Germany
2. Department of Cell Biology, University Medical Centre Rostock, Schillingallee 69, 18057 Rostock, Germany
3. AMP-Lab GmbH, Mendelstr. 11, 48149 Münster, Germany
* Correspondence: kirsten.peters@med.uni-rostock.de; Tel.: +49(0)381-494-7757
† Both authors contributed equally to this work.

Received: 4 June 2019; Accepted: 9 July 2019; Published: 10 July 2019

Abstract: Metabolic characterization of human adipose tissue-derived mesenchymal stromal/stem cells (ASCs) is of importance in stem cell research. The monitoring of the cell status often requires cell destruction. An analysis of volatile organic compounds (VOCs) in the headspace above cell cultures might be a noninvasive and nondestructive alternative to in vitro analysis. Furthermore, VOC analyses permit new insight into cellular metabolism due to their view on volatile compounds. Therefore, the aim of our study was to compare VOC profiles in the headspace above nondifferentiating and adipogenically differentiating ASCs. To this end, ASCs were cultivated under nondifferentiating and adipogenically differentiating conditions for up to 21 days. At different time points the headspace samples were preconcentrated by needle trap micro extraction and analyzed by gas chromatography/mass spectrometry. Adipogenic differentiation was assessed at equivalent time points. Altogether the emissions of 11 VOCs showed relevant changes and were analyzed in more detail. A few of these VOCs, among them acetaldehyde, were significantly different in the headspace of adipogenically differentiating ASCs and appeared to be linked to metabolic processes. Furthermore, our data indicate that VOC headspace analysis might be a suitable, noninvasive tool for the metabolic monitoring of (mesenchymal stem) cells in vitro.

Keywords: adipose tissue-derived mesenchymal stromal/stem cells (ASCs); cell differentiation; volatile organic compounds; metabolic monitoring

1. Introduction

Due to their capacity for self-renewal and multipotent differentiation, mesenchymal stem/stromal cells (MSCs) have been identified as playing an essential role in tissue homeostasis and regeneration [1]. In recent years, increasing attention has been paid to MSCs from human adipose tissue (adipose tissue-derived MSCs, referred to as ASCs), as they show promising potential as a clinical alternative to other MSCs, like bone marrow-derived MSCs (bmMSCs) [2–4]. Zuk et al. were the first to characterize the mesenchymal differentiation potential of ASCs in more detail [5,6]. Furthermore, nonmesenchymal differentiation (e.g., neuron-like morphology) of ASCs has also been demonstrated [7].

Data concerning the energy metabolism of MSCs in vitro are available but have not been worked out in detail. It has been shown that bmMSCs mainly facilitate glycolysis with subsequent lactate production rather than oxidative phosphorylation [8]. Furthermore, it was demonstrated that nondifferentiating and osteogenically differentiating bmMSCs facilitated oxidative phosphorylation as well as glycolysis in order to fulfill their energy metabolic needs [9]. It has been reported that the function of mitochondria also regulates the differentiation of MSC [10,11]. Adipogenic differentiation of ASC is accompanied by increasing mitochondrial enzyme activities, indicating a growing capacity for oxidative phosphorylation and β-oxidation and, thus, a shift towards lipid metabolism [12]. In addition, in human differentiated adipocytes, the enzymes involved in mitochondrial metabolism showed significantly higher activity rates than in the $CD34^+$ stromal vascular fraction of human adipose tissue containing the nondifferentiated progenitors of adipocytes, the ASCs [13]. Thus, in recent years the idea matured that metabolic pathways regulate cellular differentiation processes that go beyond ATP production [14]. To determine metabolic activities in different phases of differentiation, further information is needed. Ideally, gathering this data should not influence or even disturb the cell culture.

For conventional metabolomics studies in vitro, sufficient cell material is necessary. Especially when working with human stem cells, often low cell numbers are available. In contrast to those conventional methods, an analysis of volatile organic compounds (VOCs) has the great advantage of being nondestructive and noninvasive [15]. Such a destruction-free analysis can be done by means of bidirectional preconcentration combined with a versatile, standardized set-up and has, therefore, gained more attention during the last decades. Besides the occurrence of VOCs in human breath, they are also emitted in trace concentrations by cell and bacteria cultures [16–18].

Headspace analysis by means of needle trap microextraction (NTME) coupled with gas chromatography and mass spectrometry (e.g., GC-MS with electron impact quadrupole detection) allows the identification and quantification of compounds down to the parts per trillion by volume (pptV) range. Conventional headspace techniques require larger volumes and, therefore, may affect the investigated system itself. Hence, microextraction techniques are better suited for this kind of setup [19]. In contrast to solid phase microextraction (SPME), the sensitivity of NTME can be enhanced by increasing the sampling volume, as the sample volume is usually limited. Bidirectional NTME sampling can be applied to reach a high sensitivity in the VOC extraction [20] without significant effects on volume or pressure of the in vitro system. A crucial step for a reliable and reproducible VOC headspace analysis in in vitro cultures is also a standardized set-up [21].

Data from several studies suggest that different cell lines and bacterial strains can be distinguished from each other by means of their volatile emissions [22–24]. Some volatiles have been shown to be associated with different pathways in cell metabolism [25]. For example, acetone is produced by the decarboxylation of acetoacetate, and acetaldehyde is produced by ethanol oxidation [26]. Previous work has established that volatile substances over cell cultures correlate with stem cell growth [27].

Therefore, the aim of our study was to assess VOC emissions in the headspace of cell cultures to gather complementary information on metabolic changes of ASCs during differentiation. This raises the question of whether we can detect the differences in VOC emissions from cell cultures between nondifferentiating and differentiating ASCs. This in turn leads to the next question: can the differences in VOC emission be related to metabolic changes in ASCs during differentiation?

2. Materials and Methods

2.1. Isolation, Cultivation, and Differentiation of Adipose Tissue-Derived Mesenchymal Stromal/Stem Cells (ASCs)

ASCs used in this study were isolated from human lipoaspirate. Tissue donation was approved by the ethics committee of the Rostock University Medical Center (http://www.ethik.med.uni-rostock.de/) under the registration number A2013-0112. It complies with the ethical standards of the World Medical Association Declaration of Helsinki. Informed consent was obtained from all patients. The material for the different analyses was retrieved from four patients. Data, as supplied by the surgeons, showed one male and three female patients. Patients were on average 39.5 years old (ranging from 32 to 47). Liposuction procedures were performed by waterjet-assisted liposuction or a tumescent suction technique.

ASC isolation was performed as previously described [12]. ASCs were cryopreserved in passage 2 until they were used for the experiments. To achieve this, the cell suspension was transferred into a cryovial (Greiner bio-one, Germany) containing 150 µL DMSO (Sigma-Aldrich, Germany) and 350 µL fetal calf serum (FCS, PAN Biotech, Germany). The cryovials were cooled to −80 °C overnight at 1 °C per minute in a freezing container (Thermo Fisher Scientific, Berlin, Germany). Vials were then stored in liquid nitrogen at −165 °C until further use. For use in the planned experiments, the cells were thawed stepwise by gently shaking the vial at 37 °C in a water bath for 1 min. The cell suspension was then gradually transferred into cell culture medium (Dulbecco's Modified Eagle Medium/DMEM GlutaMAX-I, Thermo Fisher Scientific, Germany), containing 10% FCS and antibiotics (100 U/mL penicillin, 100 mg/mL streptomycin, Thermo Fisher Scientific, Germany; hereinafter called maintenance medium) at room temperature and centrifuged for 5 min at 400× g. The resulting cell pellet was resuspended in maintenance medium and centrifuged again for 5 min at 400× g. Cells were resuspended in maintenance medium and seeded onto cell culture flasks for cultivation at 37 °C and 5% CO_2 in a humidified atmosphere. When confluency was reached after 5 d, cells were detached from the cell culture flasks by incubation with 0.25% Trypsin EDTA for 5 min at 37 °C. The cells were seeded into cell culture petri dishes (Greiner bio-one, Frickenhausen, Germany) at a density of 20,000 cells/cm^2. After 24 h of incubation the medium was replaced. After further 48 h (Day 0), additional to the nondifferentiating cultures, adipogenic differentiation of ASCs was induced by adding a differentiation-stimulating medium: i.e., a maintenance medium containing 1 µM dexamethasone, 500 µM IBMX, 200 µM indomethacin, and 10 µM insulin (Sigma-Aldrich, Munich, Germany). Adipogenic stimulation (AS) took place with every replacement of medium three times a week (every second or third day). The medium replacement of differentiating ASCs and undifferentiating ASCs without specific differentiation factors was performed (unstimulated/US) simultaneously. To also assess the emissions of the cell culture medium, pure culture medium without ASC (medium control) was treated and analyzed in a manner identical to the ASC cultures.

2.2. Analysis of Cell Numbers

Cell numbers were determined according to the manufacturer's instructions using the Nucleocounter NC200 and the Via1-Cassettes™ (ChemoMetec, Lillerod, Denmark).

2.3. Analysis of Adipogenic Differentiation

In order to assess the adipogenic differentiation of the ASCs over the course of the experiment, fluorescent staining of the nuclei and lipid-filled vacuoles was done at the corresponding time points of 1, 7, 14, and 21 d. Cells were seeded into 96-well µClear® cell culture plates (Greiner, Frickenhausen, Germany) at a density of 20,000 cells/cm^2. Media changes were done according to the same schedule as the VOC quantification. At the corresponding time points the cells were washed twice with PBS and fixed with 4% paraformaldehyde for 30 min at room temperature. Thereafter, the cells were incubated with a Bodipy/Hoechst-staining solution (100 µL of 1 µg/mL Bodipy (Life Technologies, California, Carlsbad, USA) and 5 µg/mL Hoechst 33,342 (AppliChem, Darmstadt, Germany) in 150 mM NaCl) for 10 min at room temperature in the dark. After incubation, the cells were washed twice with PBS and twice with water for injection. Subsequently, pictures were taken with the microscopic plate scanning system Hermes WiScan (IDEA Bio-Medical, Rehovot, Israel) with a 10-fold magnification objective.

2.4. Volatile Organic Compound (VOC) Sampling by Means of Needle Trap Micro Extraction

For headspace sampling, three cell culture dishes (without lid) containing culture medium and ASCs were introduced into a hermetically closed sampling box under a sterile hood (schematically shown in Figure 1). The sampling box was constructed from emission-free materials (Teflon® and glass) to ensure a reliable measurement of trace VOC profiles [28]. As a negative control, three cell culture dishes containing pure cell culture medium without ASCs were analyzed in parallel in a second box. After introduction of the cell culture dishes, the boxes were flushed with 3 L of clean synthetic air (containing 75% N_2, 20% O_2, and 5% CO_2; Air Liquide, Düsseldorf, Germany). After an incubation time of 60 min at 37 °C in an incubator, headspace sampling by means of NTME was done. A detailed description of the sampling setup was described before [23]. Headspace samples were taken at day 4 after seeding the cells, which means 24 h after changing from maintenance to adipogenic differentiation medium and on day 7, 14, and 21 of differentiating cultures, nondifferentiating cultures, and medium control dishes, respectively (see experimental setup in Figure 1).

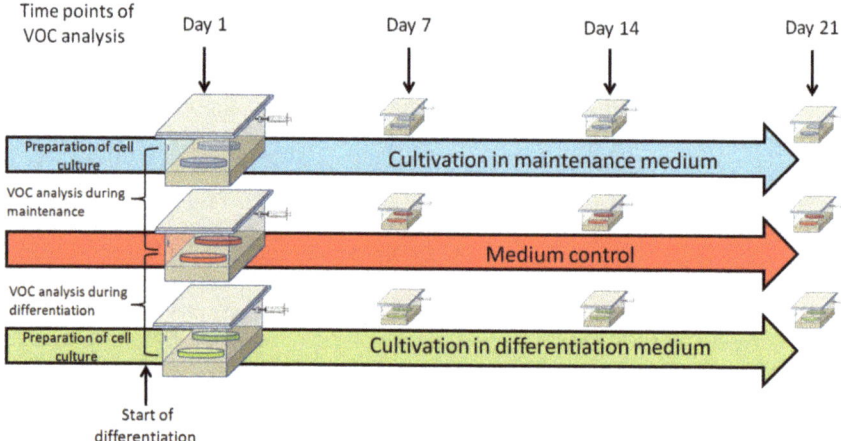

Figure 1. Schematic depiction of the experimental setup. VOC—volatile organic compound.

NTME was done with needle trap devices (NTDs, needleEX), obtained from Shinwa Ltd. (Kyoto, Japan). The NTDs were equipped with 3 cm of a copolymer of methacrylic acid and ethylene glycol dimethacrylate. Before sampling, NTDs were preconditioned for 30 min at 200 °C in a heating device (PAS Technology Deutschland GmbH, Magdala, Germany) under a helium flow. Teflon caps (PAS Technology Deutschland GmbH, Magdala, Germany) were used to seal the NTDs before and immediately after collecting the headspace samples.

For VOC preconcentration, NTDs were connected to a 1 mL sterile singleuse syringe (Omnifix-F, B. Braun Melsungen AG, Melsungen, Germany) and pierced through the septum of a Luer Lock cap (IN-Stopper, B. Braun Melsungen AG, Melsungen, Germany) at one connection port of the sampling box. Bidirectional headspace sampling was done by filling and releasing 1 mL of headspace gas 20 times, as described previously [20].

2.5. Gas Chromatography and Mass Spectrometry (GC-MS) Analysis

For VOC analysis, an Agilent 7890 A gas chromatograph coupled to an Agilent 5975 C inert XL MSD (Agilent, Santa Clara, CA, USA) with a triple axis detector was used. At an injector temperature of 200 °C, VOCs were thermally desorbed from the NTDs. Sample injection was operated in splitless mode (60 s splitless). The GC was equipped with a 60 m RTX-624 column (0.32 mm ID, 1.8 μm column thickness). Helium carrier gas flow was constant at 1.5 mL min^{-1}. The temperature program was as follows: 40 °C for 5 min, 8 °C min^{-1} to 120 °C for 2 min, 10 °C min^{-1} to 220 °C, and 20 °C min^{-1} to 240 °C for 4.5 min. Analysis of the samples was performed via electron impact ionization (EI—70 eV) in full scan mode, a mass range of 35–250 amu, and a scan rate of 2.73 scan/s. Volatile organic compounds were tentatively identified by mass spectral library search (NIST Version 2.0). Substance attribution was confirmed by comparing GC retention times and mass spectra of all selected substances with those of pure reference substances. Quantifications were made in parts per billion per volume (ppbV) and then calculated to nmol/L. To quantify the detected substances, a six-point calibration curve (from 1 to 500 ppbV) was established. Humidity-adapted standards were prepared by means of a liquid calibration unit (LCU, Ionicon Analytik GmbH, Austria). Limits of detection were calculated as a signal-to-noise ratio of 3:1, whereby limits of quantification corresponded to a signal-to-noise ratio of 10:1. Ten blank NTDs were analyzed for this purpose. Quantitative parameters (limit of detection (LOD), limit of quantification (LOQ), and standard deviation (SD)) for all identified VOCs are shown in Table S1 in the Supplementary Materials.

2.6. Reference Substances

Acetone, 2-butanone, heptanal, octanal, and acetaldehyde were acquired from Ionimed Analytik GmbH (Insbruck, Austria). Benzaldehyde and 1,3-di-tert-butylbenzene were purchased from Sigma-Aldrich (Germany); tert-butanol, ethylbenzene, as well as 2-ethylhexanol were purchased from TCI (Eschborn, Germany) and pentane from Fluka (Munich, Germany).

2.7. Statistical Analysis

Figures 2–5 show numerical data represented as medians and percentiles (25–75%). Correlation analysis and statistical testing was performed by using RStudio (version 1.0.136) and R software (version 3.3.2_ 2016-10-31). By using the Kruskal–Wallis test with the Nemenyi post hoc test, statistically significant differences in median values between all groups were identified. Values of $p < 0.05$ were considered statistically significant.

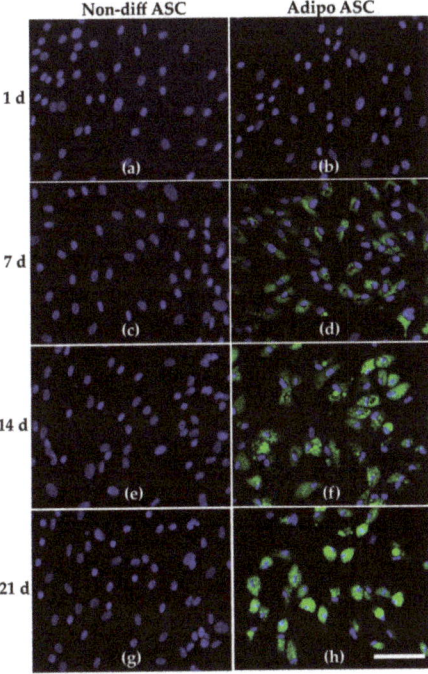

Figure 2. Depiction of adipose tissue-derived mesenchymal stromal/stem cells (ASCs) under nondifferentiating conditions (referred to as non-diff ASC, subfigures (**a,c,e,g**) for cultivation days 1, 7, 14, 21, respectively) and under adipogenic stimulation (adipo ASC, subfigures (**b,d,f,h**) for cultivation days 1, 7, 14, 21, respectively) Ffluorescence staining of nuclei (blue) and lipids (green), scale bar: 100 μm.

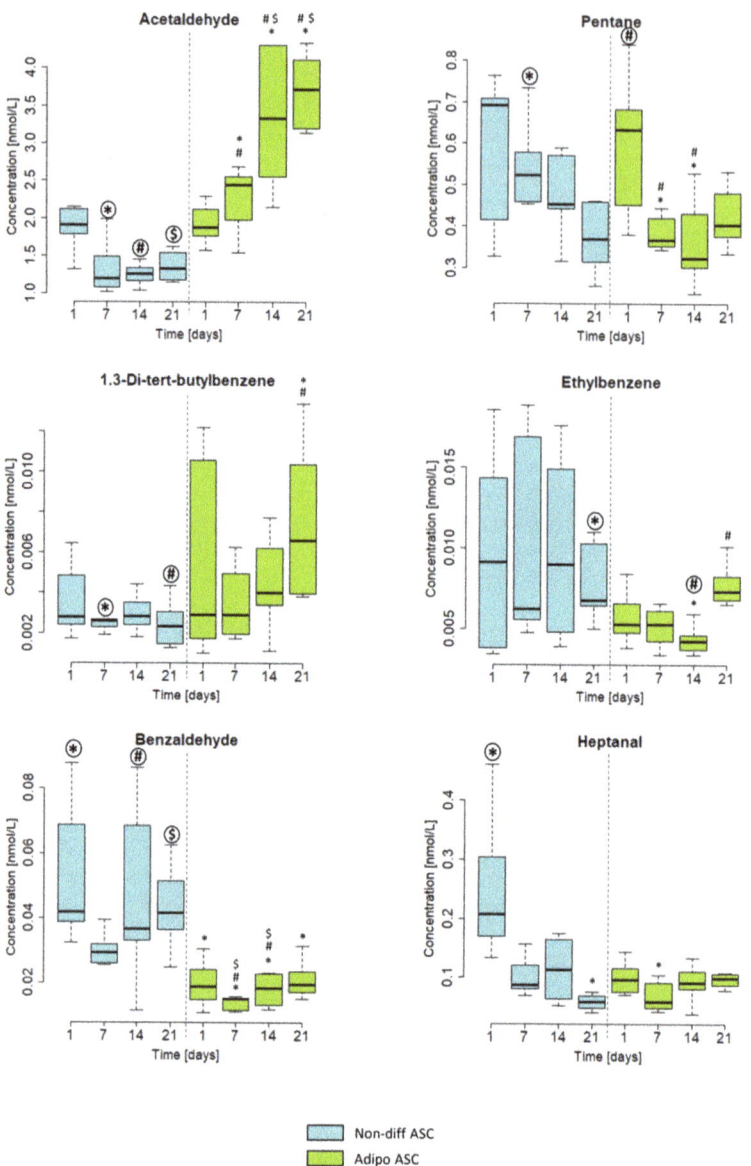

Figure 3. Emissions of acetaldehyde, pentane, 1,3-di-tert-butylbenzene, ethylbenzene, benzaldehyde, and heptanal from nondifferentiating (non-diff ASC, blue) and adipogenically differentiating ASC (adipo ASC, green). Concentrations in the headspace are shown in nmol/L on the Y-axis. The X-axis shows the time points of measurements. The boxplots represent data from three independent experiments. Significance was tested within all groups. Symbols (*, #, $) indicate significant differences to the corresponding highlighted group (p-values < 0.05).

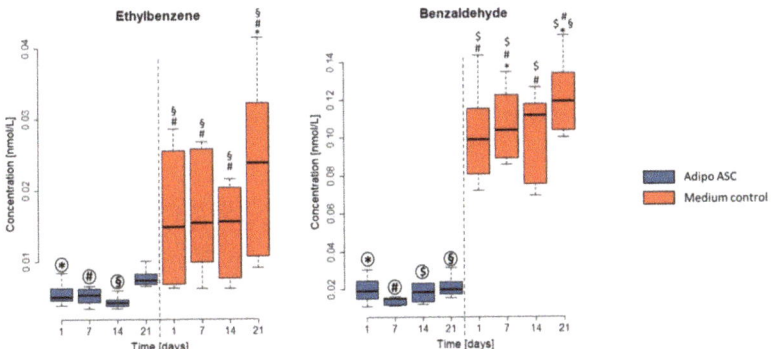

Figure 4. Example of two VOCs showing lower emissions in adipogenic differentiating ASC (adipo ASC) cultures than in the culture media controls. Concentrations in the headspace in nmol/L are shown on the Y-axis. The X-axis shows the time point of measurements. The diagram shows cell culture with adipogenically differentiating ASC (referred to as Adipo ASC, in blue) and medium controls (samples without cells, in red). Boxplots represent the data from three independent differentiation experiments. Significance was tested within all groups. Symbols (*, #, §, $) indicate significant differences to the corresponding highlighted group (p-values < 0.05).

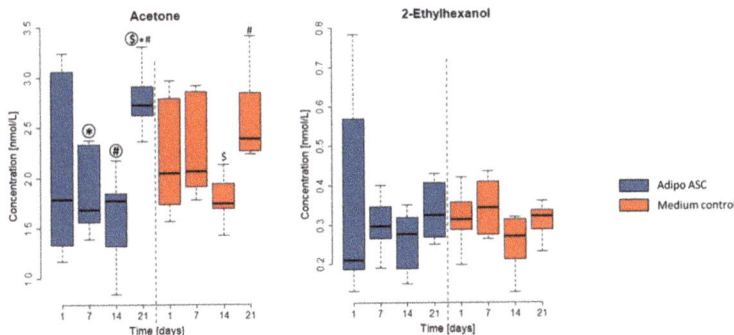

Figure 5. Acetone and 2-ethylhexanol as exemplary medium-dependent VOCs in adipogenically differentiated ASCs (referred to as Adipo ASC). The concentration in the headspace in nmol/L is shown on the Y-axis. The X-axis shows the measurement time points. The diagram shows cell culture with adipogenically differentiating ASC (referred to as Adipo ASC, in blue) and medium controls (samples without cells, in red). Boxplots represent data of three independent differentiation experiments. Significance was tested within all groups. Symbols (*, #, $) indicate significant differences to the corresponding bold highlighted group (p-values < 0.05).

3. Results

3.1. Adipogenic Differentiation of ASCs

The assessment of adipogenic differentiation by fluorescent lipid staining revealed that nondifferentiating conditions did not induce lipid accumulation in ASCs at any time point (Figure 2a,c,e,f), After 24 h, adipogenic stimulation did not lead to lipid accumulation (Figure 2b). After 7 d of adipogenic stimulation, distinct lipid vacuole formation was visible (Figure 2d). With the progression of adipogenic differentiation of ASCs (day 14 and 21), the lipid vacuoles appeared larger and showed a higher fluorescence intensity (Figure 2f,h). Thus, considerable adipogenic differentiation was clearly visible in almost all cells of the adipogenic cell culture model. This was not the case in nondifferentiating ASCs.

3.2. Comparision of VOC Emissions of Non-Differentiating and Adipogenically Differentiating ASCs

Thirty-one potential volatile marker substances were identified in the headspace above the cell cultures (concentration ranges and quantitative parameters are depicted in Table S1 of the Supplementary Materials). To focus on the most relevant substances, we excluded substances having concentrations below the limit of detection (LOD) at more than 3 time points as well as substances having concentrations in the same range (± 10%) as in pure media samples. Based on these criteria, 11 VOCs were selected for further analysis. These substances were identified and quantified by using pure reference substances. Six of these VOCs that were differentially emitted and dependent on the differentiation are depicted in Figure 3.

The compounds acetaldehyde, pentane, and 1,3-di-tert-butylbenzene displayed different trends of emission during cultivation with maintenance media compared with cultivation with differentiation medium (Figure 3).

Concentrations of the emitted acetaldehyde changed significantly between days 7, 14, and 21 of adipogenically differentiated ASCs. In nondifferentiating ASCs, no significant concentration differences could be detected between the days of cultivation.

Pentane concentrations decreased in nondifferentiating ASCs, whereas a slight increase in adipogenically differentiating ASCs was detected from day 14 to day 21 of differentiation. The production of pentane in the adipogenically differentiating cell cultures peaked on day 1 and was significantly higher than on day 7 and on day 14.

The concentration of 1,3-di-tert-butylbenzene in the headspace of nondifferentiating ASCs remained lower as well as constant over the time, whereas the emissions in the headspace of adipogenically differentiating cell cultures showed a slight increase.

Concentrations of ethylbenzene and benzaldehyde differed between nondifferentiating and adipogenically differentiating ASCs in terms of concentration and time course. Both substances showed lower emissions in adipogenically differentiating ASCs compared with nondifferentiating ASCs. For benzaldehyde, these differences were significant. Heptanal showed a significant decrease over time in nondifferentiating ACSs and an increase in adipogenically differentiating ASCs. Concentrations of heptanal on day 21 of cultivation were higher in adipogenically differentiating compared with nondifferentiating ASCs. Detailed statistical information can be found in the Supplementary Materials (Table S2).

To emphasize the differences between nondifferentiating and adipogenically differentiating ASCs, Table 1 presents concentrations of emitted VOCs normalized to the cell number at day 21. All substances other than benzaldehyde showed higher concentrations in differentiating cells than in undifferentiating ASCs. The most prominent differences were found for acetaldehyde and heptanal. In both substances, a nearly threefold increase of emitted concentrations could be detected on day 21 of the experiment.

Table 1. Ratio of VOC production in the headspace per cell from nondifferentiating and adipogenically differentiating ASCs at day 21 of cultivation. Concentrations were calculated per 1×10^6 cells from one experiment as an example. VOC concentrations are shown in pmol per L (pmol/L) ± standard deviation (SD). Statistical significance was tested by a t-test ($p < 0.05$).

Substance	Normalized VOC Concentration [pmol/L per 1×10^6 cells ± SD]		Statistically Significant
	Nondifferentiating ASCs	Adipogenically Differentiating ASCs	
Acetaldehyde	229.3 (± 34.5)	686.4 (± 14.4)	Yes
Pentane	64.2 (± 8.7)	86.9 (± 1.1)	Yes
1,3-bis-(1,1-dimethylethyl) Benzene	0.368 (± 0.04)	1.4 (± 0.2)	Yes
Ethylbenzene	0.94 (± 0.1)	1.9 (± 0.4)	Yes
Benzaldehyde	6.17 (± 2.1)	5.93 (± 1.2)	No
Heptanal	9.6 (± 1.9)	25.4 (± 5.1)	Yes
Octanal	11.5 (± 1.1)	23.8 (± 0.6)	Yes

3.3. Comparision of VOC Emissions from Medium Control and Corresponding Cell Cultures

Apart from emissions of the cells, VOCs were also emitted from the cell culture medium without cells. Therefore, the headspace of the medium without cells was used as a "medium control" for each time point tested. The detailed depictions of emissions of differentiating and nondifferentiating ASCs compared to the medium control are shown in Figures S1 and S2, respectively. In the following, exemplary results from adipogenically differentiating ASCs are presented.

Acetaldehyde, pentane, and 1,3-di-tert-butylbenzene showed medium independent emissions in adipogenically differentiating cultures. Acetaldehyde and 1,3-di-tert-butylbenzene emissions increased at every measurement time point. Most other VOCs (especially aldehydes) showed lower and decreasing concentrations compared to the medium controls.

3.3.1. VOC Consumption during Adipogenic Differentiation

The emissions of three aldehydes (heptanal, octanal, and benzaldehyde) and one aromatic hydrocarbon (ethylbenzene) were higher in the pure cell culture media compared with cell cultures. As examples, ethylbenzene and benzaldehyde of this VOC group are depicted in Figure 4 (heptanal and octanal can be found in Figure S1 of the Supplementary Materials).

Ethylbenzene concentrations were significantly higher in medium controls compared with cell culture samples at three time points analyzed. For benzaldehyde, we could find significant differences in the emissions from all cell culture samples compared with the pure medium control at all time points. In nondifferentiating ASCs, ethylbenzene and benzaldehyde emissions showed the same profile of higher emissions in the medium control compared with the cell culture (see Figure S2). Thus, the specific consumption or binding of these VOCs by the cells is indicated.

3.3.2. Culture Medium-Dependent VOCs

The emissions of 2-ethylhexanol, acetone, tert-butanol, and 2-butanone from adipogenically differentiating ASCs complied with the emissions of the medium controls. Heptanal and octanal emissions also appeared media-dependent in nondifferentiating ASCs (see Figure S2 in the Supplementary Materials).

The emissions of two exemplary VOCs, acetone and 2-ethylhexanol, over 21 days of cultivation in adipogenically differentiating ASCs are presented in Figure 5. The emissions of tert-butanol and 2-butanone for adipogenically differentiating ASCs showed a slight decreasing trend over the first two weeks of differentiation and peaked at day 21. This trend was similar in the medium control (Supplementary Figure S1). The more comprehensive depiction of adipogenically differentiating and nondifferentiating ASC VOCs from Figures 4 and 5 can also be found in the Supplemenary Figure S1.

4. Discussion

A nondestructive technique that could save time and material and gain more detailed information on cellular metabolism would be desirable. The analysis of VOCs by means of NTME preconcentration of headspace air coupled with GC-MS could be a fast and nondestructive method for the analysis of metabolic processes in cell cultures [29–31].

In this study, our previously developed versatile sampling system [28] was applied to monitor VOC emissions of cellular differentiation under standardized conditions. This method, however, presents some challenges. Physical, chemical, and biological processes (e.g., the degradation of FCS in culture medium) might affect VOC emissions. Therefore, the analysis of an adequate control—in this case pure cell culture medium without cells—is a crucial step in order to obtain reliable results. Large variations in VOC concentrations emitted from pure culture medium have been observed previously [21] and might be due to physical and chemical processes during heating and cooling as well as aging of the media. Furthermore, lipophilic VOCs (such as ethylbenzene, heptanal, or 2-ethylhexanol) might also be bound to lipids of cellular structures (e.g., membranes) in general [32].

In our study we utilized an established cell culture model that showed clear differences between nondifferentiated cells and cells in adipogenic differentiation. Analysis of the formation of lipid-filled vacuoles clearly confirmed the differentiation of the ASCs after adipogenic stimulation, whereas the nondifferentiated ASCs did not show any signs of adipogenesis. This cell culture model has already been examined for energy metabolic aspects, and it has been shown that adipogenic differentiation induces a shift towards lipid metabolism [12].

In the headspace of both ASC cultures (adipogenically differentiating and nondifferentiating), some VOC emissions seem to be related to culture media emissions rather than to emissions from the cells in culture. This applies to four substances (2-ethylhexanol, acetone, tert-butanol, and 2-butanone) in the headspace of adipogenically differentiating ASC cultures and two substances (heptanal and octanal) in the headspace of nondifferentiating ASC cultures. Whether these changes are specific and biochemically driven or merely induced by unspecific chemical conversion remains unclear. However, since the VOCs acetaldehyde, pentane, and 1,3-di-tert-butylbenzene showed clear emission differences dependent on the differentiation conditions, a specific link to metabolic processes might be possible.

Our data indicated that ASCs undergoing adipogenic differentiation increased the emission of acetaldehyde, whereas nondifferentiated ASCs reduced the emissions down to almost zero. Acetaldehyde emissions were nearly three times higher on day 21 of cultivation in adipogenically differentiating ASCs compared with nondifferentiating cultures. When taking into account the cell number, which is lower in adipogenically differentiating ASCs due to a stop in proliferation [12], this effect becomes even more distinctive. Thus, in our study, acetaldehyde is the VOC with the most variable differentiation-dependent behavior.

Acetaldehyde might be connected to mitochondrial pyruvate decarboxylation [33,34]. Whether acetaldehyde is consumed or produced could indicate the demands for intracellular acetyl-CoA. The energy metabolism of nonstimulated cells and adipogenically stimulated ASCs might be based predominantly on carbohydrate oxidation with a flux of pyruvate to acetyl-CoA. Under these conditions, it is possible that acetaldehyde can be used as well for acetyl-CoA production.

However, acetaldehyde can also be the product of ethanol degradation. Since some differentiation-inducing additives are dissolved in ethanol, a general, slightly increased level of acetaldehyde emissions compared with ASCs in maintenance medium might result from higher ethanol levels in the differentiation medium. This might be reflected in the increase of acetaldehyde emissions in the medium controls at an early time point (up to seven days). Ethanol dehydrogenase activity was detected in brown adipose tissue of rats [35]. Whether ethanol dehydrogenase is also present in the ASCs of white adipose tissue needs to be determined.

1,3-di-tert-butylbenzene emissions showed a significant increase in adipogenically differentiating ASCs compared to nondifferentiating ASCs. Tang et al. [36] found 1,3-di-tert-butylbenzene emitted differentially in cancer cells lines compared with nonmalignant cells. No further information is available about this substance in the current literature.

When normalized to cell numbers, pentane concentrations were higher in adipogenically differentiating ASCs than in nondifferentiating ones. Pentane is produced through the peroxidation of lipids and other biomolecules under the action of reactive oxygen species [37]. As shown before, adipogenic differentiation of ASCs correlates with an increase of the antioxidative defense activities of glutathione reductase [12]. This could conform with our current findings, which indicate an increase in the production of reactive oxygen species in adipogenically differentiating cells, and which could be followed by an increase in the antioxidative defense systems of ASCs.

Ethylbenzene showed higher concentrations in the headspace of medium controls than in the headspace of cultivated cells. In general, lower and less-deviating concentrations were observed in the headspaces of adipogenically differentiating ASCs compared with nondifferentiating ASCs. We, thus, conclude that cells in culture with and without differentiation stimulation consume or bind this compound. Previous studies established that ethylbenzene undergoes α- and ω-oxidation [38].

The aldehydes benzaldehyde, heptanal, and octanal were also consumed or bound by the cells from the culture media under both cultivation conditions. A consumption of aldehydes from the culture media might be based on the activity of aldehyde dehydrogenase [39,40] (e.g., benzaldehyde concentrations were reduced in the headspace of all cells but were even lower in adipogenically differentiating than in nondifferentiating cells). Zimmermann et al. [41] described NAD-aldehyde dehydrogenase as a possible enzyme for metabolizing benzaldehyde in fatty acid metabolism and tryptophan metabolism [42,43]. Amino acids are necessary for proliferation and differentiation, and their consumption was also observed in stem cell lines [27].

Heptanal and octanal showed relatively higher concentrations on day 21 in the adipogenically stimulated ASC cultures when related to the cell number. Since heptanal can be a product of lipid peroxidation [44,45], increasing enzyme activity for lipid oxidation during differentiation could lead to a higher turnover of heptanal. Other studies linked octanal to oxidative stress [46,47]. While this process includes lipid oxidation, octanal might increase during adipogenic differentiation due to an increase of the oxidation processes.

5. Conclusions

In this study we were able to identify differentially emitted VOCs, which might be linked to a changed metabolic activity in ASCs dependent on cellular differentiation. Whether these changes are driven by specific, enzyme-mediated processes or are the result of unspecific reactions has to be investigated. Irrespective of the fact that these are early stage results, the data presented are in agreement with the results of adipogenic-differentiating cells to date. Thus, further experiments might reveal if headspace VOC measurements serve as a marker for the quality and quantity of adipogenic differentiation of ASCs.

Supplementary Materials: The following are available online at http://www.mdpi.com/2073-4409/8/7/697/s1, Table S1: Quantitative parameters of VOCs: Concentration ranges, limits of detection (LOD), limits of quantification (LOQ) and standard deviation (SD) of 12 substances detected in ASC and pure culture medium, Table S2: P-values of statistical comparison between non- differentiating ASC (non-diff ASC) and adipogenically differentiating (adipo ASC), Figure S1: VOCs during the adipogenic differentiation. Figure S2: Vocs of nondifferentiating ASC.

Author Contributions: Conceptualization, A.-C.K. and K.P.; methodology, A.-C.K., S.T., J.M., and K.P.; formal analysis, A.-C.K., J.B., K.E., and J.M.; investigation, A.-C.K., J.B., S.T., J.M., and K.E.; resources, W.M., J.K.S., and K.P.; data curation, A.-C.K.; writing—original draft preparation, A.-C.K., J.B., J.M., and K.P.; writing—review and editing, A.-C.K., K.P., W.M., J.K.S., K.E., and G.K.; visualization, A.-C.K., J.M., and S.T.; supervision, K.P., W.M., J.K.S., and G.K.; funding acquisition, A.-C.K. and K.P.

Funding: This research was funded by a scholarship of the Landesgraduiertenfoerderung MV and the European Regional Development Fund (ERDF) together with the Federal State of Mecklenburg-Vorpommern ("Entwicklung eines Systems zur automatisierten Zellfraktionierung aus humanem Fettgewebe für neuartige regenerative Anwendungen und Therapien (ARENA)", TBI-V-003-VBU-001).

Acknowledgments: The authors thank Jürgen Weber (Ästhetikklinik Rostock, Germany), Klaus Ueberreiter (Park-Klinik Birkenwerder, Germany) and their patients for kindly providing liposuction tissue. Special thanks are also given to Nina Gehm and Anne Wolff for their technical support.

Conflicts of Interest: The authors declare no conflict of interest. The funders had no role in the design of the study; in the collection, analyses, or interpretation of data; in the writing of the manuscript, or in the decision to publish the results.

References

1. Valtieri, M.; Sorrentino, A. The mesenchymal stromal cell contribution to homeostasis. *J. Cell. Physiol.* **2008**, *217*, 296–300. [CrossRef] [PubMed]
2. Lee, R.H.; Kim, B.; Choi, I.; Kim, H.; Choi, H.S.; Suh, K.; Bae, Y.C.; Jung, J.S. Characterization and expression analysis of mesenchymal stem cells from human bone marrow and adipose tissue. *Cell. Physiol. Biochem. Int. J. Exp. Cell. Physiol. Biochem. Pharmacol.* **2004**, *14*, 311–324. [CrossRef] [PubMed]
3. Peroni, D.; Scambi, I.; Pasini, A.; Lisi, V.; Bifari, F.; Krampera, M.; Rigotti, G.; Sbarbati, A.; Galiè, M. Stem molecular signature of adipose-derived stromal cells. *Exp. Cell Res.* **2008**, *314*, 603–615. [CrossRef] [PubMed]

4. Spitkovsky, D.; Hescheler, J. Adult mesenchymal stromal stem cells for therapeutic applications. *Minim. Invasive Ther. Allied Technol. MITAT Off. J. Soc. Minim. Invasive Ther.* **2008**, *17*, 79–90. [CrossRef] [PubMed]
5. Zuk, P.A.; Zhu, M.; Ashjian, P.; De Ugarte, D.A.; Huang, J.I.; Mizuno, H.; Alfonso, Z.C.; Fraser, J.K.; Benhaim, P.; Hedrick, M.H. Human adipose tissue is a source of multipotent stem cells. *Mol. Biol. Cell* **2002**, *13*, 4279–4295. [CrossRef] [PubMed]
6. Zuk, P.A.; Zhu, M.; Mizuno, H.; Huang, J.; Futrell, J.W.; Katz, A.J.; Benhaim, P.; Lorenz, H.P.; Hedrick, M.H. Multilineage cells from human adipose tissue: Implications for cell-based therapies. *Tissue Eng.* **2001**, *7*, 211–228. [CrossRef]
7. De Ugarte, D.A.; Morizono, K.; Elbarbary, A.; Alfonso, Z.; Zuk, P.A.; Zhu, M.; Dragoo, J.L.; Ashjian, P.; Thomas, B.; Benhaim, P.; et al. Comparison of multi-lineage cells from human adipose tissue and bone marrow. *Cells Tissues Organs* **2003**, *174*, 101–109. [CrossRef]
8. Schop, D.; Janssen, F.W.; van Rijn, L.D.S.; Fernandes, H.; Bloem, R.M.; de Bruijn, J.D.; van Dijkhuizen-Radersma, R. Growth, metabolism, and growth inhibitors of mesenchymal stem cells. *Tissue Eng. Part A* **2009**, *15*, 1877–1886. [CrossRef]
9. Pattappa, G.; Heywood, H.K.; de Bruijn, J.D.; Lee, D.A. The metabolism of human mesenchymal stem cells during proliferation and differentiation. *J. Cell. Physiol.* **2011**, *226*, 2562–2570. [CrossRef]
10. Li, Q.; Gao, Z.; Chen, Y.; Guan, M.-X. The role of mitochondria in osteogenic, adipogenic and chondrogenic differentiation of mesenchymal stem cells. *Protein Cell* **2017**, *8*, 439–445. [CrossRef]
11. Zhang, Y.; Marsboom, G.; Toth, P.T.; Rehman, J. Mitochondrial respiration regulates adipogenic differentiation of human mesenchymal stem cells. *PLoS ONE* **2013**, *8*, e77077. [CrossRef] [PubMed]
12. Meyer, J.; Salamon, A.; Mispagel, S.; Kamp, G.; Peters, K. Energy metabolic capacities of human adipose-derived mesenchymal stromal cells in vitro and their adaptations in osteogenic and adipogenic differentiation. *Exp. Cell Res.* **2018**, *370*, 632–642. [CrossRef] [PubMed]
13. Meyer, J.; Engelmann, R.; Kamp, G.; Peters, K. Human adipocytes and CD34+ cells from the stromal vascular fraction of the same adipose tissue differ in their energy metabolic enzyme configuration. *Exp. Cell Res.* **2019**, *380*, 47–54. [CrossRef] [PubMed]
14. Mathieu, J.; Ruohola-Baker, H. Metabolic remodeling during the loss and acquisition of pluripotency. *Development* **2017**, *144*, 541–551. [CrossRef] [PubMed]
15. Capuano, R.; Spitalieri, P.; Talarico, R.V.; Domakoski, A.C.; Catini, A.; Paolesse, R.; Martinelli, E.; Novelli, G.; Sangiuolo, F.; Di Natale, C. A preliminary analysis of volatile metabolites of human induced pluripotent stem cells along the in vitro differentiation. *Sci. Rep.* **2017**, *7*, 1621. [CrossRef] [PubMed]
16. Filipiak, W.; Sponring, A.; Mikoviny, T.; Ager, C.; Schubert, J.; Miekisch, W.; Amann, A.; Troppmair, J. Release of volatile organic compounds (VOCs) from the lung cancer cell line CALU-1 in vitro. *Cancer Cell Int.* **2008**, *8*. [CrossRef]
17. Filipiak, W.; Sponring, A.; Baur, M.M.; Ager, C.; Filipiak, A.; Wiesenhofer, H.; Nagl, M.; Troppmair, J.; Amann, A. Characterization of volatile metabolites taken up by or released from Streptococcus pneumoniae and Haemophilus influenzae by using GC-MS. *Microbiology* **2012**, *158*, 3044–3053. [CrossRef]
18. Kai, M.; Haustein, M.; Molina, F.; Petri, A.; Scholz, B.; Piechulla, B. Bacterial volatiles and their action potential. *Appl. Microbiol. Biotechnol.* **2009**, *81*, 1001–1012. [CrossRef]
19. Trefz, P.; Rösner, L.; Hein, D.; Schubert, J.K.; Miekisch, W. Evaluation of needle trap micro-extraction and automatic alveolar sampling for point-of-care breath analysis. *Anal. Bioanal. Chem.* **2013**, *405*, 3105–3115. [CrossRef]
20. Bergmann, A.; Trefz, P.; Fischer, S.; Klepik, K.; Walter, G.; Steffens, M.; Ziller, M.; Schubert, J.K.; Reinhold, P.; Köhler, H.; et al. In Vivo Volatile Organic Compound Signatures of Mycobacterium avium subsp. paratuberculosis. *PLoS ONE* **2015**, *10*, e0123980. [CrossRef]
21. Filipiak, W.; Mochalski, P.; Filipiak, A.; Ager, C.; Cumeras, R.; Davis, C.E.; Agapiou, A.; Unterkofler, K.; Troppmair, J. A Compendium of Volatile Organic Compounds (VOCs) Released By Human Cell Lines. *Curr. Med. Chem.* **2016**, *23*, 2112–2131. [CrossRef] [PubMed]
22. Trefz, P.; Koehler, H.; Klepik, K.; Moebius, P.; Reinhold, P.; Schubert, J.K.; Miekisch, W. Volatile Emissions from Mycobacterium avium subsp. paratuberculosis Mirror Bacterial Growth and Enable Distinction of Different Strains. *PLoS ONE* **2013**, *8*, e76868. [CrossRef] [PubMed]

23. Acevedo, C.A.; Sanchez, E.Y.; Reyes, J.G.; Young, M.E. Volatile profiles of human skin cell cultures in different degrees of senescence. *J. Chromatogr. B Analyt. Technol. Biomed. Life. Sci.* **2010**, *878*, 449–455. [CrossRef] [PubMed]
24. Acevedo, C.A.; Sánchez, E.Y.; Reyes, J.G.; Young, M.E. Volatile organic compounds produced by human skin cells. *Biol. Res.* **2007**, *40*, 347–355. [CrossRef] [PubMed]
25. Smith, D.; Wang, T.; Spaněl, P. On-line, simultaneous quantification of ethanol, some metabolites and water vapour in breath following the ingestion of alcohol. *Physiol. Meas.* **2002**, *23*, 477–489. [CrossRef] [PubMed]
26. Miekisch, W.; Schubert, J.K.; Noeldge-Schomburg, G.F.E. Diagnostic potential of breath analysis–focus on volatile organic compounds. *Clin. Chim. Acta Int. J. Clin. Chem.* **2004**, *347*, 25–39. [CrossRef]
27. Bischoff, A.-C.; Oertel, P.; Sukul, P.; Rimmbach, C.; David, R.; Schubert, J.; Miekisch, W. Smell of cells: Volatile profiling of stem- and non-stem cell proliferation. *J. Breath Res.* **2017**, *12*. [CrossRef]
28. Traxler, S.; Bischoff, A.-C.; Trefz, P.; Schubert, J.K.; Miekisch, W. Versatile set-up for non-invasive in vitro analysis of headspace VOCs. *J. Breath Res.* **2018**, *12*, 041001. [CrossRef]
29. Mochalski, P.; Sponring, A.; King, J.L.; Unterkofler, K.; Troppmair, J.; Amann, A. Release and uptake of volatile organic compounds by human hepatocellular carcinoma cells (HepG2) in vitro. *Cancer Cell Int.* **2013**, *13*, 72. [CrossRef]
30. Küntzel, A.; Fischer, S.; Bergmann, A.; Oertel, P.; Steffens, M.; Trefz, P.; Miekisch, W.; Schubert, J.K.; Reinhold, P.; Köhler, H. Effects of biological and methodological factors on volatile organic compound patterns during cultural growth of Mycobacterium avium ssp. paratuberculosis. *J. Breath Res.* **2016**, *10*, 037103. [CrossRef]
31. Mochalski, P.; Theurl, M.; Sponring, A.; Unterkofler, K.; Kirchmair, R.; Amann, A. Analysis of volatile organic compounds liberated and metabolised by human umbilical vein endothelial cells (HUVEC) in vitro. *Cell Biochem. Biophys.* **2015**, *71*, 323–329. [CrossRef] [PubMed]
32. Odinokov, A.; Ostroumov, D. Structural Degradation and Swelling of Lipid Bilayer under the Action of Benzene. *J. Phys. Chem. B* **2015**, *119*, 15006–15013. [CrossRef] [PubMed]
33. Michoudet, C.; Baverel, G. Characteristics of acetaldehyde metabolism in isolated dog, rat and guinea-pig kidney tubules. *Biochem. Pharmacol.* **1987**, *36*, 3987–3991. [CrossRef]
34. Nelson, D.L.; Cox, M.M. *Lehninger Biochemie*; Springer: Berlin, Heidelberg, 2001; ISBN 978-3-662-08290-4.
35. Kortelainen, M.L.; Huttunen, P.; Hirvonen, J. Histochemical and biochemical detection of alcohol dehydrogenase in rat brown adipose tissue. *Alcohol Fayettev. N* **1991**, *8*, 151–154. [CrossRef]
36. Tang, H.; Lu, Y.; Zhang, L.; Wu, Z.; Hou, X.; Xia, H. Determination of volatile organic compounds exhaled by cell lines derived from hematological malignancies. *Biosci. Rep.* **2017**, *37*. [CrossRef] [PubMed]
37. Amann, A.; de Costello, B.L.; Miekisch, W.; Schubert, J.; Buszewski, B.; Pleil, J.; Ratcliffe, N.; Risby, T. The human volatilome: Volatile organic compounds (VOCs) in exhaled breath, skin emanations, urine, feces and saliva. *J. Breath Res.* **2014**, *8*, 034001. [CrossRef] [PubMed]
38. El Masry, A.M.; Smith, J.N.; Williams, R.T. Studies in detoxication. 69. The metabolism of alkylbenzenes: N-propylbenzene and n-butylbenzene with further observations on ethylbenzene. *Biochem. J.* **1956**, *64*, 50–56. [CrossRef] [PubMed]
39. Marchitti, S.A.; Brocker, C.; Stagos, D.; Vasiliou, V. Non-P450 aldehyde oxidizing enzymes: The aldehyde dehydrogenase superfamily. *Expert Opin. Drug Metab. Toxicol.* **2008**, *4*, 697–720. [CrossRef]
40. Marcato, P.; Dean, C.A.; Giacomantonio, C.A.; Lee, P.W.K. Aldehyde dehydrogenase: Its role as a cancer stem cell marker comes down to the specific isoform. *Cell Cycle Georget. Tex* **2011**, *10*, 1378–1384. [CrossRef]
41. Zimmermann, D.; Hartmann, M.; Moyer, M.P.; Nolte, J.; Baumbach, J.I. Determination of volatile products of human colon cell line metabolism by GC/MS analysis. *Metabolomics* **2007**, *3*, 13–17. [CrossRef]
42. Wermuth, B.; Münch, J.D.; von Wartburg, J.P. Purification and properties of NADPH-dependent aldehyde reductase from human liver. *J. Biol. Chem.* **1977**, *252*, 3821–3828. [PubMed]
43. Klyosov, A.A. Kinetics and Specificity of Human Liver Aldehyde Dehydrogenases toward Aliphatic, Aromatic, and Fused Polycyclic Aldehydes †. *Biochemistry* **1996**, *35*, 4457–4467. [CrossRef] [PubMed]
44. Jareño-Esteban, J.J.; Muñoz-Lucas, M.Á.; Carrillo-Aranda, B.; Maldonado-Sanz, J.Á.; de Granda-Orive, I.; Aguilar-Ros, A.; Civera-Tejuca, C.; Gutiérrez-Ortega, C.; Callol-Sánchez, L.M. Volatile Organic Compounds in Exhaled Breath in a Healthy Population: Effect of Tobacco Smoking. *Arch. Bronconeumol. Engl. Ed.* **2013**, *49*, 457–461. [CrossRef] [PubMed]

45. Kneepkens, C.M.; Lepage, G.; Roy, C.C. The potential of the hydrocarbon breath test as a measure of lipid peroxidation. *Free Radic. Biol. Med.* **1994**, *17*, 127–160. [CrossRef]
46. Corradi, M.; Pignatti, P.; Manini, P.; Andreoli, R.; Goldoni, M.; Poppa, M.; Moscato, G.; Balbi, B.; Mutti, A. Comparison between exhaled and sputum oxidative stress biomarkers in chronic airway inflammation. *Eur. Respir. J. Off. J. Eur. Soc. Clin. Respir. Physiol.* **2004**, *24*, 1011–1017. [CrossRef] [PubMed]
47. Halliwell, B. Free radicals, antioxidants, and human disease: Curiosity, cause, or consequence? *Lancet Lond. Engl.* **1994**, *344*, 721–724. [CrossRef]

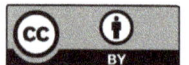

© 2019 by the authors. Licensee MDPI, Basel, Switzerland. This article is an open access article distributed under the terms and conditions of the Creative Commons Attribution (CC BY) license (http://creativecommons.org/licenses/by/4.0/).

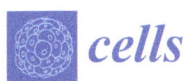

Article

Collagen I Promotes Adipocytogenesis in Adipose-Derived Stem Cells In Vitro

Nadja Zöller, Sarah Schreiner, Laura Petry, Stephanie Hoffmann, Katja Steinhorst, Johannes Kleemann, Manuel Jäger, Roland Kaufmann, Markus Meissner and Stefan Kippenberger *

Department of Dermatology, Venereology and Allergy, Johann Wolfgang Goethe University, Theodor-Stern-Kai 7, D-60590 Frankfurt/Main, Germany; Nadja.Zoeller@kgu.de (N.Z.); S_Schreiner@gmx.de (S.S.); Laura.Petry@kgu.de (L.P.); Stephanie.Hoffmann@kgu.de (S.H.); katja.Steinhorst@kgu.de (K.S.); Johannes.Kleemann@kgu.de (J.K.); Manuel.Jaeger@kgu.de (M.J.); kaufmann@em.uni-frankfurt.de (R.K.); Markus.Meissner@kgu.de (M.M.)
* Correspondence: kippenberger@em.uni-frankfurt.de; Tel.: +49-69-6301-7734

Received: 7 March 2019; Accepted: 28 March 2019; Published: 1 April 2019

Abstract: A hallmark of ageing is the redistribution of body fat. Particularly, subcutaneous fat decreases paralleled by a decrease of skin collagen I are typical for age-related skin atrophy. In this paper, we hypothesize that collagen I may be a relevant molecule stimulating the differentiation of adipose-derived stem cells (ASCs) into adipocytes augmenting subcutaneous fat. In this context lipogenesis, adiponectin, and collagen I receptor expression were determined. Freshly isolated ASCs were characterized by stemness-associated surface markers by FACS analysis and then transdifferentiated into adipocytes by specific medium supplements. Lipogenesis was evaluated using Nile Red staining and documented by fluorescence microscopy or quantitatively measured by using a multiwell spectrofluorometer. Expression of adiponectin was measured by real-time RT-PCR and in cell-free supernatants by ELISA, and expression of collagen I receptors was observed by western blot analysis. It was found that supports coated with collagen I promote cell adhesion and lipogenesis of ASCs. Interestingly, a reverse correlation to adiponectin expression was observed. Moreover, we found upregulation of the collagen receptor, discoidin domain-containing receptor 2; receptors of the integrin family were absent or downregulated. These findings indicate that collagen I is able to modulate lipogenesis and adiponectin expression and therefore may contribute to metabolic dysfunctions associated with ageing.

Keywords: adipose-derived stem cells; adipocytes; differentiation; collagen I; adiponectin; integrins; discoidin domain-containing receptor; ageing; subcutaneous fat

---

1. Introduction

Adipose-derived stem cells (ASCs), residing within fat tissue, display multilineage plasticity, which makes them interesting for regenerative medicine. Minimal invasive procedures allowing liposuction facilitate access, particularly to superficial adipose tissue. After purification and plating, the fate of native ASCs can be directed by specific culture conditions. As a result, different phenotypes can be induced that are characteristic for adipocytes [1,2], fibroblasts [3], endothelial cells [4], osteoblasts [5], chondrocytes [6], cardio-myocytes [7], neural-like cells [2], hepatocytes [8], pancreatic cells [9], and others.

Skin ageing is triggered by intrinsic and extrinsic factors, leading to a massive remodeling of the extracellular matrix (ECM) [10,11]. In this study, we hypothesize that the age-related decrease of ECM molecules also has an impact on the adipogenic differentiation potential in ASCs. In this context, we focus on the role of collagen I, which is the most prominent constituent of ECM molecules distributed throughout the interstitium, making up to 90% of the total connective tissue. Besides providing mechanical rigidity, collagen fibrils also act as guidance structures for contacting cells. Among cellular collagen receptors, the surface receptors of the integrin family are most prominent. They are composed of noncovalently associated α and β subunits forming a heterodimer that recognizes specific amino acid motifs within collagen molecules, hereby initiating intracellular signaling cascades. Besides integrins, two receptor tyrosine kinases, namely discoidin domain receptors 1 and 2 (DDR1 and DDR2), have also been identified to be activated upon collagen binding [12,13]. Particularly, DDR2 is characteristic for cells of mesenchymal origin, such as fibroblasts and smooth muscle cells [14].

In order to characterize adipogenic differentiation, we put particular emphasis on lipogenesis by measuring the lipid content. Moreover, another characteristic of adipocytes is the signature pattern of secreted factors that have been collectively termed 'adipokines'. Prominent among those are leptin, adiponectin, resistin, and visfatin, as well as cytokines and chemokines, such as tumor necrosis factor-α and interleukin-6 [15]. It is assumed that these factors contribute to a subinflammatory state that triggers the development of many chronic obesity-correlated diseases. In this present paper, we focus on adiponectin, a multifaceted adipokine, known as a modulator of inflammation [16,17].

The data presented in this paper show that the contact of ASCs to collagen I is a relevant factor in adipogenic differentiation as characterized by lipogenesis and adiponectin secretion. It could be speculated that collagen synthesis under physiological conditions might control the fate of ASCs.

2. Materials and Methods

2.1. Ethics Statement

This study was conducted according to the Declaration of Helsinki Principles and in agreement with the Local Ethic Commission of the faculty of Medicine of the Johann Wolfgang Goethe University (Frankfurt am Main, Germany). The Local Ethic Commission waived the need for consent.

2.2. Isolation and Characterization of ASCs

Isolation and initiation of human ASC cultures were performed as described [18]. As source served abdominal subcutaneous fat tissue derived from plastic surgeries, generously provided by Dr. Ulrich Rieger (Klinik für Plastische und Ästhetische Chirurgie, Wiederherstellungs und Handchirurgie, Markus Krankenhaus, Frankfurt/Main, Germany). The fat tissue was placed in PBS with 2% penicillin/streptomycin (Biochrom, Berlin, Germany) incubated overnight (4 °C). On the next day, skin and blood vessels were mechanically removed by scissors and forceps. Small pieces, with approximately 5 mm lengths, were given to a collagenase type I solution (Worthington, Lakewood, USA) and incubated for 3 h at 37 °C. Cell debris was discarded by filtration through sterile gauze. Then, the cell suspension was centrifuged (400× g, 6 min, 4 °C), the cell pellet resuspended in medium, and passed through a cell strainer (70 μm, Greiner, Frickenhausen, Germany). Next, cells were separated by density filtration using a Biocoll solution with a specific density of 1.077 g/mL. After another centrifugation (400× g, 30 min, 4 °C), ASCs were isolated from the opaque interphase and seeded in DMEM supplemented with 1% UltroSerG (Pall, Dreieich, Germany) and 1% penicillin/streptomycin. The medium was renewed every 3 days.

2.3. Flow Cytometry

Phenotypical characterization of ASCs was performed using the BD FACSCalibur and analyzed with the CellQuest software (v. 1.0.1, Becton–Dickinson, Heidelberg, Germany). The cells were trypsinized, placed on ice for 30 min, and treated with the following labeled stemness-associated antigen markers: CD31-, CD34+, CD45–, CD54–, CD90+, CD105+, CD166+, HLA-ABC+, HLA-DR–. CD34-PE, CD90–FITC, and CD105-PerCP were part of the BD Stemflow Kit (Becton Dickinson, 562245). The other antibodies with the indicated specifications were purchased separately: CD31-FITC (R & D, Systems, Wiesbaden, Germany, FAB3567F), HLA-DR-PE (Becton Dickinson, 347401), CD166-PE

(Becton Dickinson, 559263), CD34-APC (Becton Dickinson, 555824), CD54-FITC (Beckman Coulter, Krefeld, Germany, PN IM0726U), HLA-ABC-FITC (Becton Dickinson, 555552), and CD45-PE (Becton Dickinson, 555483). Table 1 shows the results from three donors. All experiments shown in this paper were performed with cells until reaching passage 5.

Table 1. Characterization of ASCs.

Surface Marker	Positive Cells [%]		
	Donor 1	Donor 2	Donor 3
CD31/PECAM-1	0.75 ± 0.29	1.30 ± 0.19	0.83 ± 0.02
CD34	53.94 ± 7.09	63.98 ± 13.67	78.00 ± 1.29
CD45	0.85 ± 0.10	1.10 ± 0.13	0.97± 0.11
CD54/ICAM-1	1.36 ± 0.36	1.88 ± 0.57	2.76 ± 1.06
CD90/Thy-1	99.96 ± 0.03	99.88 ± 0.11	99.09 ± 1.39
CD105/Endoglin	91.07 ± 4.92	90.82 ± 11.62	60.17 ± 5.36
CD166/ALCAM	98.93 ± 0.82	97.83 ± 1.80	99.12 ± 0.11
HLA-ABC	99.74 ± 0.17	99.88 ± 0.05	99.48 ± 0.27
HLA-DR	0.78 ± 0.46	0.72 ± 0.11	0.56 ± 0.10

2.4. Adhesion Assay

For the adhesion experiments, ASCs were trypsinized and seeded at a concentration of 1×10^4 cells/well onto microtiter plates coated with collagen I (Becton-Dickinson, Heidelberg, Germany). The coating procedure was performed as previously described [19]. Briefly, collagen type I was dissolved with sterile acetic acid and given in the specific vessels (5 mg/cm^2). After drying, solvent and collagen remnants were removed by washing with PBS. Regular plastic dishes served as controls. After seeding, the cells were allowed to attach for 30, 60, 90, and 120 min at 37 °C. Then, non-anchored cells were removed by two washings with PBS, and the nuclei of anchored cells were stained with the DNA-binding fluorochrome bisbenzimide (2 mg/mL, 20 min, RT). After two washing steps, fluorescence was detected using the CytoFluor multi-well plate reader (Applied Biosystems, Langen, Germany) at 360/460 nm [19,20]. Experiments were performed three times with three triplicates.

2.5. Induction of Adipogenesis

ASCs were seeded in 24-well culture dishes at a concentration 5×10^4 cells/well. Adipogenic differentiation was induced by Adi-medium consisting of DMEM supplemented with 10 µM insulin, 0.5 mM 3-isobutyl-1-methylxanthine, 1 µM dexamethasone, 200 µM indomethacine, 1% penicillin/streptomycin solution, and 2% UltroserG [2,18].

2.6. Detection of Lipids

ASCs were cultured in Adi-medium (or standard medium) on collagen I-coated and non-coated supports for 9, 11, and 15 days. Consecutively, the lipid content was quantitatively detected as described [21]. Briefly, cultures were washed with PBS and then stained with nile red (1 µg/mL, 20 min, 37 °C). After two washing steps with PBS, fluorescence documented by fluorescence microscopy or quantitatively measured using a multiwell spectrofluorometer (Cytofluor, Applied Biosystems, Langen, Germany) equipped with 485/560 nm filters for neutral lipids. Moreover, cell nuclei were stained with bisbenzimide (2 µg/mL, 20 min, 37.4 °C) and the fluorescence, as a measure for cell count, was detected at 360/460 nm. In order to normalize the lipid values to different cell counts, a ratio was formed between nile red and bisbenzimide measurements. The values derived from cells cultured on plastic were set to 100% and all other values were related to that. Experiments were performed in quadruplicate, with 4 parallel determinations for each condition.

2.7. Western Blot

Cells cultured as described above were lysed in 100 mL SDS sample buffer (62.5 mM Tris-HCl [pH 6.8], 2% SDS, 10% glycerol, 50 mM DTT, 0.1% bromphenol blue), sonicated and boiled for 5 min, and separated on SDS-polyacrylamide gels. Consecutively, proteins were immunoblotted to a PVDF membrane. The membrane was blocked in blocking buffer (TBS [pH 7.6], 0.1% Tween-20, 5% nonfat dry milk) for at least 3 h at 4 °C followed by incubation with the primary antibody in TBS (pH 7.6), 0.05% Tween-20, and 5% BSA. Bound primary antibodies were detected using anti-mouse IgG-horseradish peroxidase conjugate and visualized with the LumiGlo detection system (Cell Signaling, Frankfurt, Germany). The following primary antibodies were used: Integrin β1 (Santa Cruz, sc-6622), integrin α1 (R & D, MAB5676-SP), integrin α2 (Becton-Dickinson, 611016), integrin α11 (R & D, AF4235-SP), and discoidin domain-containing receptor 2 (DDR2) (R & D, AF2538).

2.8. Adiponectin ELISA

Cells were seeded on collagen or plastic supports and exposed to either Adi-medium (or standard medium) for 9, 11, and 15 days. Cell-free supernatants were obtained and assayed for human adiponectin using a commercial ELISA test kit (R & D) according to the manufacturers' instructions. Briefly, supernatants were placed in microwell plates coated with antibodies against adiponectin. After incubation with a biotin-labeled secondary antibody, a streptavidin horseradish-peroxidase conjugate was added. A colorimetric reaction was exerted by addition of a substrate (tetramethylbenzidine/peroxide), giving rise to a colored product measured at 450 nm in a scanning multiwell spectrophotometer (ELISA reader MR 5000, Dynatech, Guernsey, UK).

2.9. Real-Time RT-PCR Analysis

Total cellular RNA was isolated from cells cultured as described above using the ExtractMe Total RNA Kit (Blirt, Gdansk, Poland). After DNase digestion, a total amount of 25 ng RNA was used for first-strand cDNA synthesis using a QuantiTect SYBR Green RT-PCR Kit (Qiagen, Hilden, Germany). Real-time PCRs were performed on a Light Cycler system 2.0 (Roche Diagnostics, Mannheim, Germany). The following primers for adiponectin (accession no. ENST00000320741.6) and PBDG (accession no. ENST00000278715) were used:

Adiponectin-for: 5'-TGTGGTTCTGATTCCATACCAG-3'
Adiponectin-rev: 5'-CGGGCAGAGCTAATAGCAGTA-3'
PBDG-for: 5'-CCATGTCTGGTAACGGCAAT-3'
PBDG-rev: 5'-GTCTGTATGCGAGCAAGCTG-3'

The relative expression of transcripts was determined using the 2-ΔΔCT method [22].

2.10. Statistics

All data are presented as mean values ± standard deviation. Statistical significance of the data was calculated by Wilcoxon-Mann-Whitney-U-test (BIAS, Frankfurt, Germany). Data sets were statistically compared as indicated in the graphics.

3. Results

Although most cell cultures were carried out on uncoated plastic dishes, it is known that extracellular matrix molecules have impacts on cell physiology. Therefore, we initially tested the adherence of ASCs held in standard medium to collagen I in comparison to uncoated plastic (Figure 1). Representative photographs of time-dependent adhesion are shown in Figure S1. It was found that ASCs in suspension feature a significant faster adherence to collagen I-coated substrates in the first 30 min. In the further course, the cell count adherent to either plastic or collagen I was similar in the observed time span. These results indicate that naïve ASCs also express adhesion molecules with avidity to collagen I.

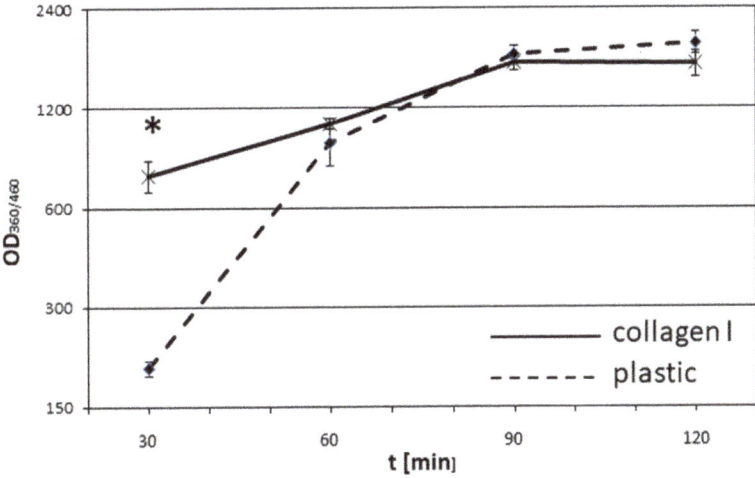

Figure 1. Quantitative adhesion of ASCs on plastic vs collagen I. ASCs were plated at a density of 1×10^4 cells per well into microtiterplates either non-coated or coated with collagen I. After 30, 60, 90, and 120 min, non-adherent cells were discarded and the remaining cells were stained with bisbenzimide. Fluorescence, as a measure for adherent cells, was quantified using a CytoFluor multi-well plate reader at 360/460 nm. Each point represents the mean of five independent experiments. The standard deviations are indicated. * $p < 0.05$. The whole experiment was repeated three times with similar results.

Furthermore, we investigated the impact of adhesion to collagen I on cell morphology and differentiation (Figure 2). Cells were seeded on supports coated with collagen I or plastic for control and then cultured for 19 days in either standard medium (DMEM) or adipogenic medium (Adi-medium). On plastic (Figure 2A), ASCs feature a domed cell center with filigree dendritic plasma extrusions in the periphery. These dendritic branches are less pronounced in cells on collagen I (Figure 2B). When cells were held in adipogenic medium, the cell morphology changed massively. Cells form a large interconnected network with many extended cell branches reminding on a network of nerve cells (Figure 2C,D). Moreover, cells accumulate tightly packed vesicles in the cell center, which putatively represent lipid droplets. In order to verify the nature of these droplets, a nile red staining was performed (Figure 2E–H). Positive nile staining was found around the cell nucleus, stained in blue with bisbenzimide, indicating the presence of lipids. Of note, on the photographs, the expression of lipids seems to be more distinct in cells cultured on collagen I.

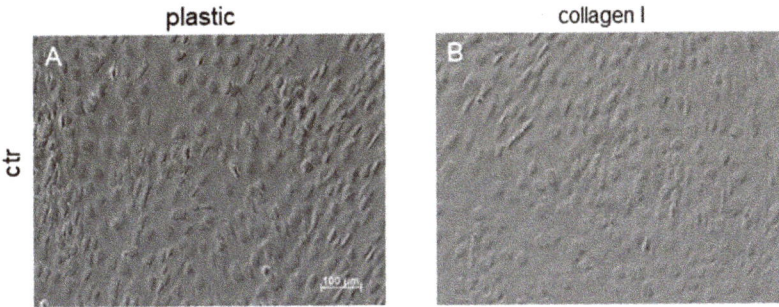

Figure 2. *Cont.*

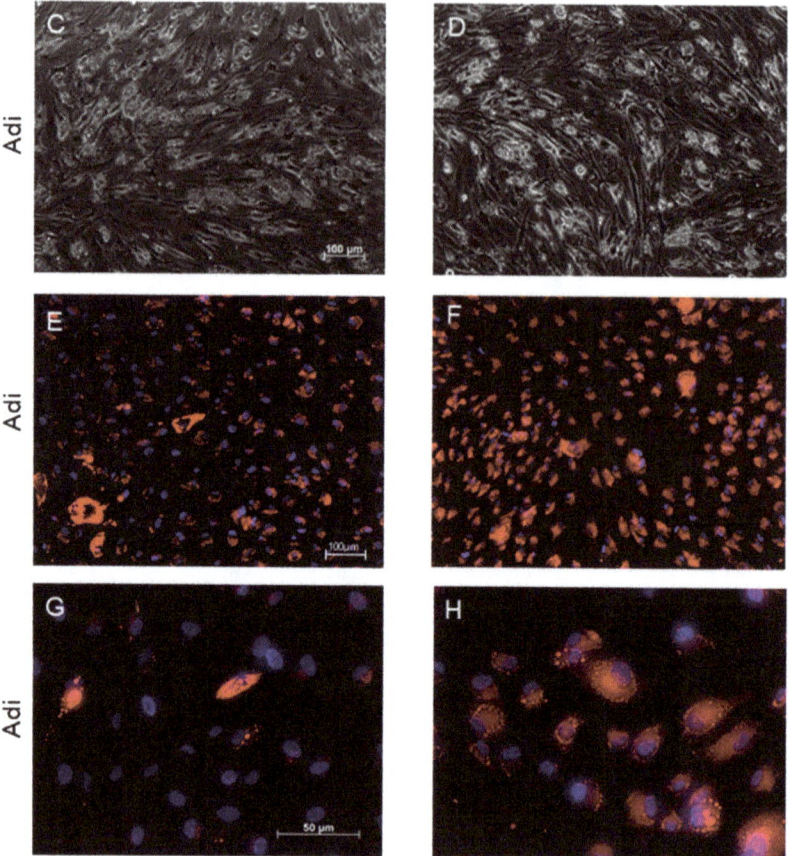

Figure 2. ASCs cultured on plastic or collagen I. (**A,B**) show the cell morphology after cultivation in ASC standard medium (ctr) for 19 days, (**C,D**) after cultivation in adipogenic medium (Adi). (**E–H**) display cellular lipids (red) after cultivation in adipogenic medium for 19 days stained with the fluorescence dye nile red; cell nuclei (blue) are stained with bisbenzimide. Photographs show representative sections.

In order to validate this first impression, nile red staining was quantified at different time points (9, 11, 15 days) by fluorometric means as described. Figure 3 shows the content of neutral lipids of ASCs in dependence to culture medium (DMEM vs Adi-medium) and cell support (plastic vs collagen I). The value determined for ASCs cultured in DMEM on plastic was set to 100%. In these cells, which are absent of lipid droplets, nile red stains showed lipid-containing membranes only. All other measured values were related to this. It was found that cultivation on collagen I led to a slight, but significant increase in lipid content at all examined time points in DMEM (black bars). Moreover, the change to Adi-medium induced the expected massive and significant increase in lipids in cells on plastic and collagen I (striped bars). Of note, cultures on collagen I showed an increase in lipids compared to their counterparts held on plastic. In sum, these results indicated a lipogenic effect of collagen I in ASCs.

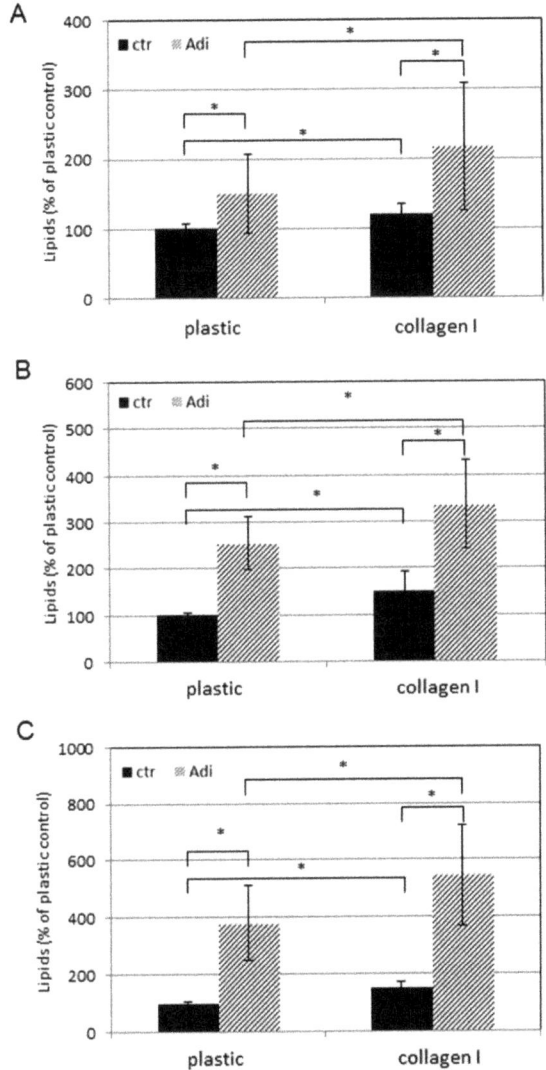

Figure 3. Quantitative lipogenesis of ASCs on plastic or collagen I. ASCs were plated at a density of 1×10^4 cells per well into microtiterplates either non-coated (plastic) or coated with collagen I. One part was held in regular DMEM medium (ctr) and the other in adipogenic medium (Adi). After (**A**) 9 days, (**B**) 11 days, and (**C**) 15 days, cells were stained with nile red and bisbenzimide and the fluorescence was measured (see Materials and Methods). Each point represents the mean of 16 independent experiments. The standard deviations are indicated. Data sets were statistically compared as indicated. * $p < 0.05$.

Next, the release of adiponectin, a prototypical adipokine, was evaluated in cell-free supernatants by ELISA after 9, 11, and 15 days (Figure 4A–C). ASCs cultured in DMEM showed no significant release of adiponectin in the period under observation regardless of whether they were cultured on plastic or collagen I (black bars). Changing the medium to Adi-medium induced a massive release of adiponectin (striped bars). Comparison of both cell substrates shows that the measured levels of adiponectin on collagen I were significantly reduced.

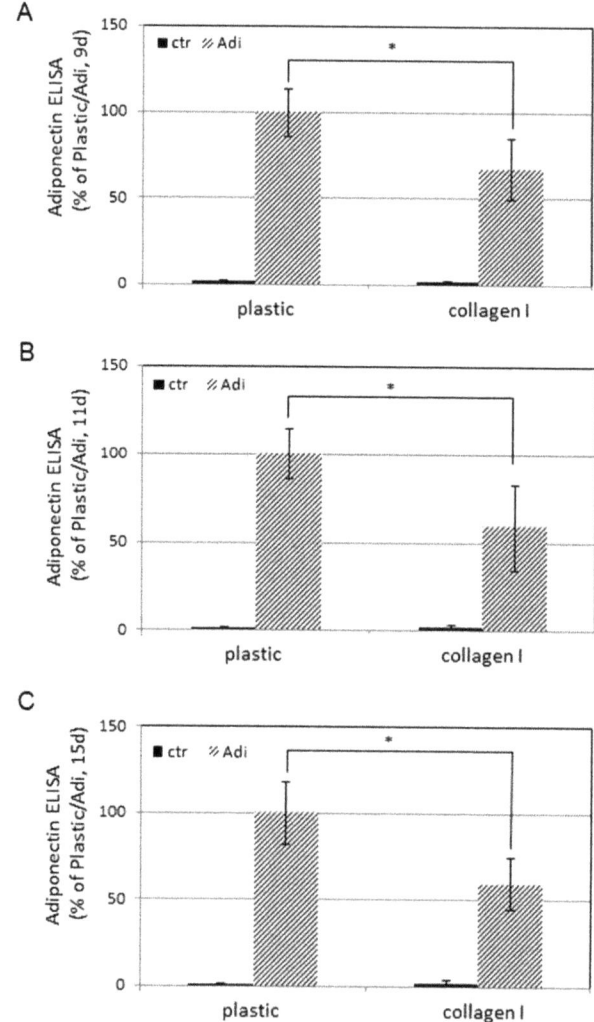

Figure 4. Adiponectin release of ASCs on plastic or collagen I. ASCs were plated at a density of 1×10^4 cells per well into microtiterplates either non-coated (plastic) or coated with collagen I. One part was held in regular DMEM medium (ctr) and the other in adipogenic medium (Adi). After (**A**) 9 days, (**B**) 11 days, and (**C**) 15 days, supernatants were examined for adiponectin by ELISA. Each point represents the mean of 20 independent experiments. The standard deviations are indicated. Data sets of Adi/plastic and Adi/collagen I were statistically compared as indicated. * $p < 0.05$.

To learn more about the level of this regulation, mRNA transcripts of adiponectin were quantified by real-time RT-PCR analysis (Figure 5). As found for the adiponectin release, almost no adiponectin mRNA expression was found in ASCs held in DMEM (black bars). In contrast, massive induction was initiated by changing the medium to Adi-medium (striped bars). Similar to the measured protein levels, this induction was gradually diminished by cultivation on supports coated with collagen I. The measured Ct values ranged from ca. (circa) 29 for non-differentiated to ca. 22 for differentiated cells. The Ct values for reference gene (PBGD) expression were ca. 27 independent from culture conditions.

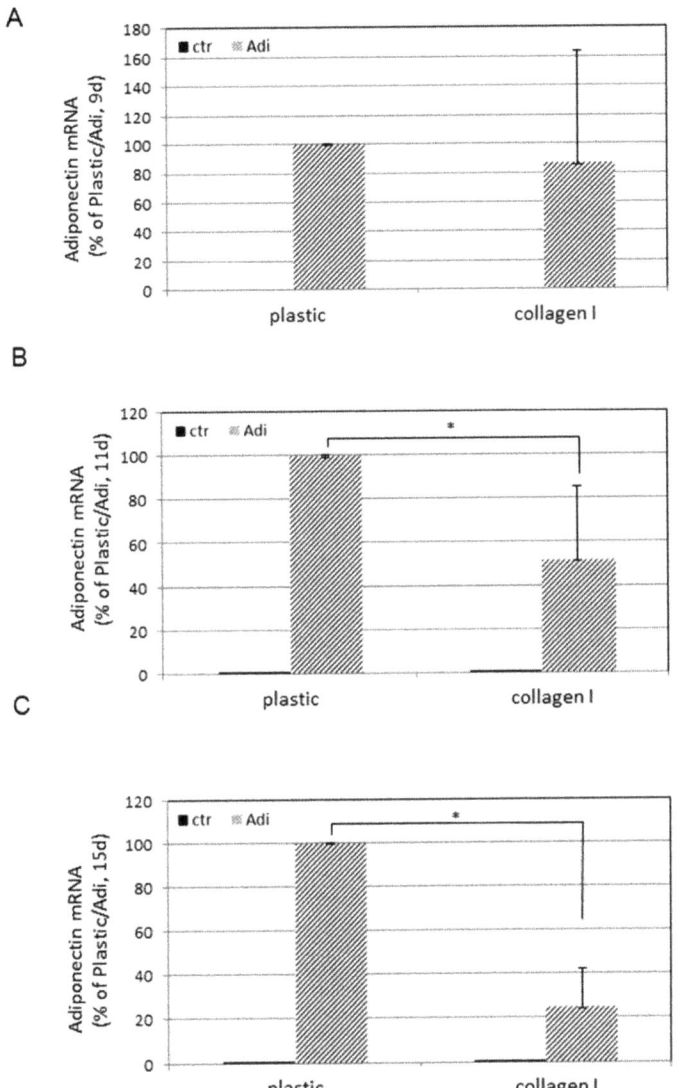

Figure 5. Adiponectin mRNA expression of ASCs on plastic or collagen I. ASCs were plated at a density of 1×10^4 cells per well into microtiterplates either non-coated (plastic) or coated with collagen I. One part was held in regular DMEM medium (ctr) and the other in adipogenic medium (Adi). After (**A**) 9 days, (**B**) 11 days, and (**C**) 15 days, total RNA was extracted and real-time RT-PCR analysis was performed. The values for ASCs in DMEM are less than 1%. Data sets of Adi/plastic and Adi/collagen I were statistically compared as indicated. * $p < 0.05$.

Our results demonstrate that collagen I has an impact on the cell physiology in ASCs. Therefore, the expression of collagen receptors was determined by western blot analysis (Figure 6). Surface receptors of the integrin family form heterodimers composed of α and β subunits, which convey substrate specific recognition. For the recognition of collagens, the α1, α2, α11, and β1 subunits are relevant. Positive controls for the detection of α1 and α11 were protein lysates derived from normal human fibroblasts; for α2 and β1, lysates from HaCaT keratinocytes were used. It was found that ASCs in DMEM produce distinct amounts of α1 on plastic as well as on collagen I (Figure 6A). A change to Adi-medium significantly reduced this expression. Likewise, α11 was massively reduced in ASCs cultured in Adi-medium. Interestingly, the basal level in ASCs held in DMEM was in the range of the positive control. Integrin α2 was only present in the positive control. The β1 subunit was even more pronounced than in the positive control, particularly in ASCs held in DMEM. A shift to Adi-medium caused a decrease in β1 expression. Moreover, DDR2, another collagen receptor present in mesenchymal cells, was investigated (Figure 6B). Here, a moderate expression in ASCs cultured in DMEM was found. Of note, a shift to Adi-medium caused a profound upregulation. Lysates derived from fibroblasts served as a positive control.

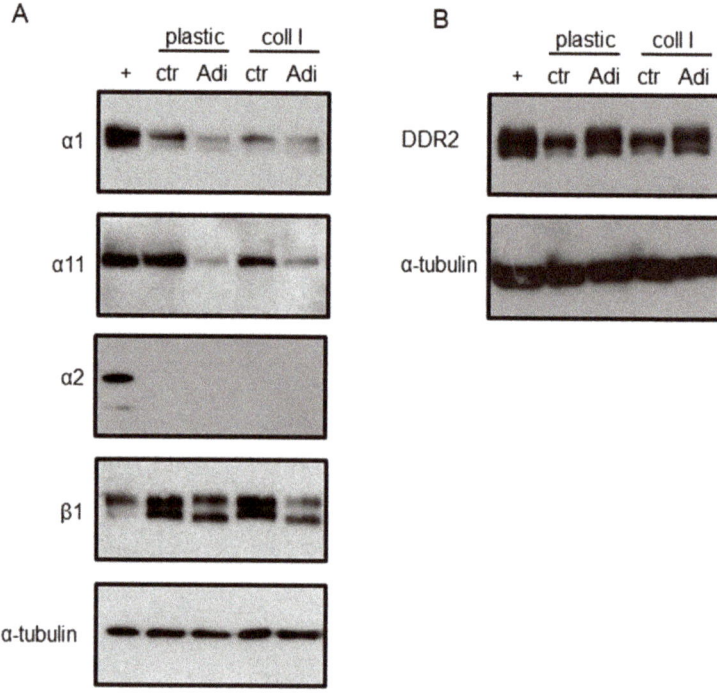

Figure 6. Expression of collagen I receptor molecules. ASCs, plated on regular plastic supports or supports coated with collagen I, were held for 9 days in standard DMEM medium (ctr) or in adipogenic medium (Adi). Protein extracts were subjected to western blot and tested for (**A**) α1, α2, α11, β1 integrin, and (**B**) DDR2. Equal loading was monitored by using antibodies directed against α-tubulin. The blots show representative results ($n = 3$). + indicates positive controls.

4. Discussion

Collagen I, as the most abundant ECM molecule, is produced by fibroblasts. It is known to provide a structural scaffold for cell attachment with impacts on tissue organization and tissue homeostasis by affecting cell growth, motility, viability, and differentiation [23]. The omnipresence of collagen in the mesenchym makes this molecule interesting as a potential trigger factor determining the cell's fate. It is known that the amount of collagen decreases during ageing with implications to the above mentioned physiological parameters [24]. An imbalance of the production and degradation leads to the accumulation of fragmented collagen molecules on which fibroblast cannot efficiently attach to. The absence of a mechanical load, which is a trigger factor for proliferation [25], marks the entry to a self-perpetuating detrimental cycle, accelerating the decrease of collagen [24]. Moreover, another hallmark of ageing is the redistribution of fat, with a decrease of peripheral subcutaneous fat [26]. It is an interesting issue if both observations are somehow functionally linked. ASCs residing in subcutaneous fat tissue have the potential to transdifferentiate into adipocytes, serving to compensate the age-dependent volume loss. In this paper, we showed that ASCs produce more lipids, a marker for adipogenic differentiation, when cultured in collagen coated dishes. This effect was measured both in cells cultured in standard medium containing no differentiation factors, and also in cells cultured in Adi-medium, described to promote adipogenic differentiation. Against this background, the stimulation of collagen synthesis by topical retinoic acid [27–29] or carbon dioxide laser resurfacing [30] may also support the differentiation of ASCs into adipocytes. Furthermore, injectable preparations containing animal collagen, which are widely used in cosmetic medicine as injectable fillers to increase lip volume, to minimize wrinkles, or to correct post-acne and traumatic scars [31], impact this differentiation process.

In addition to lipogenesis, the expression of adiponectin was also examined, a fat-derived hormone that is predominantly produced by adipocytes [32]. Corroboratively, ASCs in standard medium produce no adiponectin while cultivation in Adi-medium leads to a massive induction, indicating successful transdifferentiaton to adipocytes. Although adiponectin has pleiotropic metabolic effects, it is mainly known for its action as an insulin sensitizer with anti-apoptotic and anti-inflammatory properties [33–35]. Interestingly, the presence of collagen suppressed the expression of adiponectin. In humans, an inverse correlation between fat mass and adiponectin plasma levels was observed [36,37]. In this context, the inhibitory effect of collagen may represent a countermeasure in response to the massive induction of lipogenesis.

After we learnt that collagen impacts on metabolic parameters in ASCs, we looked at the potent receptors conveying such a signal, namely integrins and DDR2. In higher vertebrates, there are 18 α subunits and 8 β subunits, which form 24 distinct integrins. Specific for collagen binding are the following heterodimers: α1β1, α2β1, α10β1, and α11β1 [38]. Therefore, in western blot analysis, the expression of these integrins were investigated. An inverse regulation between lipogenesis/adiponectin expression and the expression of α1, α11, and β1 was found (α2 was not detectable in ASCs independent from culture conditions). In contrary, DDR2 was massively induced in ASCs when transdifferentiated to adipocytes. These findings suggest a contribution of this receptor in the collagen I-induced regulations of lipogenesis and adiponectin expression.

In sum, the presented results identified collagen I as a new regulator of adipogenic differentiation of ASCs. These findings have implications for the understanding of changes in age-related fat metabolism.

Supplementary Materials: The following are available online at http://www.mdpi.com/2073-4409/8/4/302/s1, Figure S1: Time-dependent cell adhesion of ASCs to plastic vs collagen I.

Author Contributions: Conceptualization, S.K., M.M., R.K., J.K., N.Z. and M.J.; Methodology, S.S., L.P., S.H., K.S.; Writing—Original Draft Preparation, S.K.

Acknowledgments: We are grateful to Ulrich Rieger (Klinik für Plastische und Ästhetische Chirurgie, Wiederherstellungs- und Handchirurgie, Markus Krankenhaus, Frankfurt/Main, Germany) for providing us with fat tissue.

Conflicts of Interest: The authors declare no conflict of interest.

References

1. Baer, P.C.; Bereiter-Hahn, J.; Missler, C.; Brzoska, M.; Schubert, R.; Gauer, S.; Geiger, H. Conditioned medium from renal tubular epithelial cells initiates differentiation of human mesenchymal stem cells. *Cell Prolif.* **2009**, *42*, 29–37. [CrossRef]
2. Zuk, P.A.; Zhu, M.; Ashjian, P.; De Ugarte, D.A.; Huang, J.I.; Mizuno, H.; Alfonso, Z.C.; Fraser, J.K.; Benhaim, P.; Hedrick, M.H. Human adipose tissue is a source of multipotent stem cells. *Mol. Biol. Cell* **2002**, *13*, 4279–4295. [CrossRef]
3. Adams, A.M.; Arruda, E.M.; Larkin, L.M. Use of adipose-derived stem cells to fabricate scaffoldless tissue-engineered neural conduits in vitro. *Neuroscience* **2012**, *201*, 349–356. [CrossRef] [PubMed]

4. Miranville, A.; Heeschen, C.; Sengenes, C.; Curat, C.A.; Busse, R.; Bouloumie, A. Improvement of postnatal neovascularization by human adipose tissue-derived stem cells. *Circulation* **2004**, *110*, 349–355. [CrossRef]
5. Hicok, K.C.; Du Laney, T.V.; Zhou, Y.S.; Halvorsen, Y.D.; Hitt, D.C.; Cooper, L.F.; Gimble, J.M. Human adipose-derived adult stem cells produce osteoid in vivo. *Tissue Eng.* **2004**, *10*, 371–380. [CrossRef]
6. Erickson, G.R.; Gimble, J.M.; Franklin, D.M.; Rice, H.E.; Awad, H.; Guilak, F. Chondrogenic potential of adipose tissue-derived stromal cells in vitro and in vivo. *Biochem. Biophis. Res. Commun.* **2002**, *290*, 763–769. [CrossRef]
7. Song, Y.H.; Gehmert, S.; Sadat, S.; Pinkernell, K.; Bai, X.; Matthias, N.; Alt, E. VEGF is critical for spontaneous differentiation of stem cells into cardiomyocytes. *Biochem. Biophis. Res. Commun.* **2007**, *354*, 999–1003. [CrossRef]
8. Banas, A.; Teratani, T.; Yamamoto, Y.; Tokuhara, M.; Takeshita, F.; Quinn, G.; Okochi, H.; Ochiya, T. Adipose tissue-derived mesenchymal stem cells as a source of human hepatocytes. *Hepatology* **2007**, *46*, 219–228. [CrossRef]
9. Timper, K.; Seboek, D.; Eberhardt, M.; Linscheid, P.; Christ-Crain, M.; Keller, U.; Muller, B.; Zulewski, H. Human adipose tissue-derived mesenchymal stem cells differentiate into insulin, somatostatin, and glucagon expressing cells. *Biochem. Biophis. Res. Commun.* **2006**, *341*, 1135–1140. [CrossRef] [PubMed]
10. Aldag, C.; Nogueira Teixeira, D.; Leventhal, P.S. Skin rejuvenation using cosmetic products containing growth factors, cytokines, and matrikines: A review of the literature. *Clin. Cosmet. Investig. Dermatol.* **2016**, *9*, 411–419. [CrossRef] [PubMed]
11. Baumann, L. Skin ageing and its treatment. *J. Pathol.* **2007**, *211*, 241–251. [CrossRef] [PubMed]
12. Kim, D.; You, E.; Min, N.Y.; Lee, K.H.; Kim, H.K.; Rhee, S. Discoidin domain receptor 2 regulates the adhesion of fibroblasts to 3D collagen matrices. *Int. J. Mol. Med.* **2013**, *31*, 1113–1118. [CrossRef]
13. Vogel, W.; Gish, G.D.; Alves, F.; Pawson, T. The discoidin domain receptor tyrosine kinases are activated by collagen. *Mol. Cell* **1997**, *1*, 13–23. [CrossRef]
14. Vogel, W. Discoidin domain receptors: Structural relations and functional implications. *FASEB J.* **1999**, *13*, S77–S82. [CrossRef]
15. Antuna-Puente, B.; Feve, B.; Fellahi, S.; Bastard, J.P. Adipokines: The missing link between insulin resistance and obesity. *Diabetes Metab.* **2008**, *34*, 2–11. [CrossRef]
16. Fasshauer, M.; Bluher, M. Adipokines in health and disease. *Trends Pharmacol. Sci.* **2015**, *36*, 461–470. [CrossRef] [PubMed]
17. Tsatsanis, C.; Zacharioudaki, V.; Androulidaki, A.; Dermitzaki, E.; Charalampopoulos, I.; Minas, V.; Gravanis, A.; Margioris, A.N. Peripheral factors in the metabolic syndrome: The pivotal role of adiponectin. *Ann. N. Y. Acad. Sci.* **2006**, *1083*, 185–195. [CrossRef]
18. Kroeze, K.L.; Jurgens, W.J.; Doulabi, B.Z.; van Milligen, F.J.; Scheper, R.J.; Gibbs, S. Chemokine-mediated migration of skin-derived stem cells: Predominant role for CCL5/RANTES. *J. Investig. Dermatol.* **2009**, *129*, 1569–1581. [CrossRef] [PubMed]
19. Knies, Y.; Bernd, A.; Kaufmann, R.; Bereiter-Hahn, J.; Kippenberger, S. Mechanical stretch induces clustering of beta1-integrins and facilitates adhesion. *Exp. Dermatol.* **2006**, *15*, 347–355. [CrossRef]
20. Kippenberger, S.; Loitsch, S.; Muller, J.; Guschel, M.; Kaufmann, R.; Bernd, A. Ligation of the beta4 integrin triggers adhesion behavior of human keratinocytes by an "inside-out" mechanism. *J. Investig. Dermatol.* **2004**, *123*, 444–451. [CrossRef]
21. Zouboulis, C.C.; Seltmann, H.; Hiroi, N.; Chen, W.; Young, M.; Oeff, M.; Scherbaum, W.A.; Orfanos, C.E.; McCann, S.M.; Bornstein, S.R. Corticotropin-releasing hormone: An autocrine hormone that promotes lipogenesis in human sebocytes. *Proc. Natl. Acad. Sci. USA* **2002**, *99*, 7148–7153. [CrossRef]
22. Livak, K.J.; Schmittgen, T.D. Analysis of relative gene expression data using real-time quantitative PCR and the 2(-Delta Delta C(T)) Method. *Methods* **2001**, *25*, 402–408. [CrossRef]
23. Plant, A.L.; Bhadriraju, K.; Spurlin, T.A.; Elliott, J.T. Cell response to matrix mechanics: Focus on collagen. *BBA-Mol. Cell Res.* **2009**, *1793*, 893–902. [CrossRef]
24. Fisher, G.J.; Varani, J.; Voorhees, J.J. Looking older: Fibroblast collapse and therapeutic implications. *Arch. Dermatol.* **2008**, *144*, 666–672. [CrossRef]
25. Kippenberger, S.; Bernd, A.; Loitsch, S.; Guschel, M.; Muller, J.; Bereiter-Hahn, J.; Kaufmann, R. Signaling of mechanical stretch in human keratinocytes via MAP kinases. *J. Investig. Dermatol.* **2000**, *114*, 408–412. [CrossRef]

26. Sepe, A.; Tchkonia, T.; Thomou, T.; Zamboni, M.; Kirkland, J.L. Aging and regional differences in fat cell progenitors - a mini-review. *Gerontology* **2011**, *57*, 66–75. [CrossRef] [PubMed]
27. Cho, S.; Lowe, L.; Hamilton, T.A.; Fisher, G.J.; Voorhees, J.J.; Kang, S. Long-term treatment of photoaged human skin with topical retinoic acid improves epidermal cell atypia and thickens the collagen band in papillary dermis. *J. Am. Acad. Dermatol.* **2005**, *53*, 769–774. [CrossRef] [PubMed]
28. Griffiths, C.E.; Russman, A.N.; Majmudar, G.; Singer, R.S.; Hamilton, T.A.; Voorhees, J.J. Restoration of collagen formation in photodamaged human skin by tretinoin (retinoic acid). *N. Engl. J. Med.* **1993**, *329*, 530–535. [CrossRef]
29. Kafi, R.; Kwak, H.S.; Schumacher, W.E.; Cho, S.; Hanft, V.N.; Hamilton, T.A.; King, A.L.; Neal, J.D.; Varani, J.; Fisher, G.J.; et al. Improvement of naturally aged skin with vitamin A (retinol). *Arch. Dermatol.* **2007**, *143*, 606–612. [CrossRef]
30. Orringer, J.S.; Kang, S.; Johnson, T.M.; Karimipour, D.J.; Hamilton, T.; Hammerberg, C.; Voorhees, J.J.; Fisher, G.J. Connective tissue remodeling induced by carbon dioxide laser resurfacing of photodamaged human skin. *Arch. Dermatol.* **2004**, *140*, 1326–1332. [CrossRef]
31. Marinelli, E.; Montanari Vergallo, G.; Reale, G.; di Luca, A.; Catarinozzi, I.; Napoletano, S.; Zaami, S. The role of fillers in aesthetic medicine: Medico-legal aspects. *Eur. Rev. Med. Pharmacol. Sci.* **2016**, *20*, 4628–4634. [PubMed]
32. Ye, R.; Scherer, P.E. Adiponectin, driver or passenger on the road to insulin sensitivity? *Mol. Metab.* **2013**, *2*, 133–141. [CrossRef] [PubMed]
33. Jian, L.; Su, Y.X.; Deng, H.C. Adiponectin-induced inhibition of intrinsic and extrinsic apoptotic pathways protects pancreatic beta-cells against apoptosis. *Horm. Metab. Res.* **2013**, *45*, 561–566. [CrossRef] [PubMed]
34. Yadav, A.; Kataria, M.A.; Saini, V.; Yadav, A. Role of leptin and adiponectin in insulin resistance. *Clin. Chim. Acta* **2013**, *417*, 80–84. [CrossRef] [PubMed]
35. Yamauchi, T.; Nio, Y.; Maki, T.; Kobayashi, M.; Takazawa, T.; Iwabu, M.; Okada-Iwabu, M.; Kawamoto, S.; Kubota, N.; Kubota, T.; et al. Targeted disruption of AdipoR1 and AdipoR2 causes abrogation of adiponectin binding and metabolic actions. *Nat. Med.* **2007**, *13*, 332–339. [CrossRef] [PubMed]
36. Arita, Y.; Kihara, S.; Ouchi, N.; Takahashi, M.; Maeda, K.; Miyagawa, J.; Hotta, K.; Shimomura, I.; Nakamura, T.; Miyaoka, K.; et al. Paradoxical decrease of an adipose-specific protein, adiponectin, in obesity. *Biochem. Biophis. Res. Commun.* **1999**, *257*, 79–83. [CrossRef]
37. Hoffstedt, J.; Arvidsson, E.; Sjolin, E.; Wahlen, K.; Arner, P. Adipose tissue adiponectin production and adiponectin serum concentration in human obesity and insulin resistance. *J. Clin. Endocrinol. Metab.* **2004**, *89*, 1391–1396. [CrossRef]
38. Leitinger, B. Transmembrane collagen receptors. *Annu. Rev. Cell Dev. Biol.* **2011**, *27*, 265–290. [CrossRef]

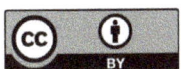

© 2019 by the authors. Licensee MDPI, Basel, Switzerland. This article is an open access article distributed under the terms and conditions of the Creative Commons Attribution (CC BY) license (http://creativecommons.org/licenses/by/4.0/).

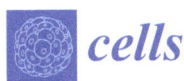

Article

Permanent Pro-Tumorigenic Shift in Adipose Tissue-Derived Mesenchymal Stromal Cells Induced by Breast Malignancy

Jana Plava [1,†], Marina Cihova [1,†], Monika Burikova [1], Martin Bohac [2,3,4], Marian Adamkov [5], Slavka Drahosova [6], Dominika Rusnakova [7], Daniel Pindak [7], Marian Karaba [7], Jan Simo [7], Michal Mego [2], Lubos Danisovic [3,6], Lucia Kucerova [1,*] and Svetlana Miklikova [1,*]

1. Cancer Research Institute, Biomedical Research Center, University Science Park for Biomedicine, Slovak Academy of Sciences, 845 05 Bratislava, Slovakia; jana.plava@savba.sk (J.P.); marina.cihova@savba.sk (M.C.); monika.burikova@savba.sk (M.B.)
2. 2nd Department of Oncology, Faculty of Medicine, Comenius University, National Cancer Institute, Klenova 1, 833 10 Bratislava, Slovakia; bohac.md@gmail.com (M.B.); misomego@gmail.com (M.M.)
3. Department of Oncosurgery, National Cancer Institute, Klenova 1, 833 10 Bratislava, Slovakia; lubos.danisovic@fmed.uniba.sk
4. Regenmed Ltd., Medena 29, 811 08 Bratislava, Slovakia
5. Comenius University Bratislava, Jessenius Faculty of Medicine Martin, Department of Histology and Embryology, 036 01 Martin, Slovakia; adamkov@jfmed.uniba.sk
6. Hermes LabSystems, s.r.o., 831 06 Bratislava, Slovakia; slavka.drahosova@hermeslab.sk
7. Institute of Medical Biology, Genetics and Clinical Genetics, Faculty of Medicine, Comenius University, 813 72 Bratislava, Slovakia; domeenica@gmail.com (D.R.); daniel.pindak@nou.sk (D.P.); marian.karaba@nou.sk (M.K.); jan.simo@nou.sk (J.S.)
* Correspondence: lucia.kucerova@savba.sk (L.K.); svetlana.miklikova@savba.sk (S.M.); Tel.: +4212-3229-5136 (S.M.)
† These authors contributed equally to this paper.

Received: 22 January 2020; Accepted: 17 February 2020; Published: 19 February 2020

Abstract: During cancer progression, breast tumor cells interact with adjacent adipose tissue, which has been shown to be engaged in cancer aggressiveness. However, the tumor-directed changes in adipose tissue-resident stromal cells affected by the tumor–stroma communication are still poorly understood. The acquired changes might remain in the tissue even after tumor removal and may contribute to tumor relapse. We investigated functional properties (migratory capacity, expression and secretion profile) of mesenchymal stromal cells isolated from healthy ($n = 9$) and tumor-distant breast adipose tissue ($n = 32$). Cancer patient-derived mesenchymal stromal cells (MSCs) (MSC-CA) exhibited a significantly disarranged secretion profile and proliferation potential. Co-culture with MDA-MB-231, T47D and JIMT-1, representing different subtypes of breast cancer, was used to analyze the effect of MSCs on proliferation, invasion and tumorigenicity. The MSC-CA enhanced tumorigenicity and altered xenograft composition in immunodeficient mice. Histological analysis revealed collective cell invasion with a specific invasive front of EMT-positive tumor cells as well as invasion of cancer cells to the nerve-surrounding space. This study identifies that adipose tissue-derived mesenchymal stromal cells are primed and permanently altered by tumor presence in breast tissue and have the potential to increase tumor cell invasive ability through the activation of epithelial-to-mesenchymal transition in tumor cells.

Keywords: mesenchymal stromal cells; adipose tissue; breast cancer; tumor microenvironment; perineural invasion

1. Introduction

The interaction of breast epithelium and stroma promotes normal breast structure and function [1]. However, adipose tissue surrounding breast tumors is no longer recognized as a passive structural element, but as a key component contributing to breast cancer progression [2,3]. Diverse stromal cells, including myofibroblasts, pericytes, endothelial cells and cancer-associated fibroblasts (CAF), are recruited from adjacent adipose tissue, and these become an integral component of the tumor microenvironment [4,5]. Mesenchymal stromal cells (MSCs) also migrate to tumors, which are commonly perceived as wounds that never heal [6]. Several studies have elucidated MSC ability to transform into a carcinoma-associated fibroblast phenotype when treated in vitro with breast cancer cell-secreted factors [7–9]. This change is demonstrated by a higher expression of αSma, Vimentin, fibroblast specific protein 1 (FSP-1), stromal-derived factor 1 (SDF1) and C-C motif chemokine ligand 5 (CCL5) [10,11]. At least five tumor-associated stromal fibroblast cell subtypes have been identified in the tumor stroma, and these are differentiated by the expression of specific markers associated with various levels of tumor aggression. The most aggressive subtype is characterized by extensive matrix remodeling and the increased expression of FSP-1 and fibroblast activating protein (FAP) [12]. We previously established that factors secreted by tumor cells alter the MSCs' molecular traits and angiogenic ability. We also confirmed that these changes correlate with their subsequent pro-tumorigenic action and that chemotherapeutically pre-treated MSCs produce a similar effect [13,14]. Additionally, Yeh et al. associated the CXCL1 secreted by stromal cells in breast adipose tissue with doxorubicin resistance mediated by ABCG2 up-regulation [15]. Although studies provide evidence that in vitro MSCs are prone to differentiation into carcinoma-associated fibroblasts induced by tumor secretome [16], there is no experimental evidence as to whether breast malignancy affects the MSCs in distant adipose tissue remaining in the breast after surgery and if those changes may persist even after the tumor removal. Since has also been suggested that interactions between tumor and normal tissue are bi-directional [17,18], we hypothesize that malignant cells and their secretome shape the normal distant tissue and alter its properties.

Herein, we performed a detailed comparison of the functional properties of MSCs from the following four origins in healthy donors and breast cancer patients to determine the influence of malignancy on normal stromal precursors: (1) the first MSC group was isolated from the breast adipose tissue of healthy donors undergoing planned aesthetic breast surgery; (2) the second group comprised MSCs from cancer patient breast adipose tissue adjacent to pre-malignant lesions; (3) the third group was MSCs obtained from adipose tissue of breast cancer patients diagnosed with invasive tumor type and (4) this group contained tissue similar to that in the third group but also harboring the BRCA gene mutation. The results establish that breast cancer patient-derived MSCs are inherently altered; they promote in vivo tumor growth and they also increase tumor cell invasiveness. Finally, identification of key functional changes in the MSCs located in the tumor micro-environment and increased understanding of the mechanisms involved in MSC-enhanced tumor growth and metastasis could initiate new methods of normalizing tumor micro-environments, and thus regulate disease progression.

2. Materials and Methods

2.1. Cell Cultures

Mesenchymal stromal cells were isolated from the breast adipose tissue of four different donor groups: Group No.1 MSC-H ($n = 9$), isolated from breast adipose tissue of healthy donors, Group No.2 MSC-DCIS ($n = 2$), isolated from adipose tissue adjacent to pre-malignant lesions, Group No.3 MSC-CA ($n = 24$), isolated from adipose tissue adjacent to malignant lesions, and Group No.4 MSC-BRCA+ ($n = 6$), isolated from adipose tissue adjacent to malignant lesions harboring the BRCA gene mutation. We used tumor-adjacent adipose tissue obtained during surgery, and the samples ranged from 1.5 to 5 cm^3. All donors provided informed consent and all procedures were approved by the Ethics Committee of the Ruzinov University Hospital and the National Cancer Institute (TRUSK-003).

The MSCs were isolated as previously described [19]. The isolated cells were maintained in low-glucose (1 g/L) Dulbecco's modified Eagle medium (DMEM, PAA Laboratories GmbH, Pasching, Austria) supplemented with 10% fetal bovine serum (FBS, Biochrom AG, Berlin, Germany). Breast cancer cell lines were cultured in high-glucose (4.5 g/L) Dulbecco's modified Eagle medium (DMEM, PAA Laboratories GmbH) supplemented with 10% fetal bovine serum (FBS, Biochrom AG). Both culture media were supplemented with 2 mM glutamine (PAA Laboratories GmbH), 10.000 IU/mL penicillin (Biotica, Part. Lupca, Slovakia), 5 µg/mL streptomycin (PAA Laboratories GmbH) and 2.5 µg/mL amphotericin B (Sigma-Aldrich, Taufkirchen, Germany). The cells were maintained at 37 °C in humidified atmosphere and 5% CO_2, and the MSCs were then expanded and used for experiments not exceeding the 10th passage.

Human mammary gland adenocarcinoma cell line MDA-MB-231 (ATCC® Number: HTB-26™), T47D (ATCC® HTB-133™) and JIMT-1 (DSMZ no.: ACC 589) were purchased from stated sources and their identity was confirmed by STR profiling in July 2018. The cells were transduced with IncuCyte® NucLight Lentivirus Reagents (Essen BioScience, Ann Arbor, MI, USA) to express nuclear red fluorescent protein (mKate2) according to manufacturer protocol. These cells are referred to as NLR-T47D, NLR-MDA-MB-231 and NLR-JIMT-1 (in manuscript shortened to NLR-T47D, NLR-MDA231 and NLR-JIMT).

2.2. MSC Differentiation

Adipogenic differentiation was evaluated in MSCs plated at 3500 cells/well density in 96-well plates and maintained in low-glucose (1 g/L) DMEM medium supplemented with 60 µM indomethacin, 0.5 mM isobutylmethylxanthine, 0.5 µM hydrocortisone and 10% fetal bovine serum, GlutaMAX and antibiotic-antimycotic mix. The medium was changed every 2–3 days. The cells were washed with PBS after the 21st day of culture, fixed in 10% formalin and stained with Oil Red O (Sigma-Aldrich) for 2–5 min. The presence of adipocytes was detected by red stained lipid droplets. Osteogenic and chondrogenic differentiation was performed by StemPro Differentiation Kit (Gibco, Life Sciences, Carlsbad, CA, USA), where osteogenic differentiation was confirmed by detection of red stained calcium deposits using Alizarin Red S (Sigma-Aldrich) and chondrogenic positivity was proven by blue stained proteoglycans synthesized by chondrocytes using Alcian Blue stain (Sigma-Aldrich). Finally, the MSCs maintained in standard culture medium served as controls.

2.3. Immunophenotype

The identification and phenotyping of cultured MSCs was based on the defined International Society for Cellular Therapy (ISCT) standards and the use of human MSC Phenotyping Kit (Miltenyi Biotec, Bergisch Gladbach, Germany) [20]. The expression of CD90, CD105, CD14, CD20, CD34 and CD45 was assessed by BD FACSCanto™ II Flow cytometer (Becton Dickinson, USA) equipped with the FacsDiva program, and the data were then analyzed by FCS Express program.

2.4. Morphology and Wound Healing Assay

For MSC morphology analysis, 5×10^3 MSCs in passage 2–4 were seeded in a 96-well plate and captured by IncuCyte ZOOM™ kinetic imaging system over 72-h period. For immunofluorescent analysis, cells were seeded on slides and, after reaching desired confluence, they were fixed with 4% PFA for 15 min, washed three times in PBS and subsequently stained with Actin-AF488 (1:500, diluted in ROTI) for 1 h at 37 °C and then with DAPI (1:500) for 15 min at 37 °C to stain the nuclei. MSC migration was evaluated in 96-well plates, where 23×10^3 MSCs per well were seeded and analyzed by IncuCyte® Scratch Wound Cell Migration and Invasion System and documented by the IncuCyte ZOOM™ kinetic imaging system. To assess the invasion capacity, 1×10^4 MSCs + 2×10^4 NLR-MDA231/NLR-T47D and 1.5×10^4 MSCs + 3×10^4 NLR-JIMT were seeded on ECM-coated 96-well plates and, after executing the scratch wound, they were immediately covered with 50% ECM

(Matrigel, Sigma-Aldrich). MSCs were stained with Vybrant™ CFDA SE Cell Tracer Kit (Thermo-Fisher Scientific, Waltham, MA, USA) according to the manufacturer protocol.

2.5. Evaluation of Proliferation

MSC doubling-time was evaluated by RealTime-Glo™ MT Cell Viability Assay (Promega Corporation, Madison, WI, USA). This was performed in a 96-well plate with 5×10^3 cells per well seeded in eight replications. Relative luminescence was determined on LUMIstar GALAXY reader (BMG Labtechnologies, Germany) approximately every 12 h for 3 days. The luminescence values were extrapolated by a graph and trend line equation, and the mean luminescence after 24 and 48 h was determined by formula. The doubling-time was calculated as follows: doubling time = duration × log (2)/log (luminescence value after 48 h) − log (luminescence value after 24 h). The experiments were repeated at least twice with similar results, and the mean results were reported.

Fluorescently labeled tumor cells and MSCs were mixed in a 2:1 ratio for co-culture experiments; 4×10^3 NLR-JIMT and 2×10^3 MSC or 2×10^3 NLR-MDA231 and 1×10^3 MSC were seeded in standard culture medium in 96-well plates. Each well was imaged every two hours by IncuCyte ZOOM™ Kinetic Imaging System (Essen BioScience, Newark Close, UK) until cells reached confluence. The tumor cell number was evaluated by IncuCyte ZOOM™ software (Essen BioScience) based on the enumeration of tumor cells' red nuclei by kinetic imaging scanning. The values are expressed as means of replicates ± SD. Three-dimensional multicellular spheroids were prepared by seeding 2×10^3 tumor cells mixed with 1×10^3 MSCs in 96-well ultra-low attachment plates (Corning 7007, Corning Inc., Corning, NY, USA) in 100 µL of culture medium. Representative pictures of spheroids were taken after 7 days of culture by IncuCyte ZOOM™ Kinetic Imaging System (Essen BioScience) and the relative luminescence of spheroids was evaluated by the CellTiter-Glo™ 3D Cell Viability Assay (Promega Corporation).

2.6. Gene Expression Array

The Human Mesenchymal Stem Cells RT2 Profiler™ PCR Array then analyzed specific human mesenchymal stem cell gene expression in individual MSC groups (PAHS-082ZD; Qiagen, Hilden, Germany). RNA from 5×10^5 MSCs was isolated by AllPrep RNA/Protein kit (Qiagen) and reverse transcribed with RT2 First Strand Kit (Qiagen). The expression of 84 human MSC-related genes was analyzed by RT2 SYBR Green Mastermix (Qiagen) and Bio-Rad CFX96™ Real-Time PCR Detection system (Bio-Rad Laboratories Ltd, Watford, UK). The CT cut-off was set at 35, and targets expressed at very low levels or undetected in MSC-H were excluded from relative expression calculations. The expression profile of MSC-H was used as a reference. Relative expression exceeding 4-fold alteration in tested samples was considered for further analysis.

2.7. Proteome Profiler

Proteome profile analysis of human cytokines and chemokines was performed with the XL Cytokine Array Kit (R&D Systems™, Minneapolis, MN, USA). ImageJ software (NIH, Bethesda, MD, USA) was used for the quantitative evaluation; the pixel density was determined and calculated. Serum-free conditioned media obtained from 2×10^5 MSC-H or MSC-CA were loaded on the membranes with blotted antibodies and evaluated as recommended by the manufacturer.

2.8. Enzyme-Linked Immunosorbent Assay (ELISA)

IGF1 and leptin levels were quantified in the conditioned media from 1×10^5 MSCs using a quantitative sandwich ELISA kit (Fine Biotech, China). The PTX3 level was quantified in the same way from the obtained media using a quantitative sandwich ELISA kit (R&D Systems).

2.9. In Vivo Experiments

Six-week-old female SCID/Beige mice from SCID/bg, Charles River in Germany were used in accordance with institutional guidelines and approved protocols. The animals were bilaterally subcutaneously injected with a mixture of 5×10^5 MSCs and 1×10^6 NLR-JIMT cells re-suspended in 100 µL serum-free DMEM diluted 1:1 with ECM gel (Sigma-Aldrich). The animals were divided into five groups according to the type of injected MSC: control group of NLR-JIMT alone ($n = 6$), MSC-H ($n = 6$), MSC-DCIS ($n = 6$), MSC-CA ($n = 6$) and MSC-BRCA+ ($n = 5$). Alternatively, a mixture of 5×10^5 NLR-JIMT cells and 2.5×10^5 MSCs in 100 µL serum-free DMEM diluted 1:1 with ECM gel (Sigma-Aldrich) was injected bilaterally into the mammary fat pad of SCID/Beige mice. The animals were also divided into five groups according to the type of injected MSC: control group of NLR-JIMT alone ($n = 3$), MSC-H ($n = 3$), MSC-CA ($n = 3$), MSC-BRCA+ (2) ($n = 3$) obtained from breast tissue where prophylactic mastectomy was performed and MSC-BRCA+ (1) ($n = 3$) from contralateral breast of the same patient with confirmed relapsed invasive ductal carcinoma (pT1bpNx). The animals were regularly inspected for tumor growth, and tumor volume was calculated according to the formula: volume = (length × width2)/2. The animals were sacrificed according to the ethical guidelines when the tumor volume exceeded 1 cm^3. The tumors were analyzed histologically and immuno-histochemically as described below.

All in vivo experiments were performed in the authorized animal facility under license No. SK UCH 02017 and approved by the institutional ethic committee and by the national competent authority of the State Veterinary and Food Administration of the Slovak Republic (Registration Number Ro:1976/17-221) in compliance with Directive 2010/63/EU of the European Parliament and the European Council and Regulation 377/2012 for the protection of animals used for scientific purposes.

2.10. The Immunofluorescence Analysis of Fresh Cryosections

Tissues were embedded in Tissue-Tek (Sakura Finetek Europe, Alphen aan den Rijn, Netherlands), snap-frozen on dry ice and then cut into 10 µm sections on cryostat. The sections were gently washed three times with phosphate-buffered saline (PBS), fixed with 4% PFA for 15 min, washed three times in PBS and then permeabilized with 0.05% Triton X-100 in PBS for 15 min. The washed sections were incubated with ROTI protein free blocking solution (Carl Roth, Germany) for 30 min at 37 °C. Staining was performed by incubation with primary antibody Actin-AF488 (1:500, diluted in ROTI) for 1 h at 37 °C and then with DAPI (1:500) for 15 min at 37 °C to stain the nuclei. Finally, the slides were washed three times with PBS, and Fluormount-G® medium (SouthernBiotech, Birmingham, AL, USA) was used to mount the coverslips. The staining patterns were analyzed using a Zeiss fluorescent microscope and automated imaging Metafer (MetaSystems GmbH, Altlussheim, Germany) (630× magnification).

2.11. Immunohistochemistry

Formalin-fixed, paraffin-embedded tumor tissues were cut into 5-µm sections. De-parafinization, rehydration and epitope retrieval via Target Retrieval solution high-pH (DAKO, Carpinteria, CA, USA) were performed under PT Link (Pre-Treatment module for tissue Specimens, DAKO) at 96 °C for 20 min. The slides were then washed in FLEX wash buffer (Tris-buffered saline solution containing Tween 20, pH 7.6) prior to loading onto the automated DAKO Autostainer_Link 48. Endogenous peroxidase was blocked by 5 min of incubation with FLEX peroxidase Block (DAKO), and sections were then incubated with primary antibodies, anti-human Ki67 MIB-1, anti-human Vimentin or anti-human smooth muscle actin (αSMA) for 20 min at RT (FLEX, DAKO). This was followed by incubation with LSAB2 System-HRP, Biotinylated Link for 15 min and then Strepatavidin-HRP for 15 min. Positive staining was visualized by the brown color from 3.3'-Diaminobenzidine (DAB substrate-chromogen solution, DAKO) after 5 min, and counterstaining was performed with hematoxylin (FLEX, DAKO) for 5–8 min. Sections with DAB-evident double-staining were incubated with other primary antibodies (Vimentin or αSMA) for 20 min, and in the same manner with LSAB2 system-HRP. Positive staining was visualized by Magenta (EnVision FLEX HRP Magenta Substrate Chromogen, DAKO) for 8 min (red color) and final sample counterstaining was with hematoxylin. The slides were washed between each incubation with 1× FLEX wash buffer and dehydrated by washing in alcohol, aceton:xylen (1:1) and xylen, each for 10 min. The slides were mounted with Q-D media (Bamed, Czech Republic) and the staining patterns were analyzed by Axio Scope A1, Zeiss microscope with Axiocam 105 color.

3. Results

3.1. Characterization of Mesenchymal Stromal Cells

Herein, we isolated mesenchymal stromal cells from breast adipose tissue and assigned each isolate to one of the following four groups schematically depicted in Figure 1: breast adipose tissue-derived MSCs from healthy donors (MSC-H), MSCs derived from breast adipose tissue from patients with pre-malignant lesions (MSC-DCIS) and adipose-derived MSCs from tissue adjacent to malignant lesions (MSC-CA and MSC-BRCA+).

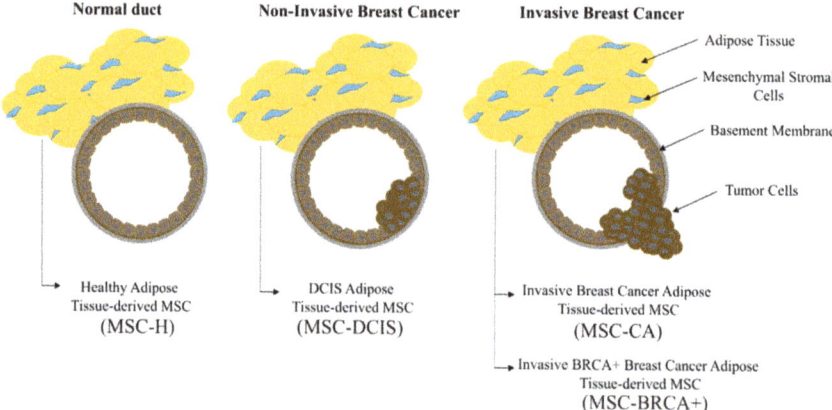

Figure 1. Mesenchymal stromal cells (MSCs) were isolated from four breast adipose tissue origins; healthy donors (MSC-H), breast cancer patients with non-invasive (MSC-DCIS) or invasive tumors (MSC-CA), and BRCA+ breast cancer patients (MSC-BRCA+). In breast cancer patients, adipose tissue at a distance of 1.5-2 cm from the tumor was used.

Each MSC isolate fulfilled the essential minimum criteria for multipotent stromal cells. MSCs were positive for CD90, CD105 and CD73 (>95%), but did not express CD14, CD20, CD34 and CD45 markers, as expected (<5% positive cells, representative sample in Figure 2A). Some MSC isolates were subjected to in vitro differentiation assay to confirm multi-lineage differentiation potential. MSCs readily differentiated into adipocytes (red stained lipid droplets), osteocytes (red stained calcium deposits) and chondrocytes (blue stained proteoglycans) under the in vitro culture conditions depicted in Figure 2B. Each MSC isolate produced actively proliferating cells which adhered to the plastic surface, and all isolates had fibroblast-like spindle-shape morphology. The phase-contrast photographs and actin immunofluorescence staining obtained 72 h after seeding revealed no morphological difference in the MSC-H, MSC-DCIS and MSC-CA groups (Figure 2C left) and also no age-dependent changes (Figure 2C right).

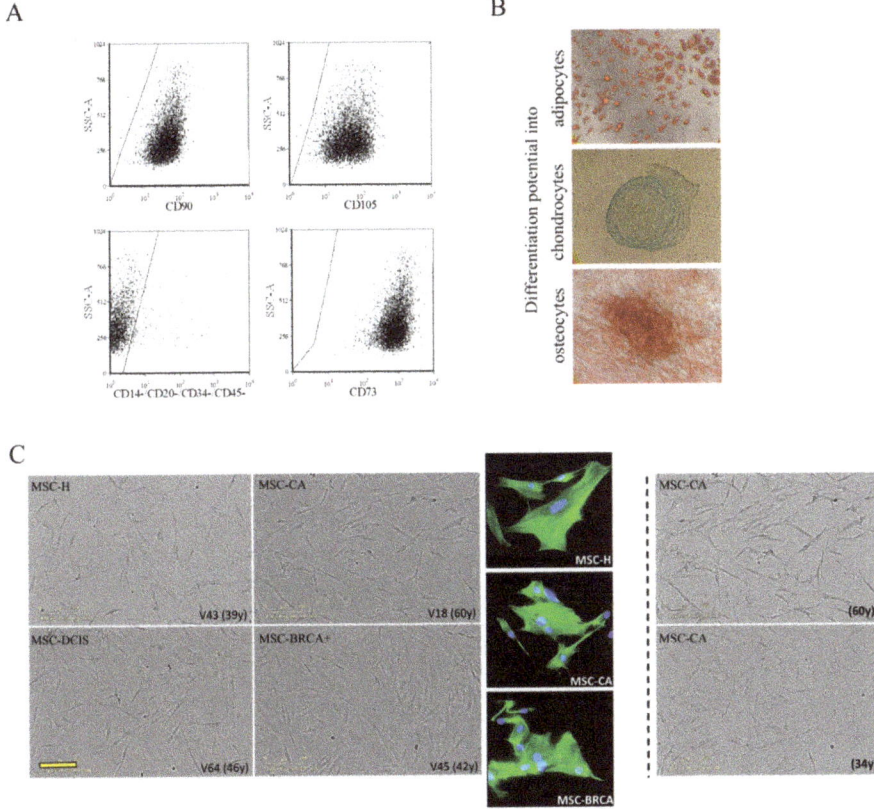

Figure 2. (**A**) MSC-specific marker expression was analyzed by flow cytometry. MSCs expressed CD73, CD90 and CD105 on their surface, but lacked hematopoietic/endothelial marker expression. (**B**) MSC multipotency was analyzed by their differentiation potential into adipocytes, osteocytes, and chondrocytes. Magnification 100×. (**C**) MSC phenotype was documented by IncuCyte ZOOM™ kinetic imaging system and actin immunofluorescent staining (actin - green, DAPI - blue). The morphology of MSCs obtained from donors with different diagnosis (left) or age (right) did not differ over the analyzed period. Scale bar 200 μm. One representative picture from each group is shown.

We also compared proliferation rates for individual MSC isolates and correlated these with patient age, BMI and diagnosis. Even though no significant difference was noted in age-related proliferation, a slightly lower proliferation trend was observed in the older MCS donors (Figure 3A left). However, the doubling-time of MSC-CA was significantly higher when compared to MSC-H (Figure 3A middle, $p < 0.05$, Mann Whitney test). This could be explained by the lower proliferation trend in older patients when solely MSC-CA doubling time was analyzed (Figure 3A right). It is well known that MSCs are endowed with the capacity to migrate towards tumors or the site of injury. Therefore, to see if this MSC trait could also be affected by tumor proximity, we compared the MSC migration in a standard wound healing assay. A wounded MSC monolayer was regularly imaged by live-cell kinetic imaging system and relative wound density was determined by wound confluence after 24 h. All MSC isolates showed high migratory capacity, with average 24-h wound confluence of 69% for 30–49-year-olds and 62% for those over 50. The migratory process, however, had no significant correlation with patient diagnosis (Figure 3B left) or age (Figure 3B middle). A moderately better wound healing process was evidenced in the MSC-DCIS, MSC-CA or MSC-BRCA+ of older patients (Figure 3B right).

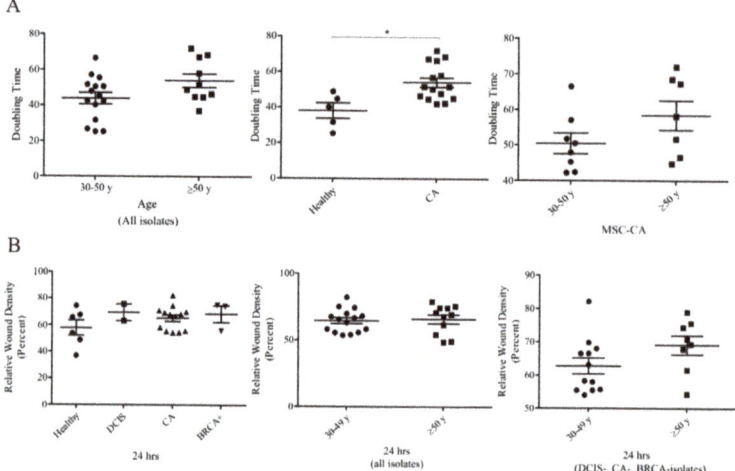

Figure 3. Functional changes in cancer patient adipose tissue-derived MSCs (**A**) Left: MSC doubling-time in all MSC isolates had increasing tendency in older donors, but this tendency was not statistically significant. Middle: Based on the diagnosis of MSC donors, we observed significantly longer doubling-time in MSCs isolated from patients with invasive cancer compared to healthy MSCs (* $p < 0.05$; Mann-Whitney test). Right: The trend of increased doubling-time was present also in the MSC-CA group. (**B**) MSC migration potential analysis based on diagnosis (left), age in all MSC groups (middle) or age in solely cancer patients (right) showed no statistically significant differences. MSCs used for analysis did not exceed 10th passage.

In an aspiration to analyze the expression profile of mesenchymal stromal cells derived from different origin, RT^2 Profiler™ PCR array for human mesenchymal stem cell expression profiles was conducted on representative isolates from each group. The common alterations were noted in the MSC-DCIS and MSC-CA expression profiles (Figure 4A). These included; (1) up-regulation of brain-derived neurotrophic factor (*BDNF*), neurogenic locus notch homolog protein 1 (*NOTCH1*) and cytoskeletal Vimentin and (2) down-regulation of growth differentiation factor 15 (*GDF15*), insulin-like growth factor 1 (*IGF1*), matrix metallopeptidase 2 (*MMP2*), platelet-derived growth factor receptor β (*PDGFRB*) and transforming growth factor β3 (*TGFB3*). In addition, the MSC-BRCA+ cells exhibited down-regulation of Bone morphogenic protein 4 (*BMP4*) and up-regulation of SRY-box 9 (*SOX9*) and vascular cell adhesion molecule 1 (*VCAM1*). To examine how the MSC isolates within each group resemble each other in terms of expression profile, two different patient isolates from each group were compared. While the expression of mesenchymal stem cell markers in healthy donors was similar, with only a few genes being expressed differentially (Figure 4B left), the expression profiles in the MSC-CA (Figure 4B middle) and MSC-BRCA+ groups (Figure 4B right) were considerably different. This suggests that not only adjacent stroma but distant adipose tissue is affected by the presence of tumor mass as well and these changes remain in the MSCs even after the tumor-secreted factors are no longer present, as suggested by the altered expression profiles even after a certain time of culturing. However, if these tumor-caused changes are permanently retained in MSCs, such altered MSCs may later contribute to (or even cause) tumor recurrence.

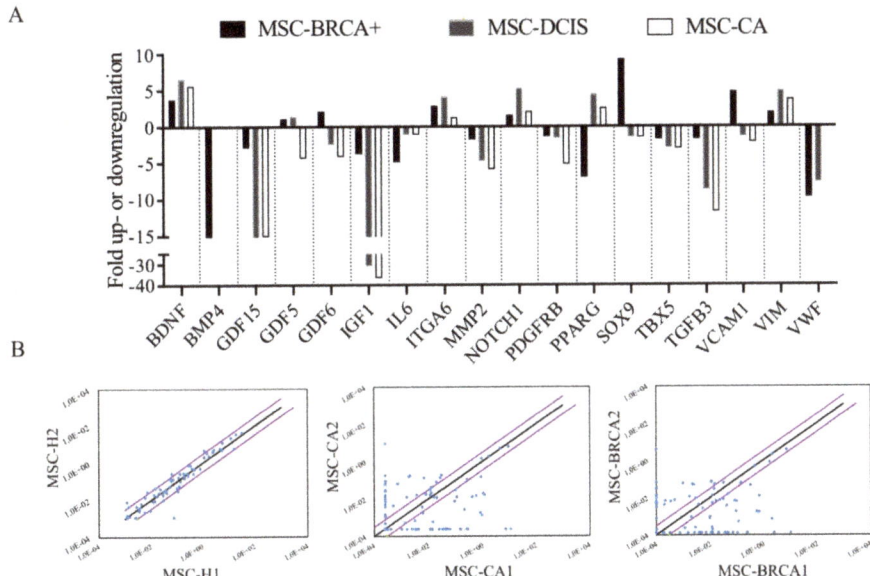

Figure 4. Expression profiles of healthy and cancer patient adipose tissue-derived MSCs. (**A**) RT^2 Profiler™ PCR human mesenchymal stem cells array of individual MSC isolates used in in vivo study revealed several gene expression changes. (**B**) Scatter plot of mesenchymal stem cell gene expression at the mRNA level comparing two different healthy (left), cancer (middle) and BRCA+ isolates (right). Lateral diagonal lines indicate a 2-fold increase or decrease. Results were obtained using the RT2 Profiler PCR Array Data Analysis software (at Qiagen data analysis web portal). MSCs used for analysis did not exceed 10th passage.

Further, we performed ELISA assays on more isolates to prevent misleading results caused by differences between individual MSC isolates. We have shown significantly lower concentrations of IGF1 in MSC-CA and MSC-BRCA+ (Figure 5A). As the molecular interplay between IGF1 and leptin, as well as its association with the pathogenesis of breast cancer, was shown previously, we have also analyzed the level of leptin which was significantly decreased in the group of MSC-CA (Figure 5B). After observing that the secretion of analyzed factors was decreased in cancer patient-derived MSCs, we were intrigued to see whether MSC-CA generally release less cytokines compared to MSC-H. The relative levels of human cytokines and chemokines in MSC culture medium were determined via a cytokine array kit. We were able to detect only nine out of 105 cytokines in MSC-CA media after 48-h culture compared to 20 out of 105 in MSC-H (Figure 5C). To see if this halted cytokine production could be connected to the tumor-released factors present in the tumor-adjacent adipose tissue used for MSC-CA isolation, we cultured healthy MSCs in NLR-MDA231 conditioned medium (CM-BCC) for 2 weeks. The analysis of the exemplary cytokine PTX3 concentration released to the media showed that it was decreased in MSC-H cultured in CM-BCC compared to the same isolate cultured in standard growth control media (Figure 5D).

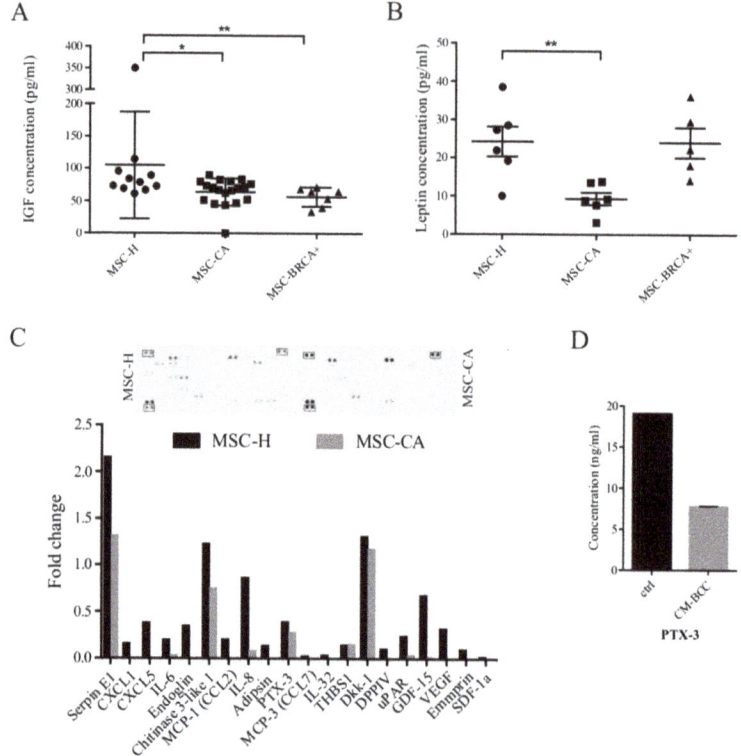

Figure 5. Secretion profile of cancer patient adipose tissue-derived MSCs is halted by tumor cell-secreted factors. (**A**) Decreased expression of IGF1 correlated with decreased IGF1 concentration detected in MSC-CA cell media (* $p < 0.05$; ** $p < 0.01$; Mann–Whitney test). (**B**) Leptin concentration in MSC-CA was also lower compared to MSC-H. The IGF1 and leptin concentration was measured by ELISA test in MSC medium after 48 h of culture (* $p < 0.05$; ** $p < 0.01$; Mann–Whitney test). (**C**) Cytokine analysis revealed a decreased release of cytokines and chemokines in MSC-CA isolate. The relative change in analyte level between MSC groups was determined by subtraction of each pair of capture antibody from the reference spot signal on the corresponding membrane. (**D**) The PTX3 concentration was decreased in healthy MSCs cultured for 2 weeks in NLR-MDA231 conditioned media. The concentration of PTX3 was measured by ELISA test in MSC medium after 48 h. MSCs used for analysis did not exceed 10th passage.

3.2. MSC Interactions with Breast Cancer Cells

After seeing that the cytokine production in MSC-CA is seemingly halted, we speculated different ways of communication between MSCs and tumor cells. We looked at the presence of direct cell-to-cell contacts in MSC-breast cancer cell co-culture and observed thin plasma membrane structures formed between cancer cells and MSC, which could allow cellular cross-talk leading to alteration of cell properties (Figure 6A). The altered functions and phenotype of breast cancer cells were analyzed in co-culture with MSCs of different origins. Direct co-culture of MSCs with breast cancer cells resulted in a more mesenchymal-like morphology of NLR-T47D and NLR-JIMT cells (Figure 6B) and their proliferation, regardless of the co-cultured MSC origin, was increased (Figure 6C middle, right). The NLR-MDA231 cell proliferation in vitro, however, was not affected by direct contact with MSCs (Figure 6C left).

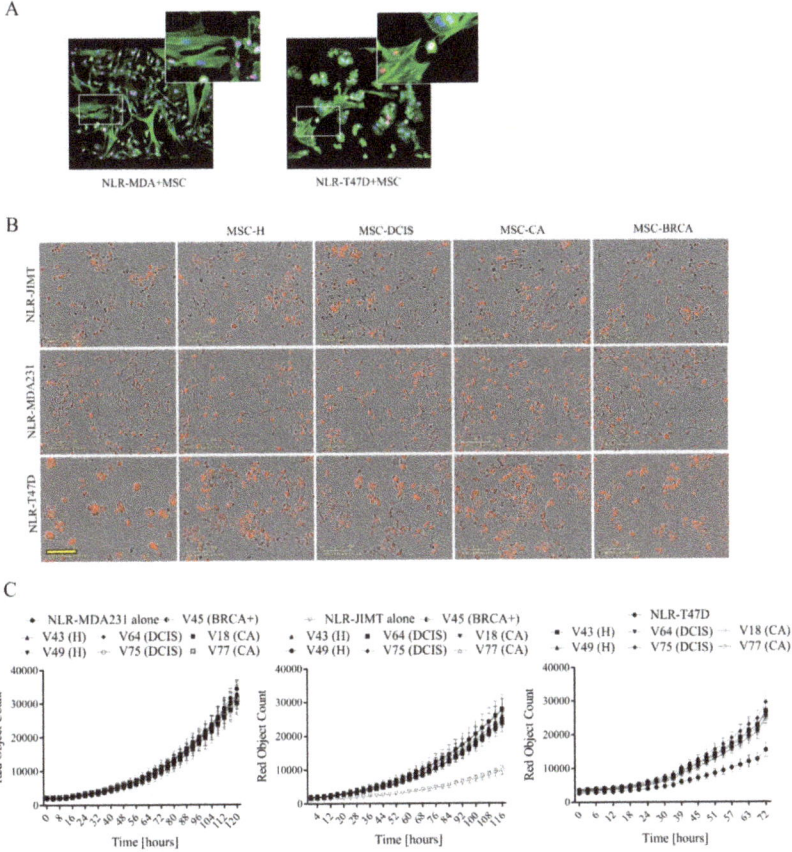

Figure 6. MSC–tumor cell interactions in 2D in vitro conditions. (**A**) Thin plasma membrane structures are formed between cancer cells and MSCs in co-culture allowing cell-to-cell communication and signaling. Magnification 200×. Cytoplasmic actin was stained green, nuclei were stained with DAPI (blue). The nuclei of tumor cells also expressed red fluorescent protein, therefore they appear as magenta colored. (**B**) MSC co-culture with tumor cells expressing red fluorescent nuclear protein resulted in more mesenchymal-like cell morphology of co-cultured NLR-T47D and NLR-JIMT cells. Scale bar: 200 µm. (**C**) Direct 7-day co-culture of NLR-JIMT and NLR-T47D breast cancer cells with MSCs of different origins highlighted the supportive role of MSCs in tumor cell proliferation, but no diagnosis-specific effects on proliferation were observed. NLR-MDA231 proliferation was not enhanced by the presence of MSCs.

To test the MSCs' effect on NLR-JIMT and NLR-T47D cell proliferation in a more relevant in vitro model, we proceeded to co-culture in 3D non-adherent culture conditions (Figure 7A). Although in NLR-T47D co-culture the spheroid size was bigger, the structure was less compact, and the luminescent assay showed significantly less ATP in all MSC groups (Figure 7B left). NLR-JIMT-MSC co-culture in 3D conditions showed MSC support of tumor cell proliferation, and this was also confirmed by luminescent assay (Figure 7B right). While this leads to the assumption that the MSC-mediated augmentation of cancer cell proliferation is cell-line specific, there was no difference in effect regarding whether the MSCs were isolated from the adipose tissue of healthy donors or cancer patients. To gain deeper insight into how the MSCs affect breast tumor cells, the invasion profiles of both MSC populations in co-culture with tumor cells were evaluated in IncuCyte® Scratch Wound Invasion assay. Interestingly,

MSC-CA invaded the 50% ECM much more rapidly than MSC-H and, moreover, they augmented the invasion of NLR-MDA231 cells as well (Figure 7C).

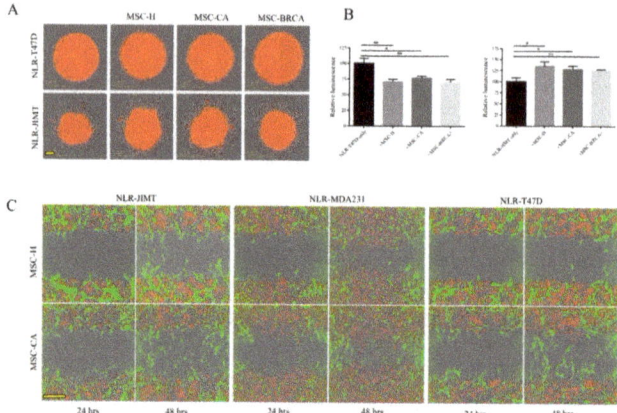

Figure 7. Faster invading cancer patient-derived MSCs are followed by more rapidly invading tumor cells. (**A**) Monoculture vs. co-culture in 3D non-adherent culture conditions showed less compact NLR-T47D-MSC spheroids and bigger NLR-JIMT-MSC spheroids, but no difference between MSC isolates was observed. Scale bar: 100 µm. Breast cancer cells—red color, MSCs—unstained. (**B**) Luminometric measurement of spheroid cultures after 7 days revealed significantly lower ATP amount in NLR-T47D-MSC co-culture and higher ATP amount in NLR-JIMT-MSC co-culture (* $p <$ 0.05; ** $p < 0.01$; Mann–Whitney test). In the control group (only breast cancer cells without MSC), 8 samples were analyzed. In each group with MSC, 4 spheroids were analyzed. (**C**) MSC-CA exhibited increased invasion potential in Scratch wound invasion assay after 24 or 48 h. The invasion of tumor cells was also increased in co-culture with MSC-CA compared to MSC-H (1×10^4 MSCs + 2×10^4 NLR-MDA231/NLR-T47D and 1.5×10^4 MSCs + 3×10^4 NLR-JIMT were seeded on Matrigel coated 96-well plates and covered with 50% Matrigel). Scale bar: 200 µm. MSCs used for analysis did not exceed 10th passage. MSCs were stained with Vybrant™ CFDA SE Cell Tracer Kit (green color), breast cancer cell lines expressed red fluorescent protein.

3.3. The Effect of MSCs on Tumor Growth In Vivo

To evaluate the effects of MSCs on tumorigenicity in vivo, immuno-compromised SCID/Beige mice were subcutaneously injected solely with NLR-JIMT cells or with NLR-JIMT cells mixed with MSCs from different origins (Figure 8A). The NLR-JIMT cell line represents the HER2-enriched non-luminal tumor type characterized by aggressive growth with intermediate prognosis. The confirmed insensitivity to HER-2 inhibiting drugs (trastuzumab and pertuzumab) makes it a valuable experimental model for studies of resistance mechanisms. Subsequent tumor volume analysis on Day 15 revealed the supportive effect of MSCs on tumor growth in the co-injected xenografts compared to those composed solely of tumor cells (Figure 8B). In addition, the NLR-JIMT co-injected with cancer patient-derived MSC-BRCA+, MSC-DCIS and MSC-CA produced a significantly higher tumor volume than NLR-JIMT co-injected with healthy donor-derived MSC-H ($p < 0.01$ in MSC-H vs. MSC-CA and MSC-H vs. MSC-BRCA+; $p < 0.05$ in MSC-H vs. MSC-DCIS). The highest pro-tumorigenic effect, however, was observed in xenografts formed by NLR-JIMT cells co-injected with invasive cancer patient-derived MSC-CA. When the NLR-JIMT were co-injected with MSC-CA, the average tumor volume on Day 15 was 338.3 mm^3 compared to 76.6 mm^3 volume of the MSC-H co-injected tumors. This demonstrates a striking MSC-CA pro-tumorigenic effect. The experimental mice were sacrificed when tumors reached more than 11 mm in any dimension. Subsequent histological analysis of the tumor xenografts showed decreased Ki67 expression in the center of xenografts formed by NLR-JIMT co-injected with cancer patient-derived MSC-BRCA+, MSC-DCIS and MSC-CA than in NLR-JIMT co-injected with healthy donor-derived MSC-H, or NLR-JIMT alone (Figure 8C, 1st column). This is explained by MSC localization in the xenograft center, and the subsequent denser micro-environment surrounding the tumor cells.

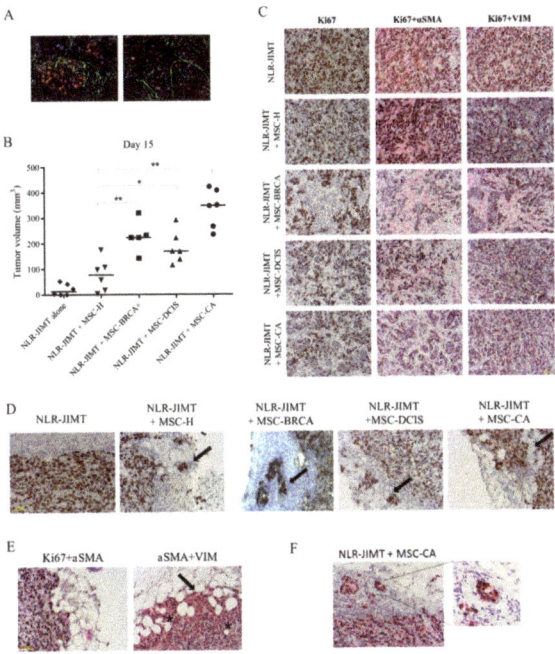

Figure 8. Cancer patient adipose tissue-derived MSCs showed a pro-tumorigenic effect on subcutaneous tumor xenografts in vivo. (**A**) Actin immunofluorescence staining of mice xenograft cryosection shows xenograft composition formed by tumor cells and MSCs (left—xenograft periphery, right—xenograft center; red—cancer cell nuclei, green—actin cytoplasm staining, blue - nuclei staining with DAPI. Magnification 630×.) (**B**) 5×10^5 MSCs of different origin were subcutaneously co-injected with 1×10^6 NLR-JIMT cells in immuno-compromised SCID/Beige mice. Tumor volume examination on Day 15 revealed profound supportive effect of MSCs on tumor growth in the co-injected xenografts. Xenografts composed solely of tumor cells failed to induce significant tumor volume in the analyzed period. Tumor volume was calculated by formula: volume = (length × width2)/2 (* $p < 0.05$, ** $p < 0.01$, Man-Whitney test). The significantly most supportive effect was observed in mice injected with NLR-JIMT + MSC-CA. (**C**) Detection of Ki67, αSMA and VIM markers by immuno-histochemistry in tumor tissue sections. Mice were sacrificed when the tumor xenograft reached 1 cm^3. Xenografts were fixed with formaldehyde, embedded in paraffin and processed for immuno-histochemical staining with monoclonal antibodies. Representative images of tumors formed by NLR-JIMT co-injected with cancer patient-derived MSCs (BRCA+, DCIS, CA) showed lower Ki67 positivity in the tumor center than in NLR-JIMT co-injected with healthy donor-derived MSC-H. The αSMA and Vimentin (VIM) staining showed that mainly the MSC-CA and MSC-BRCA+ attempted to form aligned pathway-like structures around the tumor cells. Magnification 200×. (**D**) Representative Ki67-stained pictures of xenograft periphery showed clusters of tumor cells invading surrounding stroma in tumors formed by NLR-JIMT co-injected with MSCs (MSC-H, -DCIS, -BRCA) and collective cell migration with a distinguishable invasive front was observed in the group co-injected with MSC-CA. (**E**) Immuno-histochemical staining of αSMA and Vimentin revealed up-regulation in tumor cells located in the invasive front of the xenografts co-injected with MSC-CA. This suggests the epithelial-to-mesenchymal transition of tumor cells. Asterisks identify smaller adipocytes with dilated inter-cellular spaces near the tumor invasive front. (**F**) Detail of the xenograft periphery showing Vimentin positivity in tumor cells.

The αSMA and Vimentin staining in Figure 8C suggests that in tumors injected with cancer patient-derived MSCs, and particularly in those with MSC-BRCA+, the MSCs attempt to form aligned structures around the tumor cells that resemble cellular pathways. α-SMA was used to visualize the localization of MSCs within the tumor xenografts, and although human αSMA antibody was used, the mouse endothelial cells in xenografts formed by NLR-JIMT cells were stained as well. Therefore, additional staining with the MSC marker Vimentin was performed, and confirmed that the αSMA positive cells were indeed MSCs. This was independently evaluated by a pathologist (MA) and histology specialist (MBu) who confirmed specific MSC-positive staining in the carcinoma-associated MSC-containing xenografts. In addition, Figure 8D confirms that Ki67 staining of the xenograft periphery depicts clusters of tumor cells invading surrounding tissue in NLR-JIMT co-injected with MSC-H, MSC-BRCA and MSC-DCIS xenografts. This manifest substantial effect of these MSCs on tumor cell invasiveness and also highlights collective cell-scattering, where the tumor cells detach and spread in small clusters. In contrast, the histological analysis of tumors formed by NLR-JIMT co-injected with MSC-CA showed collective cell migration with a distinguishable invasive front (Figure 8E; indicated with arrow). These tumor cells were in immediate proximity to adipocytes and spread along adipocyte intercellular spaces. Moreover, the adipocytes closest to the tumor invasive front are clearly smaller and have wider intercellular spaces (Figure 8E; indicated with asterisks). Finally, Vimentin staining in these tumor cells suggested epithelial-to-mesenchymal transition (EMT). Vimentin staining was positive in the tumor cell cytoplasm of xenografts co-injected with MSC-CA located in the invasive front (Figure 8F). Ki67 staining quantification revealed its uneven distribution throughout the tissue section, but its expression in all groups proved similar when a greater number of zones was investigated (Table 1).

Table 1. Ki67 score in tumor xenografts. Ki67 expression analysis in several areas of tissue section revealed its uneven distribution throughout the xenograft. When a higher number of zones was investigated, the Ki67 staining quantification showed similar expression in all groups.

Injected Cells (NLR-JIMT)	Ki67 Positivity in Analyzed Area (%)	Average Ki67 Positivity (%)
alone	59.59 66.53 92.46	72.9
+MSC-H	77.55 59.34 75.88	70.9
+MSC-BRCA	76.77 69.41 73.9	73.4
+MSC-DCIS	95.35 68.45 94.57	86.1
+MSC-CA	64.95 65.91 86.71	72.5

In order to verify the observed effects in a clinically more relevant model, an orthotopic model of mammary carcinogenesis was used (Figure 9A). The mixture of NLR-JIMT and MSC-CA resulted in a higher tumor volume in the mammary glands of injected mice compared to the mixture of NLR-JIMT and MSC-H. The co-injection of tumor cells with MSC-BRCA (2) obtained from patient breast tissue where prophylactic mastectomy was performed and MSC-BRCA (1) from contralateral breast of the same patient with confirmed relapsed invasive ductal carcinoma (pT1bpNx) demonstrated that MSCs isolated from the adipose tissue adjacent to a tumor mass have a more aggressive phenotype and augmented tumor volume in NLR-JIMT + MSC-BRCA (1) (Figure 9B). Ki67 staining of the xenograft periphery confirmed the invasive character of tumor cells co-injected with MSCs isolated from tumor-adjacent adipose tissue. Interestingly, the increased metastatic potential in the presence of MSC-CA was confirmed also by the increased innervation of tumor xenografts. The perineural and intraneural invasion of CK7- and vimentin-positive tumor cells was detected (Figure 9C), as well as the presence of tumor cells inside the blood vessels (Figure 9D).

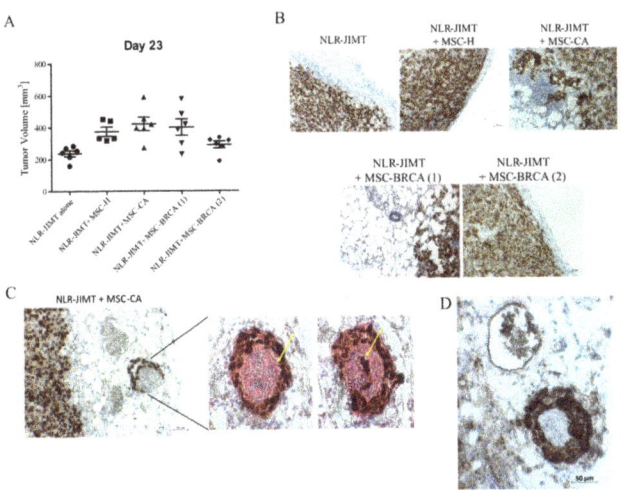

Figure 9. Pro-tumorigenic effect of MSC-CA in orthotopic mouse model. (**A**) Mixture of 5 × 10^5 NLR-JIMT cells and 2.5 × 10^5 MSCs in 100 µL serum-free DMEM diluted 1:1 with ECM gel (Sigma-Aldrich) was injected bilaterally into mammary fat pad of SCID/Beige mice. The animals were divided into five groups according to the type of injected MSC: control group of NLR-JIMT alone ($n = 6$), MSC-H ($n = 6$), MSC-CA ($n = 6$), MSC-BRCA (2) ($n = 6$) obtained from breast tissue where prophylactic mastectomy was performed and MSC-BRCA (1) ($n = 6$) from contralateral breast of the same patient with confirmed relapsed invasive ductal carcinoma. Tumor volume was calculated according to the formula: volume = (length × width2)/2. The animals were sacrificed when the tumor volume exceeded 1 cm^3. The most supportive effect was observed in mice injected with NLR-JIMT + MSC-CA and MSC-BRCA (1). (**B**) Ki67 staining of xenograft periphery showed collective cell invasion in the group co-injected with MSC-CA. This manner of invasion was also observed in the MSC-BRCA (1), but was lacking in the MSC-BRCA (2) co-injected group. While both MSC-BRCA isolates come from the same patient, the former were isolated from a breast with relapsed ductal carcinoma and the later from a contralateral healthy breast where prophylactic mastectomy was performed. MSCs derived from breast adipose tissue with confirmed presence of tumor (MSC-BRCA (1)) increased the invasion of tumor cells in xenograft periphery. (**C**) Nerve fibers were detected in serial sections of NLR-JIMT + MSC-CA orthotopic xenografts using IHC staining with specific neuronal marker PGP9.5. The perineural and intraneural tumor cell invasion (yellow arrow pointing at invading single tumor cell in the left picture and group of tumor cells in the right picture) was present only in the MSC-CA group. (**D**) CK7 antibody (breast cancer marker) staining confirmed the presence of tumor cells in the perineural space and also inside the blood vessel.

4. Discussion

Tumor–stroma interaction, and particularly the cytokine–cytokine receptor interaction pathway, is significantly altered in highly aggressive tumors [21]. While many studies have evaluated the role of mesenchymal stromal cells in the tumor microenvironment [22], the majority were based on adipose MSCs from non-breast origins [23,24]. In contrast, we compared normal breast adipose tissue-derived

MSCs and their tumor-activated counterparts and revealed phenotypic, molecular and functional changes which determined the stromal cell activation status.

There is a growing substantial interest in identifying MSC proliferation properties for future application in cell therapy and tissue engineering [25,26]. Herein, the growth kinetics and population doubling-time were influenced by age when younger and older donors were compared, as shown by others [27,28]. While the correlation between MSC doubling-time and age or BMI status in MSC donors was not significant at first sight, the separate analysis of doubling-time in younger and older patient groups for healthy and cancer patient-derived MSCs highlighted an increased doubling-time in the older group. Apparently, the conflicting observations are likely related to increased doubling-time in MSC-CA compared to MSC-H.

MSC morphological analysis did not reveal any changes related to diagnosis or age. The changes might be evident only when MSCs differentiate into CAF in the tumor micro-environment [10], while adjacent adipose tissue-derived MSC morphology remains unaffected or the tumor cell influence in the culture is lacking.

In addition to doubling-time changes, we also identified altered gene expression and cytokine production in breast cancer-derived MSCs. The most evident was the down-regulation of *GDF5*, *GDF6*, *IGF1*, *PDGFRB* and *TGFB3* genes in MSC-CA compared to MSC-H. Morales et al. [21] identified 76 differentially expressed genes associated with the metastasis of relapsed primary tumors. Two of these, down-regulated *GDF5* and *TGFB3*, corresponded to the results observed in our analysis. *NOTCH1* expression has also been implicated in cancer cell metastasis, and breast cancer patients positive for *NOTCH1* have experienced shorter disease-free survival [29,30]. Here, it is most likely that adipose tissue's close proximity to a breast tumor correlates with the observed MSC expression changes, and these could well explain the increased in vivo invasion of NLR-JIMT + MSC-CA tumor xenografts.

It was reported that BMP4 possesses both tumor-suppressive and oncogenic properties in breast cancer and that it is a potent suppressor of breast cancer metastasis [31,32]. Therefore, the decreased *BMP4* expression in MSC-BRCA+ could contribute to the in vivo cell cluster migration we observed in the more distant parts of tumors. In addition, BMP4 down-regulation in the tumor micro-environment could lead to the formation of these clusters and thus increase tumor cell metastatic ability. Furthermore, increased *SOX9* expression in MSC-BRCA+ correlates with prognostic significance in invasive ductal carcinoma and metastatic breast cancer [33]. Therefore, we assume it can also be associated with the observed invasive nature of NLR-JIMT + MSC-BRCA+ tumors. We also suggest that the up-regulation of brain-derived neurotrophic factor (BDNF), which supports innervation in tumor xenografts, could be a promising determinant of tumor cell invasion and metastasis. We propose that mesenchymal stromal cells in the tumor proximity are pushed by tumor cells to help in nerve recruitment and, interestingly, these alterations in MSCs become permanent as they remain even when the tumor is not present anymore.

In MSC-CA and MSC-DCIS, here we determined the decreased expression of *GDF15* and *IGF*, but this conflicts with published results which show increased expression of these genes in the tumor micro-environment [34].

We propose that the decreased cytokine production by MSC-CA could correlate with tumor presence in adipose tissue, as also healthy MSCs cultured in NLR-MDA231 conditioned media showed altered cytokine production. However, tumor cells co-cultured with MSC-CA exhibited a more aggressive phenotype in vitro and in vivo, which could be associated with direct cell-to-cell communication and connections, indicating the presence of nanotubes in MSC–tumor cell cultures. Moreover, histological tumor xenograft analysis revealed functional changes associated with epithelial-to-mesenchymal transition induction and increased tumor cell invasion in co-culture with MSC-CA. While the collective migration of tumor cells was combined with high Ki67 and VIM positivity in the invasive front, the cell invasion differed in tumor cells co-injected with MSC-DCIS compared to MSC-CA. This identifies that MSC-CA have a more aggressive phenotype.

Vimentin up-regulation is an EMT-specific marker of increased cancer cell motility and migration [35,36]; therefore, its positive staining in NLR-JIMT-MSC-CA xenograft suggests significant functional changes in cancer patients' MSCs where breast adipose tissue has close proximity to the tumor. The functional changes are also suggested by the smaller adipocytes and wider intercellular spaces in close proximity to the xenograft invasive front, suggesting additional extracellular matrix alterations [37].

Finally, the combined data provide the conclusion that MSCs in cancer patient adipose tissue have inherently altered expression profiles and functional characteristics which enhance their ability to support in vivo tumor cell propagation. Moreover, the adipose tissue MSCs derived from closely adjacent tumor tissue increased the volume of tumor xenografts when co-injected with NLR-JIMT subcutaneously and orthotopically, and also supported the release of tumor cell clusters. Orthotopic model confirmed the pro-tumorigenic phenotype of MSC-CA which induced the perineural invasion of tumor cells. Our data suggest the capacity of cancer patient-derived MSCs to support cell scattering and invasion by involving tumor cell epithelial-to-mesenchymal transition.

5. Conclusions

To the best of our knowledge, we have described permanent proliferative and functional changes in tumor-adjacent adipose tissue-derived MSCs for the first time. The analysis of MSCs isolated from breast cancer patients provides improved understanding of the changes provoked in adipose tissue by close proximity to the tumor and also identifies MSCs' role in the promotion and progression of tumor growth.

Herein, we showed that the micro-environment of adipose tissue closely adjacent to breast tumor tissue is composed of tumor-exposed MSCs which differ in doubling-time, expression profile, cytokine production and tumor-promoting ability shown by perineural invasion in vivo compared to the MSCs in healthy adipose tissue. Further study focused on the specific molecular pathways responsible for the activation and re-programming of MSCs exposed to tumor micro-environment should reveal potential therapeutic strategies which will block the tumor-induced alterations caused to adjacent adipose tissue.

Author Contributions: S.M., L.K. and M.B. (Martin Bohac), discussed and designed this study; S.M., J.P., M.C., M.B. (Monika Burikova), and L.K. analyzed data and wrote manuscript; J.P., M.C., S.M., M.B. (Monika Burikova), L.K. performed all experiments; M.A., M.B. (Monika Burikova), S.D. performed and analyzed histology of tumor xenografts and D.R. analyzed the data from breast cancer patients; M.B. (Martin Bohac), M.M., D.P., M.K. and J.S. provided material for MSC isolation; S.M., J.P., M.C. and L.D. isolated MSC, and S.M., M.C. and L.K. revised the manuscript. All authors have read and approved the final manuscript.

Funding: This work was supported by the Slovak Research and Development Agency under contracts APVV-16-0178, APVV 16-0010, APVV 15-0697 and VEGA grants 1/0271/17, 2/0087/15. This work was financially supported also by the 7FP platform ERA-NET program EuroNanoMed II Innocent.

Acknowledgments: We thank L.Rojikova for assistance with in vivo experiments, D. Manasova, S. Schmidtova, L. Demkova for sample collection, M. Dubrovcakova and S. Balentova for technical assistance and A. Babelova for help with immunofluorescence analysis.

Conflicts of Interest: The authors declare no conflict of interest.

References

1. Jena, M.K.; Janjanam, J. Role of extracellular matrix in breast cancer development: A brief update. *F1000Research* **2018**, *7*, 274. [CrossRef] [PubMed]
2. Cozzo, A.J.; Fuller, A.M.; Makowski, L. Contribution of Adipose Tissue to Development of Cancer. *Compr. Physiol.* **2017**, *8*, 237–282. [PubMed]
3. Martins, D.; Schmitt, F. Microenvironment in breast tumorigenesis: Friend or foe? *Histol. Histopathol.* **2018**, *34*, 18021.
4. Kidd, S.; Spaeth, E.; Watson, K.; Burks, J.; Lu, H.; Klopp, A.; Andreeff, M.; Marini, F.C. Origins of the tumor microenvironment: Quantitative assessment of adipose-derived and bone marrow-derived stroma. *PLoS ONE* **2012**, *7*, e30563. [CrossRef] [PubMed]

5. Turley, S.J.; Cremasco, V.; Astarita, J.L. Immunological hallmarks of stromal cells in the tumour microenvironment. *Nat. Rev. Immunol.* **2015**, *15*, 669–682. [CrossRef] [PubMed]
6. Berger, L.; Shamai, Y.; Skorecki, K.L.; Tzukerman, M. Tumor Specific Recruitment and Reprogramming of Mesenchymal Stem Cells in Tumorigenesis. *Stem. Cells* **2016**, *34*, 1011–1026. [CrossRef]
7. Jotzu, C.; Alt, E.; Welte, G.; Li, J.; Hennessy, B.T.; Devarajan, E.; Krishnappa, S.; Pinilla, S.; Droll, L.; Song, Y.-H. Adipose tissue derived stem cells differentiate into carcinoma-associated fibroblast-like cells under the influence of tumor derived factors. *Cell Oncol. (Dordr)* **2011**, *34*, 55–67. [CrossRef]
8. Mishra, P.J.; Humeniuk, R.; Medina, D.J.; Alexe, G.; Mesirov, J.P.; Ganesan, S.; Glod, J.W.; Banerjee, D. Carcinoma-associated fibroblast-like differentiation of human mesenchymal stem cells. *Cancer Res.* **2008**, *68*, 4331–4339. [CrossRef]
9. Ridge, S.M.; Sullivan, F.J.; Glynn, S.A. Mesenchymal stem cells: Key players in cancer progression. *Mol. Cancer* **2017**, *16*, 31. [CrossRef]
10. Visweswaran, M.; Keane, K.N.; Arfuso, F.; Dilley, R.J.; Newsholme, P.; Dharmarajan, A. The Influence of Breast Tumour-Derived Factors and Wnt Antagonism on the Transformation of Adipose-Derived Mesenchymal Stem Cells into Tumour-Associated Fibroblasts. *Cancer Microenviron. Off. J. Int. Cancer Microenviron. Soc.* **2018**, *11*, 71–84. [CrossRef]
11. Spaeth, E.L.; Dembinski, J.L.; Sasser, A.K.; Watson, K.; Klopp, A.; Hall, B.; Andreeff, M.; Marini, F. Mesenchymal stem cell transition to tumor-associated fibroblasts contributes to fibrovascular network expansion and tumor progression. *PLoS ONE* **2009**, *4*, e4992. [CrossRef] [PubMed]
12. Bussard, K.M.; Mutkus, L.; Stumpf, K.; Gomez-Manzano, C.; Marini, F.C. Tumor-associated stromal cells as key contributors to the tumor microenvironment. *Breast Cancer Res. BCR* **2016**, *18*, 84. [CrossRef] [PubMed]
13. Kucerova, L.; Zmajkovic, J.; Toro, L.; Skolekova, S.; Demkova, L.; Matuskova, M. Tumor-driven Molecular Changes in Human Mesenchymal Stromal Cells. *Cancer Microenviron. Off. J. Int. Cancer Microenviron. Soc.* **2015**, *8*, 1–14. [CrossRef]
14. Skolekova, S.; Matuskova, M.; Bohac, M.; Toro, L.; Durinikova, E.; Tyciakova, S.; Demkova, L.; Gursky, J.; Kucerova, L. Cisplatin-induced mesenchymal stromal cells-mediated mechanism contributing to decreased antitumor effect in breast cancer cells. *Cell Commun. Signal. CCS* **2016**, *14*, 4. [CrossRef]
15. Yeh, W.L.; Tsai, C.F.; Chen, D.R. Peri-foci adipose-derived stem cells promote chemoresistance in breast cancer. *Stem. Cell Res. Ther.* **2017**, *8*, 177. [CrossRef]
16. Kucerova, L.; Skolekova, S.; Matuskova, M.; Bohac, M.; Kozovska, Z. Altered features and increased chemosensitivity of human breast cancer cells mediated by adipose tissue-derived mesenchymal stromal cells. *BMC Cancer* **2013**, *13*, 535. [CrossRef]
17. Borriello, L.; Nakata, R.; Sheard, M.A.; Fernandez, G.E.; Sposto, R.; Malvar, J.; Blavier, L.; Shimada, H.; Asgharzadah, S.; Seeger, R.C.; et al. Cancer-Associated Fibroblasts Share Characteristics and Protumorigenic Activity with Mesenchymal Stromal Cells. *Cancer Res.* **2017**, *77*, 5142–5157. [CrossRef]
18. Melzer, C.; von der Ohe, J.; Hass, R. Concise Review: Crosstalk of Mesenchymal Stroma/Stem-Like Cells with Cancer Cells Provides Therapeutic Potential. *Stem. Cells* **2018**, *36*, 951–968. [CrossRef]
19. Kucerova, L.; Altanerova, V.; Matuskova, M.; Tyciakova, S.; Altaner, C. Adipose tissue-derived human mesenchymal stem cells mediated prodrug cancer gene therapy. *Cancer Res.* **2007**, *67*, 6304–6313. [CrossRef]
20. Dominici, M.; Le Blanc, K.; Mueller, I.; Slaper-Cortenbach, I.; Marini, F.; Krause, D.; Deans, R.; Keating, A.; Prockop, D.; Horwitz, E. Minimal criteria for defining multipotent mesenchymal stromal cells. The International Society for Cellular Therapy position statement. *Cytotherapy* **2006**, *8*, 315–317. [CrossRef]
21. Morales, M.; Planet, E.; Arnal-Estape, A.; Pavlovic, M.; Tarragona, M.; Gomis, R.R. Tumor-stroma interactions a trademark for metastasis. *Breast* **2011**, *20*, S50–S55. [CrossRef]
22. Nwabo Kamdje, A.H.; Kamga, P.T.; Simo, R.T.; Vecchio, L.; Etet, P.F.S.; Muller, J.M.; Bassi, G.; Lukong, E.; Goel, R.C.; Amvene, J.M.; et al. Mesenchymal stromal cells' role in tumor microenvironment: Involvement of signaling pathways. *Cancer Biol. Med.* **2017**, *14*, 129–141. [CrossRef] [PubMed]
23. El-Haibi, C.P.; Bell, G.W.; Zhang, J.; Collmann, A.Y.; Wood, D.; Scherber, C.M.; Csizmadia, E.; Mariani, O.; Zhu, C.; Campagne, A.; et al. Critical role for lysyl oxidase in mesenchymal stem cell-driven breast cancer malignancy. *Proc. Natl. Acad. Sci. USA* **2012**, *109*, 17460–17465. [CrossRef] [PubMed]

24. Melzer, C.; von der Ohe, J.; Hass, R. Enhanced metastatic capacity of breast cancer cells after interaction and hybrid formation with mesenchymal stroma/stem cells (MSC). *Cell Commun. Signal. CCS* **2018**, *16*, 2. [CrossRef] [PubMed]
25. Altaner, C.; Altanerova, V.; Cihova, M.; Hunakova, L.; Kaiserova, K.; Klepanec, A.; Vulev, I.; Madaric, J. Characterization of mesenchymal stem cells of "no-options" patients with critical limb ischemia treated by autologous bone marrow mononuclear cells. *PLoS ONE* **2013**, *8*, e73722. [CrossRef] [PubMed]
26. Moravcikova, E.; Meyer, E.M.; Corselli, M.; Donnenberg, V.S.; Donnenberg, A.D. Proteomic Profiling of Native Unpassaged and Culture-Expanded Mesenchymal Stromal Cells (MSC). *Cytom. Part. A Int. Soc. Anal. Cytol.* **2018**, *93*, 894–904. [CrossRef] [PubMed]
27. Choudhery, M.S.; Badowski, M.; Muise, A.; Pierce, J.; Harris, D.T. Donor age negatively impacts adipose tissue-derived mesenchymal stem cell expansion and differentiation. *J. Transl. Med.* **2014**, *12*, 8. [CrossRef]
28. Maredziak, M.; Marycz, K.; Tomaszewski, K.A.; Kornicka Henry, B.M. The Influence of Aging on the Regenerative Potential of Human Adipose Derived Mesenchymal Stem Cells. *Stem. Cells Int.* **2016**, *2016*, 2152435. [CrossRef]
29. Zhong, Y.; Shen, S.; Zhou, Y.; Mao, F.; Lin, Y.; Guan, J.; Xu, Y.; Zhang, S.; Liu, X.; Sun, Q. NOTCH1 is a poor prognostic factor for breast cancer and is associated with breast cancer stem cells. *Oncotargets Ther.* **2016**, *9*, 6865–6871. [CrossRef]
30. Reedijk, M.; Odorcic, S.; Chang, L.; Zhang, H.; Miller, N.; McCready, D.R.; Lockwood, G.; Egan, S.E. High-level coexpression of JAG1 and NOTCH1 is observed in human breast cancer and is associated with poor overall survival. *Cancer Res.* **2005**, *65*, 8530–8537. [CrossRef]
31. Cao, Y.; Slaney, C.Y.; Bidwell, B.N.; Parker, B.S.; Johnstone, C.N.; Rautela, J.; Eckhardt, B.L.; Anderson, R.L. BMP4 inhibits breast cancer metastasis by blocking myeloid-derived suppressor cell activity. *Cancer Res.* **2014**, *74*, 5091–5102. [CrossRef] [PubMed]
32. Ketolainen, J.M.; Alarmo, E.L.; Tuominen, V.J.; Kallioniemi, A. Parallel inhibition of cell growth and induction of cell migration and invasion in breast cancer cells by bone morphogenetic protein 4. *Breast Cancer Res. Treat.* **2010**, *124*, 377–386. [CrossRef] [PubMed]
33. Chakravarty, G.; Moroz, K.; Makridakis, N.M.; Lloyd, S.A.; Galvez, S.E.; Canavello, P.R.; Lacey, M.R.; Agrawal, K.; Mondal, D. Prognostic significance of cytoplasmic SOX9 in invasive ductal carcinoma and metastatic breast cancer. *Exp. Biol. Med. (Maywood)* **2011**, *236*, 145–155. [CrossRef] [PubMed]
34. Daubriac, J.; Han, S.; Grahovac, J.; Smith, E.; Hosein, A.; Buchanan, M.; Basik, M.; Boucher, Y. The crosstalk between breast carcinoma-associated fibroblasts and cancer cells promotes RhoA-dependent invasion via IGF-1 and PAI-1. *Oncotarget* **2018**, *9*, 10375–10387. [CrossRef] [PubMed]
35. Brabletz, T.; Kalluri, R.; Nieto, M.A.; Weinberg, R.A. EMT in cancer. *Nat. Rev. Cancer.* **2018**, *18*, 128–134. [CrossRef] [PubMed]
36. Bill, R.; Christofori, G. The relevance of EMT in breast cancer metastasis: Correlation or causality? *Febs. Lett.* **2015**, *589*, 1577–1587. [CrossRef]
37. Dirat, B.; Bochet, L.; Dabek, M.; Daviaud, D.; Dauvillier, S.; Majed, B.; Wang, Y.Y.; Meulle, A.; Salles, B.; Le Gonidec, S.; et al. Cancer-associated adipocytes exhibit an activated phenotype and contribute to breast cancer invasion. *Cancer Res.* **2011**, *71*, 2455–2465. [CrossRef]

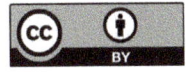 © 2020 by the authors. Licensee MDPI, Basel, Switzerland. This article is an open access article distributed under the terms and conditions of the Creative Commons Attribution (CC BY) license (http://creativecommons.org/licenses/by/4.0/).

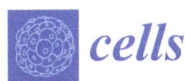

Article

Assessment of the Immunosuppressive Potential of INF-γ Licensed Adipose Mesenchymal Stem Cells, Their Secretome and Extracellular Vesicles

Teresa Raquel Tavares Serejo [1], Amandda Évelin Silva-Carvalho [1],
Luma Dayane de Carvalho Filiú Braga [1], Francisco de Assis Rocha Neves [1],
Rinaldo Wellerson Pereira [2], Juliana Lott de Carvalho [2] and Felipe Saldanha-Araujo [1,*]

[1] Laboratório de Farmacologia Molecular, Departamento de Ciências da Saúde, Universidade de Brasília, Brasília 70910-900, Brazil; raquelserejo@yahoo.com.br (T.R.T.S.); amanddaevelin@hotmail.com (A.É.S.-C.); luma.filiu@gmail.com (L.D.d.C.F.B.); nevesfar@gmail.com (F.d.A.R.N.)
[2] Pós-graduação em Ciências Genômicas e Biotecnologia, Universidade Católica de Brasília, Brasília 70790-160, Brazil; rinaldo.pereira@catolica.edu.br (R.W.P.); julianalott@gmail.com (J.L.d.C.)
* Correspondence: felipearaujo@unb.br; Tel./Fax: +55-61-3107-2008

Received: 10 December 2018; Accepted: 29 December 2018; Published: 5 January 2019

Abstract: There is an active search for the ideal strategy to potentialize the effects of Mesenchymal Stem-Cells (MSCs) over the immune system. Also, part of the scientific community is seeking to elucidate the therapeutic potential of MSCs secretome and its extracellular vesicles (EVs), in order to avoid the complexity of a cellular therapy. Here, we investigate the effects of human adipose MSCs (AMSCs) licensing with INF-γ and TLR3 agonist over AMSCs proliferation, migration, as well as the immunomodulatory function. Furthermore, we evaluated how the licensing of AMSCs affected the immunomodulatory function of AMSC derived-secretome, including their EVs. INF-γ licensed-AMSCs presented an elevated expression of indoleamine 2,3-dioxygenase (IDO), accompanied by increased ICAM-1, as well as a higher immunosuppressive potential, compared to unlicensed AMSCs. Interestingly, the conditioned medium obtained from INF-γ licensed-AMSCs also revealed a slightly superior immunosuppressive potential, compared to other licensing strategies. Therefore, unlicensed and INF-γ licensed-AMSCs groups were used to isolate EVs. Interestingly, EVs isolated from both groups displayed similar capacity to inhibit T-cell proliferation. EVs isolated from both groups shared similar TGF-β and Galectin-1 mRNA content but only EVs derived from INF-γ licensed-AMSCs expressed IDO mRNA. In summary, we demonstrated that INF-γ licensing of AMSCs provides an immunosuppressive advantage both from a cell-cell contact-dependent perspective, as well as in a cell-free context. Interestingly, EVs derived from unlicensed and INF-γ licensed-AMSCs have similar ability to control activated T-cell proliferation. These results contribute towards the development of new strategies to control the immune response based on AMSCs or their derived products.

Keywords: mesenchymal stem cells; T-cells; conditioned medium; extracellular vesicles; TLR; INF-γ

1. Introduction

Mesenchymal Stem-Cells (MSCs) are adult multipotent cells, which present a series of important biological properties, rendering them promising tools for cell-based therapy. One of the critical properties of these cells—which has attracted the attention of the scientific community decades ago—is the ability of MSCs to control the immune response. Specifically, regarding T-cells, MSCs exert their immunomodulatory effects through a broad range of mechanisms, including cell contact, secretion of anti-inflammatory molecules and induction of regulatory T-cells [1].

Over the last few years, the field of cellular therapy using MSCs to control immune-related diseases has grown enormously [2]. The use of MSCs to treat steroid-refractory acute Graft Versus Host Disease (aGVHD) represents one of the many explored applications of MSC-based therapy. Nevertheless, despite the promising potential of MSCs, there is a consensus that the clinical response to this therapeutic modality is not homogenous [3–5]. Therefore, in order to enhance the immunomodulatory function of MSCs and achieve more consistent results, several strategies have been sought. Among them, the activation and licensing of MSCs [6] with inflammatory cytokines such as INF-γ [7,8] and Toll-like receptor (TLR) agonists [9,10] has been heavily investigated.

In addition to the search for MSCs licensing strategies, another strategy that has also been subject of intensive discussion is the possibility of establishing cell-free therapies, in which the effects of MSCs are guaranteed without the need for cellular infusion. Emerging data suggest that MSCs-mediated effects appear to be partly dependent on paracrine factors, such as proteins and hormones, as well as on the transference of extracellular vesicles (EVs) to target cells [11,12]. In this scenario, several researchers are investigating the effects of MSCs-derived secretome and -EVs in various contexts, in which their parental cells effectively revealed their therapeutic potential. However, information concerning the influence of MSCs licensing over the immunosuppressive potential of their secretome and derived EVs is still scarce in the literature.

With this in mind, in the present work we evaluated whether human adipose MSCs (AMSCs) licensing with INF-γ alone or in combination with Poly (I:C) (a TLR3 agonist) influenced their phenotype, proliferation, migration capacity and immunosuppressive potential. Furthermore, we collected the conditioned medium from licensed and unlicensed AMSCs and investigated their immunosuppressive capacity. Finally, we isolated, characterized and analyzed the immunomodulatory potential of licensed and unlicensed AMSCs-derived EVs.

2. Materials and Methods

2.1. AMSCs Obtention, Culture and Characterization

AMSCs (n = 3) were kindly obtained from Cellseq Solutions, as control cell batches. Each lot of these cells was obtained from a single, healthy donor after lipoaspiration procedure. The cells were cultured in Minimum Essential Medium alpha (alpha-MEM) supplemented with 15% v.v. fetal bovine serum (FBS—HyClone, Logan, UT, USA), 2 mM glutamine and 100 U/mL penicillin/streptomycin (Sigma, St. Louis, MO, USA), at 37 °C and 5% CO_2. Medium was changed every two days and the cells were split when they reached 80–90% confluence.

AMSCs were phenotypically characterized at 3rd passage by flow cytometry (FACSVerse, BD Biosciences), using the BD Stemflow™ hMSC Analysis Kit, following manufacturer's instructions (Pharmingen, BD Biosciences, Franklin Lakes, NJ, USA). Briefly, control and licensed AMSCs were incubated with CD105-PerCP-Cy5.5, CD73-APC, CD90-FITC, CD44-PE and with the negative cocktail markers, which included CD45/CD34/CD11b/CD19/HLA-DR antibodies, all conjugated with PE.

The cells were used between the 3rd to 6th passages for all experiments. This study was conducted with the approval of the Institutional Ethics Committee of the Faculty of Health Sciences of the University of Brasilia (35640514.5.0000.0030) and written informed consent was obtained from all participants.

2.2. AMSCs Licensing

For all performed experiments, we included a control group of untreated AMSCs. Licensing was performed following three different treatment strategies, which included 48h incubation of AMSCs with (i) 50 ng/mL of INF-γ; (ii) 1 μg/mL of Poly (I:C); or 50 ng/mL of INF-γ and 1 μg/mL of Poly (I:C) [13,14]. After treatment, cells were washed with PBS for three times before the beginning of the experiments.

2.3. AMSCs Viability and Proliferation

The effect of AMSCs licensing over cellular growth (proliferation and/or viability) was assessed by MTT [3-(4.5-dimethylthiazol-2-yl)-2,5-diphenyl tetrazolium bromide] assay, as previously described [15]. Briefly, cells were plated at 2×10^3 in 96-well plates and submitted to the different licensing protocols, as described above. Then, cells were washed 3 times with PBS and received basal medium. Cell viability assay was performed at days 1, 3 and 5, counted from the end of the licensing procedure. In these time-points, 20 µL of MTT (5 mg/mL) was added in each well and the plates incubated for 3 h. After this period, MTT and medium were removed and replaced by DMSO and the plate was homogenized for 15 min. The optical density was read on a DTX 800 Series Multimode Detector (Beckman Coulter, Brea, CA, USA) at 570 nm.

2.4. AMSCs Migration

AMSCs migration was investigated following the licensing procedure, by wound scratch assay [16]. To this end, 2×10^5 AMSCs were seeded in 6 well plates and licensed for 48 h, under the different licensing conditions. Next, AMSCs monolayers were washed with PBS and then scratched across the center of the well using a 200 µL pipette tip. AMSCs were maintained in alpha-MEM without FBS or in alpha-MEM containing 2% FBS, as a positive control. The scratch zones were photographed at 0, 12 and 24 h post-scratch using a Zeiss Primo Vert microscope equipped with a digital camera (Carl Zeiss, Heidelberg, Germany). The open area post-scratch was measured using the software ImageJ (National Institutes of Health, Bethesda, MD, USA).

2.5. Isolation and Activation of Peripheral Blood Mononuclear Cells (PBMCs)

Peripheral Blood Mononuclear Cells (PBMCs) were obtained from healthy volunteers by centrifugation using Ficoll-Paque PLUS (Amersham Biosciences, Uppsala, Sweden). After isolation, PBMCs were activated with 5 µg/mL of Phytohaemagglutinin (PHA, Sigma-Aldrich, St. Louis, MO, USA) and stained with 2.5 µM carboxyfluorescein succinimidyl ester (CFSE), as previously described [17–19]. T-cell proliferation was analyzed by Flow Cytometry (BD Biosciences, San Jose, CA, USA) after culturing PBMCs for 5 days with either AMSCs, AMSCs-conditioned medium or EVs isolated from unlicensed and licensed AMSCs, as detailed below.

2.6. AMSCs Co-Culture with PBMCs

The immunosuppressive effect of licensed and unlicensed AMSCs was determined by flow cytometry. Following AMSCs licensing, the medium was removed, cells were washed 3 times with PBS and immediately co-cultured with 3×10^5 PHA-activated PBMCs (1:10 ratio) for 5 days [17,18]. Then, PBMCs were recovered and stained with APC-conjugated anti-CD3 antibody and assessed for T-cell proliferation.

2.7. PBMCs Culture with AMSCs-Derived Conditioned Medium

To analyze the effects of the medium obtained from the different strategies of AMSCs licensing over T-cell proliferation, we removed the supernatants after the AMSCs licensing protocols and added fresh RPMI medium supplemented with 10% FBS to AMSCs cultures. After 24 h, the medium was collected, centrifuged and used to culture 3×10^5 PBMCs activated with 5 µg/mL PHA [19]. In the 5th day of culture, PBMCs were collected, stained with anti-CD3 and T-cell proliferation determined by Flow Cytometry.

2.8. Vascular Cell Adhesion Protein 1 (VCAM-1) and Intercellular Adhesion Molecule 1 (ICAM-1) Expression on AMSCs

Considering the importance of the adhesion molecules in MSCs-mediated immunosuppression, we investigated the expression of ICAM-1 (CD54) and VCAM-1 (CD106) in licensed and unlicensed

AMSCs, using monoclonal antibodies. Briefly, after licensing, cells were washed with PBS, harvested and stained with anti-CD54 (conjugated with allophycocyanin—APC), anti-CD106 (conjugated with fluorescein isothiocyanate—FITC) or isotype controls (eBioscience, San Diego, CA, USA). After incubation with the antibodies, the cells were analyzed by Flow Cytometry.

2.9. EVs Isolation and Characterization

After observing that the most suppressive conditioned medium was obtained from INF-γ licensed AMSCs, we isolated EVs from this group, as well as from unlicensed AMSCs, in order to assess their capacity of controlling activated T-cell proliferation. Briefly, AMSCs were cultured until confluence in 75 cm^5 flasks containing 10 mL basal medium supplemented with 10% v.v. of microvesicles-free FBS. When AMSCs reached confluence they were licensed for 24 h, the supernatant was collected and, EV isolation was immediately performed using total exosome isolation reagent (Invitrogen, Life Technologies, Carlsbad, CA, USA), as described by the manufacturer. Cell culture medium was centrifuged at 2000 g for 30 min to remove cellular debris, mixed with 5 mL of total exosome isolation reagent and incubated at 4 °C overnight. After incubation, samples were centrifuged at 10,000× g for 1 h and the pellets containing EVs were resuspended in PBS. Protein concentration was determined by Bradford method [20].

EVs were initially characterized according to average diameter using Zetasizer Nano ZS (Malvern Instruments, Malvern, UK), following to manufacturer's instructions. EVs diameter was also determined by transmission electron microscopy (TEM). For this, 5 µL of EVs samples were mounted on formvar copper grids and fixed in Karnovsky EM fixative solution (2% formaldehyde and 2.5% glutaraldehyde in 0.1 mol/L sodium cacodylate buffer, pH 7.4). Samples were then negatively stained using 2% aqueous phosphotungstic acid (PTA), examined and photographed with a JEOL JEM1011 transmission electron microscope operating at 80 kV.

EVs were also phenotypically characterized by flow cytometry using CD105-PerCP-Cy5.5 and CD90- FITC antibodies. For this, EVs were coupled with 4-µm-diameter aldehyde/sulfate latex beads and then blocked by incubation with FBS. EVs-coated beads were washed three times in PBS and resuspended in 50 µL of PBS. Next, beads were incubated with the aforementioned antibodies and analyzed by Flow Cytometry.

2.10. Immunosuppressive Effects of AMSCs-Derived EVs

To access the immunosuppressive potential of AMSCs-derived EVs, 3×10^5 PBMCs were activated with 5 µg/mL of PHA and cultured for 5 days with 0.25, 0.75 or 3.0 µg of EVs isolated from both unlicensed and INF-γ licensed AMSCs [21]. After this period, PBMCs were collected, stained with anti-CD3 and T-cell proliferation was determined by Flow Cytometry.

2.11. RNA Isolation and Real-Time PCR

Gene expression analysis was performed in unlicensed and licensed AMSCs, as well as their EVs. RNA samples were obtained using Trizol reagent. RNA amount and quality were determined by NanoDrop 1000 spectrophotometer (Wilmington, DE, USA). One microgram of RNA was converted to single-stranded cDNA, using the High Capacity Kit (Applied BioSystems, Foster City, CA, USA) according to manufacturer's recommendations. Real-time PCR was performed using TaqMan probes and MasterMix (Applied BioSystems, Foster City, CA, USA), following manufacturer's instructions.

Real time PCR for TNF (Hs01113624), TGF-β (Hs00998133), IDO (Hs00984148), Galectin-1 (Hs00355202), IL-1β (Hs00174097) and IL-10 (Hs00961622) was run in duplicates and the relative fold change obtained by the $2^{-\Delta\Delta Ct}$ method [22]. GAPDH was used as internal reference. The median Ct values of unlicensed AMSCs and their EVs were used as reference. Cycling parameters were 95 °C for 10 min followed by 40 cycles of 95 °C for 15 s and 60 °C for 1 min.

2.12. Statistical Analysis

The results are presented as mean ± SEM of three independent experiments. Statistical analyses were performed using Prism 7 software (GraphPad Software Inc., San Diego, CA, USA). Statistical significance was calculated using *t*-test analyses, considering $p < 0.05$.

3. Results

3.1. INF-γ and/or Poly (I:C) Licensing Maintain AMSCs Phenotype

AMSCs had a typical MSCs immunophenotype, with positive expression of CD44, CD73, CD90 and CD105 markers and negative expression of CD34, CD45, CD11b, CD19 and HLA-DR. We also investigated if the licensing treatments with INF-γ and/or Poly (I:C) would alter AMCSs immunophenotype, however, the phenotypic pattern was maintained in all samples, regardless of the licensing strategy adopted (Supplementary Figure S1).

3.2. INF-γ and/or Poly (I:C) Licensing did not Influence AMSCs Proliferation

Considering that MSCs immunosuppressive effects are dose-dependent, we evaluated if INF-γ and/or Poly (I:C) licensing could modulate AMSCs proliferation. Obtained results revealed that none of the licensing strategies tested modified AMSCs proliferation (Figure 1).

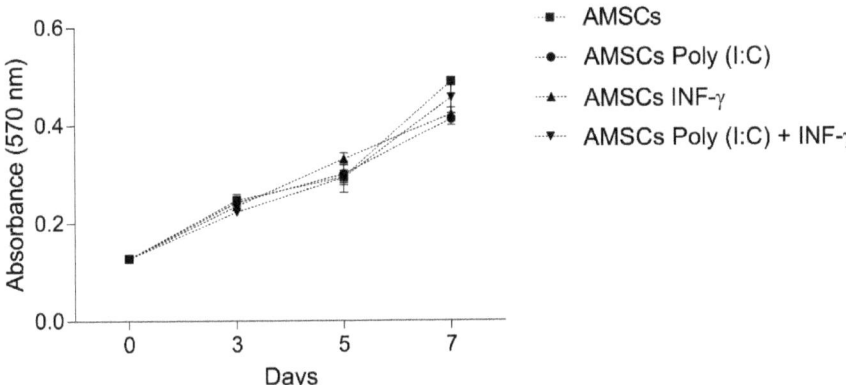

Figure 1. Proliferative capacity of licensed and unlicensed AMSCs. Control AMSCs, AMSCs licensed with 1 μg/mL of Poly (I:C), AMSCs licensed with 50 ng/mL of INF-γ; and AMSCs licensed with 50 ng/mL of INF-γ and 1 μg/mL of Poly (I:C) were cultured and cell proliferation was assessed by MTT in the days 3, 5 and 7 of the culture. No difference of proliferation/viability was observed among the groups. Values represent the means ± SEM. Three independent experiments were performed.

3.3. INF-γ and/or Poly (I:C) Licensing Did not Alter AMSCs Migration

Control and licensed AMSCs were investigated regarding their migration potential by wound scratch assay, but, once again, we observed that the licensing regimes did not affect the migratory behavior of AMSCs after 12 h and 24 h (Figure 2).

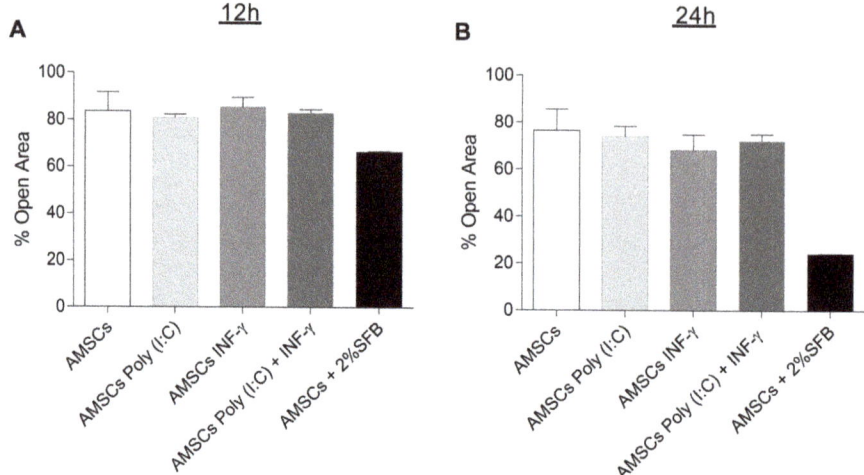

Figure 2. Migratory potential of licensed and unlicensed AMSCs. (**A**) Wound scratch assays for unlicensed AMSCs, as well as licensed AMSCs treated with either 1 µg/mL Poly (I:C), 50 ng/mL INF-γ or with both 50 ng/mL of INF-γ and 1 µg/mL of Poly (I:C). Confluent cells were wounded by a scratch with a pipette tip and cell migration was assessed under the microscope at 12 h and 24 h (**B**). Results are presented as mean ± SEM of three independent experiments.

3.4. INF-γ Enhances AMSCs-Mediated Immunomodulation

Consistent with published literature [23], our data revealed that AMSCs co-culture markedly decreased activated T-cell proliferation ($p = 0.0003$). Wondering whether licensed AMSCs presented different immunosuppression effect compared to unlicensed cells, we performed the same co-culture assay with licensed AMSCs. Interestingly, INF-γ licensed AMSCs presented significantly higher capacity to inhibit activated T-cell proliferation ($p = 0.003$). On the other hand, licensing with Poly (I:C) alone did not influence AMSCs-mediated immunosuppression capacity. Even though we did not detect a statistically significant difference, the licensing of AMSCs with both Poly (I:C) and INF-γ increased their suppressive potential in 35% (mean), compared to unlicensed AMSCs (Figure 3A,B).

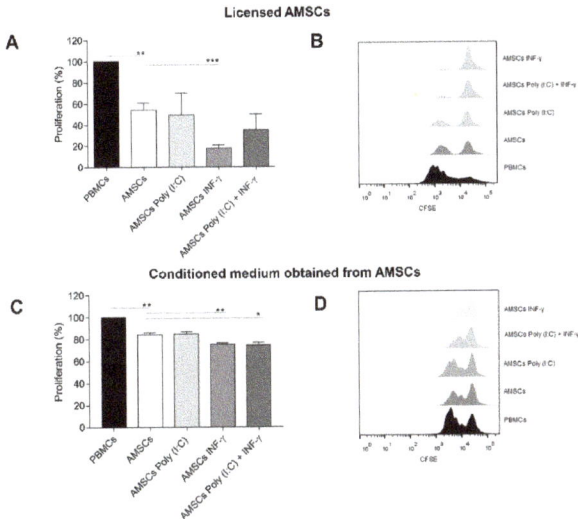

Figure 3. Immunosuppressive capacity of licensed AMSCs and their conditioned medium. (**A**) unlicensed AMSCs, as well as AMSCs licensed with either 1 µg/mL of Poly (I:C), 50 ng/mL of INF-γ or with both 50 ng/mL of INF-γ and 1 µg/mL of Poly (I:C) were cocultured with PHA-activated PBMCs (1:10 ratio) and T-cell proliferation was determined by Flow Cytometry after 5 days. Results are presented as mean ± SEM of three independent experiments; (**B**) Representative CFSE histograms of one AMSCs sample investigated; (**C**) After AMSCs licensing, medium were discarded, cells were washed 3 times with PBS and fresh medium was added to each condition. After 24 h, the AMSCs conditioned medium (from licensed and unlicensed samples) were harvested and used to culture PHA-activated PBMCs, so that T-cell proliferation could be analyzed after 5 days of treatment. Results are presented as mean ± SEM of three independent experiments; (**D**) Representative CFSE histograms from conditioned medium from one AMSCs sample investigated. * $p < 0.05$. ** $p < 0.01$. *** $p < 0.001$.

3.5. Conditioned Medium from INF-γ Licensed AMSCs Has Increased Capacity to Control the T-Cell Response

Aiming to further investigate the possible use of the AMSCs secretome in a cell free perspective, we isolated the conditioned medium of licensed and unlicensed AMSCs and investigated their immunosuppressive potential. We observed that the conditioned medium obtained from unlicensed AMSCs suppress T-cell proliferation ($p = 0.004$). The conditioned medium derived from AMSCs licensed with Poly (I:C) and INF-γ presented a slightly increased capacity to suppress T-cell proliferation ($p = 0.01$) compared to conditioned medium obtained from unlicensed AMSCs ($p = 0.01$). Importantly, the conditioned medium isolated from INF-γ licensed AMSCs showed the highest capacity to inhibit activated T-cell proliferation ($p = 0.005$) among tested groups (Figure 3C,D).

3.6. INF-γ Enhances ICAM-1 Expression on AMSCs

Considering the importance of adhesion molecules in the context of contact-dependent MSCs-immunosuppression, we investigated the expression of VCAM-1 and ICAM-1 on licensed and unlicensed AMSCs. Flow cytometry data of unlicensed AMSCs presented a mean expression of VCAM-1 and ICAM-1 of 14.38 and 54%, respectively (Figure 4A,C). While none of the licensing strategies altered the expression of VCAM-1 on AMSCs (Figure 4A,B), ICAM-1 expression was increased in INF-γ licensed AMSCs ($p = 0.01$), as well as in INF-γ and Poly (I:C) licensed cells ($p = 0.03$) (Figure 4C,D). Interestingly, when we licensed AMSCs using 25, 50 and 100 ng/mL of INF-γ, we noticed that the effect of this inflammatory factor over the AMSCs expression of ICAM-1 is increased

($p < 0.01$) between lower (25 ng/mL; mean value 95.4%) and higher concentrations (50/100 ng/mL; mean values 98.3/98.2%) (Figure 4E).

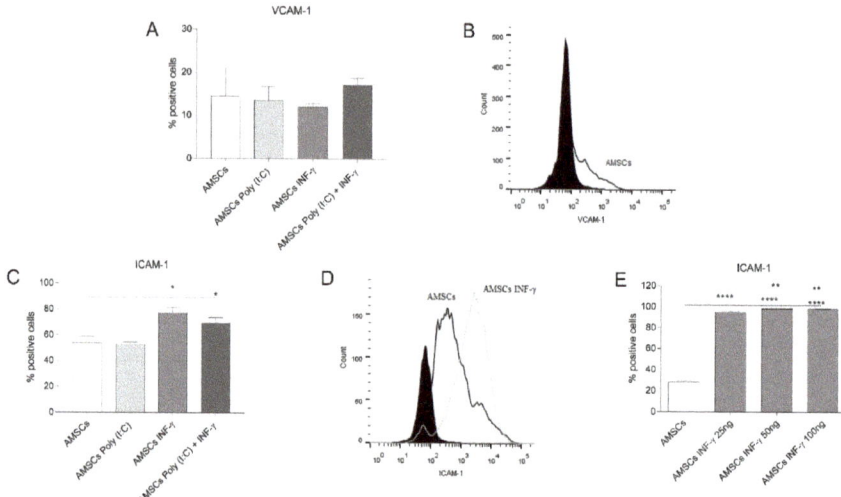

Figure 4. VCAM-1 and ICAM-1 expression of licensed and unlicensed AMSCs. (**A**) unlicensed AMSCs, as well as AMSCs licensed with either 1 µg/mL of Poly (I:C), 50 ng/mL of INF-γ or with both 50 ng/mL of INF-γ and 1 µg/mL of Poly (I:C), were used to assess VCAM-1 expression by Flow Cytometry. Results are presented as mean ± SEM of three independent experiments; (**B**) Representative histogram showing VCAM-1 expression of one sample of unlicensed AMSCs;. (**C**) unlicensed AMSCs, as well as AMSCs licensed with either 1 µg/mL of Poly (I:C), 50 ng/mL of INF-γ or with both 50 ng/mL of INF-γ and 1 µg/mL of Poly (I:C) were also used to investigate ICAM-1 expression by Flow Cytometry. Results are presented as mean ± SEM of three independent experiments; (**D**) The influence of INF-γ over ICAM-1 expression on AMSCs was confirmed using three different concentrations of this inflammatory factor. (**E**) ICAM-1 expression on unlicensed AMSCs and AMSCs licensed with 25, 50 and 100 ng/mL of INF-γ. * $p < 0.05$, ** $p < 0.01$, **** $p < 0.0001$.

3.7. EVs Characterization

EVs isolated from unlicensed AMSCs showed the mean size of 262.4 nm, as determined by Zetasizer Nano ZS measurement (Figure 5A) and TEM (Figure 5B). INF-γ licensed AMSCs did not present significant differences regarding average size, which was 264.2 nm (data not shown). EVs characterization was also performed by Flow Cytometry, being that the isolated EVs were immunophenotypically characterized and showed positive expression of MSCs markers CD90 (76.5%) and CD105 (60.7%) (Figure 5C,D).

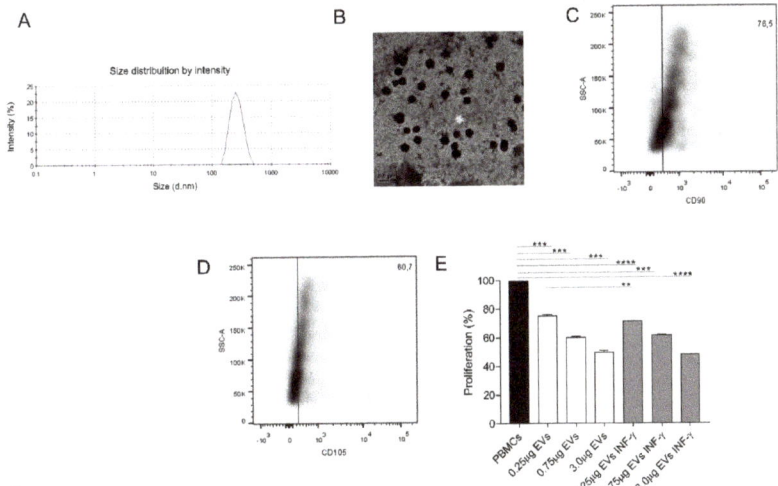

Figure 5. Characterization of EVs isolated from unlicensed and INF-γ licensed AMSCs and their capacity to control T-cell proliferation. (**A**) EVs average size estimated using Zetasizer Nano ZS; (**B**) Transmission electron microscopy of EVs (representative image of one unlicensed sample); CD90 (**C**) and CD105 (**D**) expression of EVs isolated from unlicensed AMSCs were determined by Flow Cytometry; (**E**) EVs isolated from unlicensed and INF-γ licensed AMSCs were quantified according to their protein concentration by Bradford assay and used in different concentrations (0.25, 0.75 and 3.0 µg) to treat PHA-activated PBMCs, in order to access their immunosuppressive capacity. Results are presented as mean ± SEM of three independent experiments. ** $p < 0.01$, *** $p < 0.001$ **** $p < 0.0001$.

3.8. AMSCs-Derived EVs Present Immunosuppressive Potential

After characterization, we evaluated if EVs derived from unlicensed and INF-γ licensed AMSCs presented immunoregulatory potential of inhibiting activated PBMCs proliferation. Notably, PBMCs incubation with 0.25, 0.75 and 3.0 µg of unlicensed AMSCs-derived EVs successfully suppressed activated T-cell proliferation ($p = 0.0005$; $p = 0.0002$ and $p < 0.0003$, respectively). Likewise, PBMCs incubation with 0.25, 0.75 and 3.0 µg of INF-γ licensed AMSCs also suppressed T-cell proliferation ($p < 0.0001$; $p = 0.0002$ and $p < 0.0001$, respectively). Importantly, even though both groups effectively promoted immunosuppression at all concentrations tested, when used at 0.25 µg, we detected a slight increase in the suppressive potential of EVs isolated from INF-γ licensed AMSCs compared to EVs from unlicensed AMSCs ($p = 0.004$) (Figure 5E).

3.9. Expression of Inflammatory Transcripts in Licensed and Unlicensed AMSCs and in Their EVs

Gene expression of TNF, TGF-β, IDO, Galectin-1, IL-1β and IL-10 was assessed in licensed and unlicensed AMSCs by Real Time PCR. Compared to unlicensed AMSCs, INF-γ treatment increased the expression of TNF ($p = 0.002$), IL-1β ($p = 0.001$) and IDO ($p < 0.0001$), the latter with more intensity. Interestingly, this licensing protocol abrogated IL-10 transcription. AMSCs licensing with Poly (I:C) induced a higher expression of TNF ($p = 0.04$), IL-1β ($p = 0.008$) and IDO ($p = 0.001$), as well. Interestingly, AMSCs licensing with both Poly (I:C) and INF-γ induced the most intense transcriptional differences compared to unlicensed AMSCs, leading to the highest expression of TNF ($p = 0.0003$), IL-1β ($p = 0.0003$) and IDO ($p = 0.001$). Of note, none of the tested strategies of AMSCs licensing influenced Galectin-1 and TGF-β expression (Figure 6A). We also assessed the transcriptional levels of TGF-β, IDO, Galectin-1 and IL-10 in EVs isolated from unlicensed and INF-γ licensed AMSCs. Interestingly, EVs from INF-γ licensed AMSCs showed decreased expression of Galectin-1 transcript ($p = 0.0002$). However, IDO was detected only in EVs isolated from INF-γ licensed AMSCs ($p = 0.0001$).

No statistically significant difference was detected regarding TGF-β expression between groups (Figure 6B). IL-10 expression was not detected in the analyzed EV transcripts.

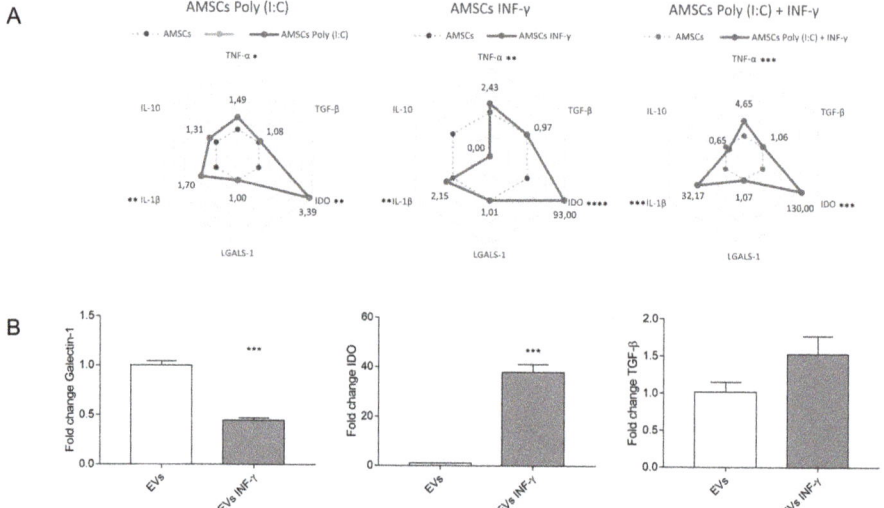

Figure 6. Gene expression analysis of selected transcripts in unlicensed and licensed AMSCs. (A) Radial plot demonstrating the differences in overall transcripts between unlicensed AMSCs, as well as AMSCs licensed with 1 μg/mL of Poly (I:C), AMSCs licensed with 50 ng/mL INF-γ and AMSCs licensed with both 50 ng/mL of INF-γ and 1 μg/mL of Poly (I:C). Solid vertices represent the mean fold change of individual transcripts. Median Ct value of unlicensed AMSCs was used as a reference. Results are presented as the mean of three independent experiments; (B) Expression of Galectin-1, IDO, IL-10 and TGF-β transcripts in EVs isolated from unlicensed and INF-γ licensed AMSCs. To analyze IDO expression in EVs, the CT value of EVs obtained from unlicensed AMSCs was arbitrarily defined as 40. *** $p < 0.001$.

4. Discussion

In the present study, we have demonstrated that the licensing of AMSCs with INF-γ and/or Poly (I:C) maintain the classic AMSCs phenotypic pattern and does not significantly alter AMSCs proliferative capacity and migratory behavior. Importantly, though, our data reveal that INF-γ licensing markedly induces AMSCs to produce higher levels of IDO, increased the expression of ICAM-1 adhesion molecule and potentializes the capacity of licensed cells to suppress activated T-cell proliferation, compared to unlicensed counterparts. On the other hand, we have also clearly demonstrated that under a perspective of a cell free therapy, the strategy of licensing of AMSCs with INF-γ was effective in promoting immunoregulatory advantages when compared to unlicensed cell samples. Finally, our data reveal that AMSCs present a constitutive potential to inhibit activated T-cell proliferation and to secrete biologically active EVs, which harbor the capacity of effectively controlling T-cell response.

Several processes contribute for MSCs immunoregulatory potential. For instance, to exert their immunoregulatory effects with the greatest potential, MSCs must survive and reach sites of injury. However, it is currently established that only a small number of infused cells can achieve this goal, following stem cell therapy. Therefore, the search for strategies capable of enhancing the suppressive capacity of MSCs is paramount to guarantee the efficacy and commercial viability of such therapy [24,25]. In this sense, among the several strategies under investigation to boost MSC therapy efficacy, lie the licensing protocols. According to this rationale, it may be possible to stimulate

MSCs to boost their pro-survival and immunomodulation properties, by treating them with specific molecules prior to treatment. Several licensing strategies have been tested so far, such as the treatment of MSCs with INF-γ and Poly (I:C). According to previous reports, INF-γ signaling did not improve the migratory capacity of bone marrow and cord blood-derived MSCs [26]. Accordingly, we have not found any effect of INF-γ regarding the migratory capacity of AMSCs. Considering the role of TLR signaling in MSCs migration, it has been showed that Poly (I:C) stimulation enhanced the migratory capacity of MSCs derived from bone marrow [27]. In contrast to previous reports, we have not noticed any impact of TLR3 signaling over AMSCs migratory behavior. In part, these discrepant results can be explained by the fact that MSCs present different migratory capacity depending on their source of obtention, as described recently [28] and probably also differ in the response to variable stimuli. This hypothesis may be subsidized by the observation that circulating MSCs are derived from bone marrow [29,30], suggesting that MSCs from other tissues may not respond to the same migration stimuli similarly.

The development of strategies to enhance MSCs proliferation has particular relevance considering that their immunomodulatory effects are dose-dependent [31]. In this context, data concerning the influence of TLR3 and INF-γ signaling on human AMSCs proliferation are markedly scarce in the literature. Our results showed that the licensing of these cells with TLR3 and/or INF-γ did not change AMSCs proliferation. In agreement with our observation, others also failed to detect any influence of TLR3 signaling in AMSCs proliferative capacity [32,33]. Long term stimulation with INF-γ, on the other hand, has been documented to reduce the proliferation of bone marrow derived MSCs [34]. More recently, it has been demonstrated that 5 days stimulation of bone marrow-derived MSCs with low a concentration of INF-γ (i.e., 0.1 ng/mL), actually increased cell proliferation but also that, when stimulated with higher levels of INF-γ (i.e., 10 ng/mL), cell proliferation was markedly compromised. In this conflicting scenario, it is important to note that, in contrast to our experimental design, MSCs were continuously maintained in the presence of INF-γ in the studies mentioned above [35].

Since the demonstration that murine MSCs licensing with INF-γ could completely prevent GVHD mortality [36], several efforts have been made to better understand the effects of this inflammatory factor over MSCs-mediated immunomodulation. Here, we have shown that AMSCs licensing with INF-γ was indeed an effective strategy to enhance AMSCs' capacity to control activated T-cell proliferation. Interestingly, this licensing protocol increased the expression of ICAM-1 protein expression and of IDO transcript levels in AMSCs, both of which have important roles in the immunomodulation exerted by these cells [37,38].

Another important strategy that has been explored to enhance MSCs-mediated immunomodulation is the stimulation of such cells with TLR3 agonists. In this sense, the results presented in the literature indicate that the positive effects of this strategy seem to be inconsistent and dependent on the MSCs source under investigation. While TLR3 signaling improves the immunosuppressive effects of MSCs isolated from the umbilical cord [39] and bone marrow [40], we have not noticed any influence on AMSCs. Accordingly, Lombardo and colleagues reported that TLR3 signaling in AMSCs did not influence their immunoregulatory phenotype [33]. In our hands, we have also explored the effects of AMSCs licensing with a combination of INF-γ and Poly (I:C). Surprisingly, though, we have observed only a slight reduction in lymphocyte PHA-induced proliferation. Besides, even though the combined INF-γ and Poly (I:C) licensing strategy significantly enhanced ICAM-1 and IDO expression, it also promoted a substantial increase in TNF and IL-1b transcript levels, two critical proinflammatory factors [41,42]. We noticed that AMSCs licensing with INF-γ abrogated IL-10 transcription, in contrast to the licensing with Poly (I:C), where IL-10 transcription was stimulated. Importantly, IL-10, as well as PGE2, TGF-β, IGF and HLA-G5, play an important role to generate Tregs, which enhance MSCs-mediated immunosuppression [43–46].

Importantly, the conditioned medium from unlicensed AMSCs showed capacity to control T-cell proliferation. In accordance with this data, Matula and colleagues also showed that conditioned medium from unlicensed AMSCs has immunosuppressive potential [47]. More importantly, we demonstrated that this immunomodulatory potential can be enhanced by INF-γ licensing. Given that AMSCs licensing with INF-γ was able to potentialize the intrinsic capacity of AMSCs conditioned medium to control activated T-cell proliferation, we continued our investigation with the isolation of EVs from this group and from unlicensed AMSCs, considering that the analysis of such EVs could provide new insights to the field of cell free technologies. In fact, the conditioned medium and the EVs isolated from MSCs are currently being explored for the most varied applications and already showed promising effects in animal models of acute myocardial infarct, as well as lung, kidney and brain injuries [48]. Interestingly, isolated EVs showed positive expression of MSCs markers and an average size compatible with previous results reported by Blazquez et al. [21]. These authors also demonstrated that EVs derived from AMSCs are able to control T-cell proliferation. In addition, we showed that both EVs isolated from unlicensed and INF-γ licensed AMSCs showed potential to significantly suppress activated T-cell proliferation and that in lower EVs concentrations, INF-γ licensed group presented a greater immunoregulatory effect. A previous work failed to detect any differences regarding the immunosuppressive potential of EVs derived from unlicensed and INF-γ licensed MSCs [49]. However, it is important to point that, despite being performed with murine bone marrow MSCs, the licensing strategy used in this study was performed with lower concentrations of INF-γ. In order to investigate molecular mechanisms that could be involved in the immunosuppressive effects observed, we investigated the presence of anti-inflammatory factors in EVs from unlicensed and INF-γ licensed AMSCs. Importantly, we demonstrated that these EVs carry transcripts of anti-inflammatory genes, involved in MSCs mediated immunoregulation, such as galectin-1 [50] and TGF-B [44]. IDO transcripts were detected only in EVs derived from INF-γ licensed AMSCs, however, we did not observe any striking immunosuppressive advantage in this group, suggesting that other anti-inflammatory players may have more significant roles in the immunosuppressive potential of AMSCs-derived EVs. The demonstration that both AMSCs conditioned medium and derived EVs are immunologically active has particular relevance, especially when taking into consideration the significant advantages of cell-free components compared to their cellular counterparts. For instance, cell-free material obtention, handling and production yields are more attractive compared to cell products, as well as the elimination of the risks associated to cellular infusion.

5. Conclusions

In summary, in the present work, we sought to comprehensively investigate the immunosuppressive potential of AMSCs under different licensing strategies, considering their direct use, as well as their conditioned medium and derived EVs. Our results clearly show that the licensing of AMSCs with INF-γ increases their immunoregulatory potential, which is accompanied by an increase in the expression of IDO and ICAM. Additionally, we have shown that conditioned medium obtained from INF-γ licensed AMSCs display a higher capacity to control T-cell proliferation compared to conditioned medium from unlicensed counterparts. Finally, our data clearly demonstrated that both EVs isolated from unlicensed and INF-γ licensed AMSCs are also capable to control the T-cell proliferation. These results contribute to the better elucidation of the suppressive potential of AMSCs and their products, serving as the basis for the development of new therapeutic approaches to control the immune response.

Supplementary Materials: The following is available online. Figure S1: Immunophenotypic characterization of AMSCs.

Author Contributions: Conceptualization, F.d.A.R.N., R.W.P., J.L.d.C. and F.S.-A.; Data curation, T.R.T.S. and A.É.S.-C.; Formal analysis, T.R.T.S., A.É.S.-C., J.L.d.C and F.S.-A.; Investigation, T.R.T.S., A.É.S.-C., L.D.d.C.F.B. and F.S.-A.; Methodology, T.R.T.S., A.É.S.-C. and L.D.d.C.F.B.; Supervision, F.d.A.R.N., R.W.P., J.L.d.C. and F.S.-A.; Validation, T.R.T.S. and A.É.S.-C.; Writing-original draft, J.L.d.C. and F.S.-A.; Writing—review & editing, F.d.A.R.N., R.W.P., J.L.d.C. and F.S.-A.

Funding: This study was supported by Conselho Nacional de Desenvolvimento Científico e Tecnológico (CNPq) and Fundação de Amparo à Pesquisa do Distrito Federal (FAPDF).

Acknowledgments: We would like to thank the technical support of the Laboratory of Microscopy and Microanalysis of the Institute of Biological Sciences of the University of Brasília.

Conflicts of Interest: The authors declare that they have no conflict of interest.

References

1. Haddad, R.; Saldanha-Araujo, F. Mechanisms of T-cell immunosuppression by mesenchymal stromal cells: What do we know so far? *Biomed. Res. Int.* **2014**, *2014*, 216806. [CrossRef] [PubMed]
2. Sharma, R.R.; Pollock, K.; Hubel, A.; McKenna, D. Mesenchymal stem or stromal cells: A review of clinical applications and manufacturing practices. *Transfusion* **2014**, *54*, 1418–1437. [CrossRef] [PubMed]
3. Munneke, J.M.; Spruit, M.J.A.; Cornelissen, A.S.; van Hoeven, V.; Voermans, C.; Hazenberg, M.D. The potential of mesenchymal stromal cells as treatment for severe steroid-refractory acute graft-versus-host disease: A critical review of the literature. *Transplantation* **2016**, *100*, 2309–2314. [CrossRef] [PubMed]
4. Rizk, M.; Monaghan, M.; Shorr, R.; Kekre, N.; Bredeson, C.N.; Allan, D.S. Heterogeneity in studies of mesenchymal stromal cells to treat or prevent graft-versus-host disease: A scoping review of the evidence. *Biol. Blood Marrow Transplant.* **2016**, *22*, 1416–1423. [CrossRef] [PubMed]
5. Gao, F.; Chiu, S.M.; Motan, D.A.L.; Zhang, Z.; Chen, L.; Ji, H.-L.; Tse, H.-F.; Fu, Q.-L.; Lian, Q. Mesenchymal stem cells and immunomodulation: Current status and future prospects. *Cell Death Dis.* **2016**, *7*, e2062. [CrossRef] [PubMed]
6. Najar, M.; Krayem, M.; Merimi, M.; Burny, A.; Meuleman, N.; Bron, D.; Raicevic, G.; Lagneaux, L. Insights into inflammatory priming of mesenchymal stromal cells: Functional biological impacts. *Inflamm. Res.* **2018**, *67*, 467–477. [CrossRef] [PubMed]
7. Chinnadurai, R.; Copland, I.B.; Patel, S.R.; Galipeau, J. IDO-Independent Suppression of T Cell Effector Function by IFN--Licensed Human Mesenchymal Stromal Cells. *J. Immunol.* **2014**, *192*, 1491–1501. [CrossRef]
8. Liang, C.; Jiang, E.; Yao, J.; Wang, M.; Chen, S.; Zhou, Z.; Zhai, W.; Ma, Q.; Feng, S.; Han, M. Interferon-γ mediates the immunosuppression of bone marrow mesenchymal stem cells on T-lymphocytes in vitro. *Hematology* **2018**, *23*, 44–49. [CrossRef]
9. Sangiorgi, B.; Panepucci, R.A. Modulation of immunoregulatory properties of mesenchymal stromal cells by Toll-like receptors: Potential applications on GVHD. *Stem Cells Int.* **2016**, *2016*, 9434250. [CrossRef]
10. Najar, M.; Krayem, M.; Meuleman, N.; Bron, D.; Lagneaux, L. Mesenchymal stromal cells and Toll-like receptor priming: A critical review. *Immune Netw.* **2017**, *17*, 89–102. [CrossRef]
11. Konala, V.B.R.; Mamidi, M.K.; Bhonde, R.; Das, A.K.; Pochampally, R.; Pal, R. The current landscape of the mesenchymal stromal cell secretome: A new paradigm for cell-free regeneration. *Cytotherapy* **2016**, *18*, 13–24. [CrossRef]
12. Fatima, F.; Ekstrom, K.; Nazarenko, I.; Maugeri, M.; Valadi, H.; Hill, A.F.; Camussi, G.; Nawaz, M. Non-coding RNAs in mesenchymal stem cell-derived extracellular vesicles: Deciphering regulatory roles in stem cell potency, inflammatory resolve and tissue regeneration. *Front. Genet.* **2017**, *8*. [CrossRef]
13. Klinker, M.W.; Marklein, R.A.; Lo Surdo, J.L.; Wei, C.-H.; Bauer, S.R. Morphological features of IFN-γ–stimulated mesenchymal stromal cells predict overall immunosuppressive capacity. *Proc. Natl. Acad. Sci. USA* **2017**, *114*, E2598–E2607. [CrossRef] [PubMed]
14. Sangiorgi, B.; De Freitas, H.T.; Schiavinato, J.L.D.S.; Leão, V.; Haddad, R.; Orellana, M.D.; Faça, V.M.; Ferreira, G.A.; Covas, D.T.; Zago, M.A.; et al. DSP30 enhances the immunosuppressive properties of mesenchymal stromal cells and protects their suppressive potential from lipopolysaccharide effects: A potential role of adenosine. *Cytotherapy* **2016**, *18*, 846–859. [CrossRef] [PubMed]
15. Oliveira-Bravo, M.; Sangiorgi, B.B.; Schiavinato, J.L.D.S.; Carvalho, J.L.; Covas, D.T.; Panepucci, R.A.; Neves, F.d.A.R.; Franco, O.L.; Pereira, R.W.; Saldanha-Araujo, F. LL-37 boosts immunosuppressive function of placenta-derived mesenchymal stromal cells. *Stem Cell Res. Ther.* **2016**, *7*. [CrossRef]
16. Liang, C.-C.; Park, A.Y.; Guan, J.-L. In vitro scratch assay: A convenient and inexpensive method for analysis of cell migration in vitro. *Nat. Protoc.* **2007**, *2*, 329–333. [CrossRef]
17. Saldanha-Araujo, F.; Ferreira, F.I.S.; Palma, P.V.; Araujo, A.G.; Queiroz, R.H.C.; Covas, D.T.; Zago, M.A.; Panepucci, R.A. Mesenchymal stromal cells up-regulate CD39 and increase adenosine production to suppress activated T-lymphocytes. *Stem Cell Res.* **2011**, *7*, 66–74. [CrossRef] [PubMed]

18. Saldanha-Araujo, F.; Haddad, R.; Farias, K.C.; Souza, A.P.; Palma, P.V.; Araujo, A.G.; Orellana, M.D.; Voltarelli, J.C.; Covas, D.T.; Zago, M.A.; et al. Mesenchymal stem cells promote the sustained expression of CD69 on activated T lymphocytes: Roles of canonical and non-canonical NF-κB signalling. *J. Cell. Mol. Med.* **2012**, *16*, 1232–1244. [CrossRef] [PubMed]
19. Vellasamy, S.; Tong, C.K.; Azhar, N.A.; Kodiappan, R.; Chan, S.C.; Veerakumarasivam, A.; Ramasamy, R. Human mesenchymal stromal cells modulate T-cell immune response via transcriptomic regulation. *Cytotherapy* **2016**, *18*, 1270–1283. [CrossRef]
20. Kruger, N.J. The Bradford method for protein quantitation. *Methods Mol. Biol.* **1994**, *32*, 9–15. [PubMed]
21. Blazquez, R.; Sanchez-Margallo, F.M.; de la Rosa, O.; Dalemans, W.; Alvarez, V.; Tarazona, R.; Casado, J.G. Immunomodulatory potential of human adipose mesenchymal stem cells derived exosomes on in vitro stimulated T cells. *Front. Immunol.* **2014**, *5*. [CrossRef] [PubMed]
22. Pfaffl, M.W. A new mathematical model for relative quantification in real-time RT-PCR. *Nucleic Acids Res.* **2001**, *29*, e45. [CrossRef] [PubMed]
23. Quaedackers, M.E.; Baan, C.C.; Weimar, W.; Hoogduijn, M.J. Cell contact interaction between adipose-derived stromal cells and allo-activated T lymphocytes. *Eur. J. Immunol.* **2009**, *39*, 3436–3446. [CrossRef] [PubMed]
24. De Becker, A.; Riet, I.V. Homing and migration of mesenchymal stromal cells: How to improve the efficacy of cell therapy? *World J. Stem Cells* **2016**, *8*, 73–87. [CrossRef] [PubMed]
25. Maijenburg, M.W.; van der Schoot, C.E.; Voermans, C. Mesenchymal stromal cell migration: Possibilities to improve cellular therapy. *Stem Cells Dev.* **2012**, *21*, 19–29. [CrossRef] [PubMed]
26. Hemeda, H.; Jakob, M.; Ludwig, A.-K.; Giebel, B.; Lang, S.; Brandau, S. Interferon-γ and tumor necrosis factor-α differentially affect cytokine expression and migration properties of mesenchymal stem cells. *Stem Cells Dev.* **2010**, *19*, 693–706. [CrossRef] [PubMed]
27. Tomchuck, S.L.; Zwezdaryk, K.J.; Coffelt, S.B.; Waterman, R.S.; Danka, E.S.; Scandurro, A.B. Toll-like receptors on human mesenchymal stem cells drive their migration and immunomodulating responses. *Stem Cells* **2008**, *26*, 99–107. [CrossRef] [PubMed]
28. Kim, J.; Shin, J.M.; Jeon, Y.J.; Chung, H.M.; Chae, J.-I. Proteomic validation of multifunctional molecules in mesenchymal stem cells derived from human bone marrow, umbilical cord blood and peripheral blood. *PLoS ONE* **2012**, *7*, e32350. [CrossRef]
29. He, Q.; Wan, C.; Li, G. Concise review: Multipotent mesenchymal stromal cells in blood. *Stem Cells* **2006**, *25*, 69–77. [CrossRef]
30. Xu, L.; Li, G. Circulating mesenchymal stem cells and their clinical implications. *J. Orthop. Transl.* **2014**, *2*, 1–7. [CrossRef]
31. Di Nicola, M. Human bone marrow stromal cells suppress T-lymphocyte proliferation induced by cellular or nonspecific mitogenic stimuli. *Blood* **2002**, *99*, 3838–3843. [CrossRef] [PubMed]
32. Cho, H.H.; Bae, Y.C.; Jung, J.S. Role of Toll-like receptors on human adipose-derived stromal cells. *Stem Cells* **2006**, *24*, 2744–2752. [CrossRef] [PubMed]
33. Lombardo, E.; DelaRosa, O.; Mancheño-Corvo, P.; Menta, R.; Ramírez, C.; Büscher, D. Toll-like receptor–mediated signaling in human adipose-derived stem cells: Implications for immunogenicity and immunosuppressive potential. *Tissue Eng. Part A* **2009**, *15*, 1579–1589. [CrossRef] [PubMed]
34. Croitoru-Lamoury, J.; Lamoury, F.M.J.; Caristo, M.; Suzuki, K.; Walker, D.; Takikawa, O.; Taylor, R.; Brew, B.J. Interferon-γ regulates the proliferation and differentiation of mesenchymal stem cells via activation of indoleamine 2,3 dioxygenase (IDO). *PLoS ONE* **2011**, *6*, e14698. [CrossRef] [PubMed]
35. Vigo, T.; Procaccini, C.; Ferrara, G.; Baranzini, S.; Oksenberg, J.R.; Matarese, G.; Diaspro, A.; Kerlero de Rosbo, N.; Uccelli, A. IFN-γ orchestrates mesenchymal stem cell plasticity through the signal transducer and activator of transcription 1 and 3 and mammalian target of rapamycin pathways. *J. Allergy Clin. Immunol.* **2017**, *139*, 1667–1676. [CrossRef] [PubMed]
36. Polchert, D.; Sobinsky, J.; Douglas, G.W.; Kidd, M.; Moadsiri, A.; Reina, E.; Genrich, K.; Mehrotra, S.; Setty, S.; Smith, B.; et al. IFN-γ activation of mesenchymal stem cells for treatment and prevention of graft versus host disease. *Eur. J. Immunol.* **2008**, *38*, 1745–1755. [CrossRef]
37. Kronsteiner, B.; Wolbank, S.; Peterbauer, A.; Hackl, C.; Redl, H.; van Griensven, M.; Gabriel, C. Human mesenchymal stem cells from adipose tissue and amnion influence T-cells depending on stimulation method and presence of other immune cells. *Stem Cells Dev.* **2011**, *20*, 2115–2126. [CrossRef]

38. Rubtsov, Y.; Goryunov, K.; Romanov, A.; Suzdaltseva, Y.; Sharonov, G.; Tkachuk, V. Molecular mechanisms of immunomodulation properties of mesenchymal stromal cells: A new insight into the role of ICAM-1. *Stem Cells Int.* **2017**, *2017*. [CrossRef]
39. Chen, D.; Ma, F.; Xu, S.; Yang, S.; Chen, F.; Rong, L.; Chi, Y.; Zhao, Q.; Lu, S.; Han, Z.; et al. Expression and role of Toll-like receptors on human umbilical cord mesenchymal stromal cells. *Cytotherapy* **2013**, *15*, 423–433. [CrossRef]
40. Opitz, C.A.; Litzenburger, U.M.; Lutz, C.; Lanz, T.V.; Tritschler, I.; Köppel, A.; Tolosa, E.; Hoberg, M.; Anderl, J.; Aicher, W.K.; et al. Toll-like receptor engagement enhances the immunosuppressive properties of human bone marrow-derived mesenchymal stem cells by inducing indoleamine-2,3-dioxygenase-1 via interferon-beta and protein kinase R. *Stem Cells* **2009**, *27*, 909–919. [CrossRef]
41. Sims, J.E.; Smith, D.E. The IL-1 family: Regulators of immunity. *Nat. Rev. Immunol.* **2010**, *10*, 89–102. [CrossRef] [PubMed]
42. Kalliolias, G.D.; Ivashkiv, L.B. TNF biology, pathogenic mechanisms and emerging therapeutic strategies. *Nat. Rev. Rheumatol.* **2016**, *12*, 49–62. [CrossRef]
43. Hsu, P.; Santner-Nanan, B.; Hu, M.; Skarratt, K.; Lee, C.H.; Stormon, M.; Wong, M.; Fuller, S.J.; Nanan, R. IL-10 potentiates differentiation of human induced regulatory T cells via STAT3 and Foxo1. *J. Immunol.* **2015**, *195*, 3665–3674. [CrossRef] [PubMed]
44. English, K.; Ryan, J.M.; Tobin, L.; Murphy, M.J.; Barry, F.P.; Mahon, B.P. Cell contact, prostaglandin E(2) and transforming growth factor beta 1 play non-redundant roles in human mesenchymal stem cell induction of CD4 + CD25 (High) forkhead box P3+ regulatory T cells. *Clin. Exp. Immunol.* **2009**, *156*, 149–160. [CrossRef] [PubMed]
45. Selmani, Z.; Naji, A.; Zidi, I.; Favier, B.; Gaiffe, E.; Obert, L.; Borg, C.; Saas, P.; Tiberghien, P.; Rouas-Freiss, N.; et al. Human leukocyte antigen-G5 secretion by human mesenchymal stem cells is required to suppress T lymphocyte and natural killer function and to induce CD4 + CD25highFOXP3+ regulatory T cells. *Stem Cells* **2008**, *26*, 212–222. [CrossRef] [PubMed]
46. Miyagawa, I.; Nakayamada, S.; Nakano, K.; Yamagata, K.; Sakata, K.; Yamaoka, K.; Tanaka, Y. Induction of regulatory T cells and its regulation with insulin-like growth factor/insulin-like growth factor binding protein-4 by human mesenchymal stem cells. *J. Immunol.* **2017**, *199*, 1616–1625. [CrossRef]
47. Matula, Z.; Németh, A.; Lőrincz, P.; Szepesi, Á.; Brózik, A.; Buzás, E.I.; Lőw, P.; Német, K.; Uher, F.; Urbán, V.S. The Role of extracellular vesicle and tunneling nanotube-mediated intercellular cross-talk between mesenchymal stem cells and human peripheral T cells. *Stem Cells Dev.* **2016**, *25*, 1818–1832. [CrossRef]
48. Phinney, D.G.; Pittenger, M.F. Concise review: MSC-derived exosomes for cell-free therapy. *Stem Cells* **2017**, *35*, 851–858. [CrossRef] [PubMed]
49. Cosenza, S.; Toupet, K.; Maumus, M.; Luz-Crawford, P.; Blanc-Brude, O.; Jorgensen, C.; Noël, D. Mesenchymal stem cells-derived exosomes are more immunosuppressive than microparticles in inflammatory arthritis. *Theranostics* **2018**, *8*, 1399–1410. [CrossRef] [PubMed]
50. Gieseke, F.; Böhringer, J.; Bussolari, R.; Dominici, M.; Handgretinger, R.; Müller, I. Human multipotent mesenchymal stromal cells use galectin-1 to inhibit immune effector cells. *Blood* **2010**, *116*, 3770–3779. [CrossRef] [PubMed]

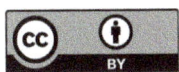

© 2019 by the authors. Licensee MDPI, Basel, Switzerland. This article is an open access article distributed under the terms and conditions of the Creative Commons Attribution (CC BY) license (http://creativecommons.org/licenses/by/4.0/).

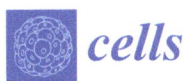

Communication

Tracking of Infused Mesenchymal Stem Cells in Injured Pulmonary Tissue in *Atm*-Deficient Mice

Patrick C. Baer [1,*], Julia Sann [1], Ruth Pia Duecker [2], Evelyn Ullrich [3,4,5], Helmut Geiger [1], Peter Bader [3], Stefan Zielen [2] and Ralf Schubert [2,*]

1. Division of Nephrology, Department of Internal Medicine III, University Hospital, Goethe-University, 60596 Frankfurt am Main, Germany; julia.sann@t-online.de (J.S.); h.geiger@em.uni-frankfurt.de (H.G.)
2. Division for Allergy, Pneumology and Cystic Fibrosis, Department for Children and Adolescents, University Hospital, Goethe-University, 60596 Frankfurt am Main, Germany; ruthpia.duecker@kgu.de (R.P.D.); stefan.zielen@kgu.de (S.Z.)
3. Division of Pediatric Stem Cell Transplantation and Immunology, Department for Children and Adolescents Medicine, University Hospital Frankfurt, Goethe University, 60596 Frankfurt am Main, Germany; evelyn.ullrich@kgu.de (E.U.); peter.bader@kgu.de (P.B.)
4. Experimental Immunology, Department for Children and Adolescents Medicine, University Hospital Frankfurt, Goethe University, 60596 Frankfurt am Main, Germany
5. German Cancer Consortium (DKTK) partner site Frankfurt/Mainz, 60596 Frankfurt am Main, Germany
* Correspondence: p.baer@em.uni-frankfurt.de (P.C.B.); ralf.schubert@kgu.de (R.S.); Tel.: +49-69-6301-5554 (P.C.B.); +49-69-6301-83611 (R.S.); Fax: +49-69-6301-4749 (P.C.B.); +49-69-6301-83349 (R.S.)

Received: 7 May 2020; Accepted: 8 June 2020; Published: 10 June 2020

Abstract: Pulmonary failure is the main cause of morbidity and mortality in the human chromosomal instability syndrome Ataxia-telangiectasia (A-T). Major phenotypes include recurrent respiratory tract infections and bronchiectasis, aspiration, respiratory muscle abnormalities, interstitial lung disease, and pulmonary fibrosis. At present, no effective pulmonary therapy for A-T exists. Cell therapy using adipose-derived mesenchymal stromal/stem cells (ASCs) might be a promising approach for tissue regeneration. The aim of the present project was to investigate whether ASCs migrate into the injured lung parenchyma of *Atm*-deficient mice as an indication of incipient tissue damage during A-T. Therefore, ASCs isolated from luciferase transgenic mice (mASCs) were intravenously transplanted into *Atm*-deficient and wild-type mice. Retention kinetics of the cells were monitored using in vivo bioluminescence imaging (BLI) and completed by subsequent verification using quantitative real-time polymerase chain reaction (qRT-PCR). The in vivo imaging and the qPCR results demonstrated migration accompanied by a significantly longer retention time of transplanted mASCs in the lung parenchyma of *Atm*-deficient mice compared to wild type mice. In conclusion, our study suggests incipient damage in the lung parenchyma of *Atm*-deficient mice. In addition, our data further demonstrate that a combination of luciferase-based PCR together with BLI is a pivotal tool for tracking mASCs after transplantation in models of inflammatory lung diseases such as A-T.

Keywords: tracking; mesenchymal stromal/stem cells; bio imaging; bioluminescence; qRT-PCR; Ataxia telangiectasia; Atm

1. Introduction

Pulmonary failure is a frequent cause of morbidity and mortality in Ataxia-telangiectasia (A-T). At present, no effective pulmonary therapy for A-T exists [1]. Thus, the development of new strategies to preserve lung function in A-T is urgently needed due to limited clinical intervention options. Aside from immunodeficiency and inflammation, fibrotic changes are a major factor leading to progressive lung destruction. A direct connection between the ATM protein (A-T Mutated) and TGF-β_1, one of the key mediators responsible for fibrotic changes in the lung, has been described [2]. In addition, we provided evidence for reduced lung function and increased inflammation in the lung of *Atm*-deficient mice displaying the human pulmonary A-T phenotype [3]. Therefore, inhibition of inflammation and fibrosis might open new avenues in the treatment of the lung disorder in A-T. Recently, we demonstrated that bone marrow transplantation (BMT) significantly improves the immunological phenotype and inhibits tumorigenesis in *Atm*-deficient mice [4]. Donor bone marrow derived cells (BMDCs) migrated into bone marrow, blood, thymus, spleen, and lung tissue of *Atm*-deficient mice. However, although the BMT overcame the immunodeficiency, migration of the donor cells into the lung tissue was low, and most of the cells were of hematopoietic origin. To improve cellular migration and to provide anti-inflammatory, anti-fibrotic, and anti-oxidative activity, a promising approach could be transplantation of mesenchymal stromal/stem cells (MSCs).

In principle, MSCs have been detected throughout the body as immature, undifferentiated cells. For the first time, their isolation from bone marrow was described, but in the meantime, they have also been described from almost all adult tissues (e.g., fatty tissue) and solid organs (e.g., liver, kidney) [5,6]. More recent data show that MSCs represent a rare population (or populations) in the perivascular niche of all tissues. A number of studies have demonstrated that MSCs preferentially migrate to injured lung tissue where they are involved in lung repair and control of injury [7]. MSCs provide both structural and functional support to the parenchymal cells of multiple organs and possess immunomodulatory, anti-fibrotic properties and relative immune privilege [8]. MSCs release a number of anti-inflammatory, proangiogenic, regeneration-promoting, and immunomodulating factors that can improve regeneration in injured cells in tissues and organs [9]. Furthermore, MSCs preferentially migrate into injured or inflamed tissues. Therefore, we investigated in this study whether infused murine adipose-derived MSCs (mASCs) displayed an increased retention in injured pulmonary tissue of *Atm*-deficient mice compared to wild type mice, which could then result in an increased regeneration of the damaged lung tissue.

2. Materials and Methods

2.1. Animals

Atm-deficient mice ($Atm^{tm1(Atm)Awb}$; 8 to 10 weeks old) and corresponding wild-type mice, in a 129S6/SvEv background, were used as the animal model. A total of 24 *Atm*-deficient mice were included in the study (histological lung sections, $n = 4$; lung function testing, $n = 12$; bioluminescence imaging and PCR, $n = 8$). The experiments were performed using respective wildtype controls (littermates). Transgenic Luc^+ mice with C57BL/6 background were used to isolate mesenchymal stromal/stem cells from murine inguinal fat. All animal procedures were performed according to the protocols approved by the Animal Care and Use Committee of the state of Hessen (RP Darmstadt (Gen. Nr. FK/1034)).

2.2. Cell Isolation and Culture

Adipose tissue was harvested from transgenic Luc^+ C57BL/6 mice (Janvier, France) as described earlier [10]. Briefly, mice were killed by cervical dislocation, and adipose tissue from inguinal fat pads was immediately dissected to isolate adipose-derived stromal/stem cells (mASCs). Tissue was minced with two scalpels (crossed blades) and then incubated in a 0.5% collagenase/phosphate buffered saline (PBS) solution (Collagenase Type: CLS; Biochrom, Berlin, Germany; PBS; Sigma, Taufkirchen, Germany) for 1 h at 37 °C with constant shaking. The digested tissue solution was then separated through a 100 μm strainer, and the resulting filtrate was centrifuged at $300 \times g$ for 5 min. The resulting pellet was washed twice with medium and centrifuged again at $300 \times g$ for 5 min. Finally, cells were plated and cultured at 37 °C in an atmosphere of 5% CO_2 in 100% humidity. Dulbecco's Modified Eagle's Medium (DMEM; Sigma, Taufkirchen, Germany) with a physiological glucose concentration (100 mg/dL) was supplemented with 10% fetal bovine serum (Biochrom, Berlin, Germany) and used as standard culture medium (DF10). The medium was replaced every three days. Subconfluent cells (90%) were passaged by trypsinization. Cells between passages 2 and 5 were used throughout the experiments. Cell morphology was examined by phase contrast microscopy and flow cytometry, as described earlier [10].

2.3. Immunohistochemistry

Mice were anesthetized with an intraperitoneal injection of a Ketamin–Rompun mixture (20% Ketamin, CuraMED GmbH, Karlsruhe, Germany; 8% Rompun, Bayer Vital GmbH, Leverkusen, Germany). They were perfused transcardially with 4% paraformaldehyde in PBS. Lung tissue sections were prepared from fixed, paraffin-embedded organs and stained with hematoxylin/eosin or with chloracetate esterase staining as neutrophil-specific marker [4,11].

2.4. Pulmonary Function

Pulmonary function was tested in *Atm*-deficient mice and wild-type mice using a computer-controlled piston ventilator (flexiVent, SCIREQ Inc., Montreal, QC, Canada). Briefly, mice were anesthetized, a tracheotomy was performed, and the trachea was cannulated. After that, the mice were placed on a temperature controlled heat blanket, the trachea was exposed, and the previously calibrated cannula (1.2 cm, 18 gauges) was inserted and fixed using a suture. Ventilation was maintained at a rate of 150 breaths/min, a tidal volume of 10 mL/kg, and a positive end-expiratory pressure of 3 cm of water. Mice were allowed to acclimate to the ventilator for 2–3 min before measurement. Lung function parameters were calculated by fitting pressure and volume data to the single compartment model by measuring respiratory system resistance (Rrs), dynamic compliance (Crs) and elastance (Ers) and by analyzing with flexiWare 7 Software [3].

2.5. Transplantation

Three wildtype mice and 4 *Atm*-deficient mice were transplanted with 0.5×10^5 Luc$^+$ mASCs in DMEM containing Heparin (10 U/100 µL). Viability of the cells was checked by trypan blue exclusion immediately before transplantation. A single injection of 100 µL was conducted via the tail vein into each mouse. Cells were tracked via bioluminescence imaging (BLI) on days 1, 3, 6, and 9 and via qRT-PCR at the indicated endpoints (day 15 and 50). The mice were weighed every two to three days, and no significant weight changes could be detected. The mice were sacrificed at the end of the experiment by cervical dislocation under anesthesia with ketamine-xylazine, and the organs were collected.

2.6. In Vivo Bioimaging

Tracking of the transplanted Luc$^+$ mASC was performed in vivo using the PerkinElmer IVIS Lumina II Imaging Chamber System. For this purpose, the mice were injected i.p. with 100 µL D-luciferin. They were then placed under anesthesia with isoflurane. After 10 min, the mice were placed dorsally or ventrally next to one another in the heated measuring chamber of the bioimaging system. Anesthesia was maintained during the measurement via a breathing mask. Images of the detectable luminescence signal were acquired at 1, 30, 60, 180, and 360 s and then evaluated using the "LivingImage" software with Region of Interest (ROI) placed over the thorax. In addition, a background field was placed on the dark border. The quantification was done in photons/s (total flux), and the background was subtracted from the measured values.

2.7. PCR Analyses

Total RNA extraction was performed using single-step RNA isolation from cultured cells by a standard protocol, as described earlier [10]. After RNA extraction, cDNAs were synthesized for 30 min at 37 °C using 1 µg of RNA, 50 µM random hexamers, 1 mM of deoxynucletide-triphosphate-mix,

50 units of reverse transcriptase (Fermentas, St. Leon-Rot, Germany) in 10× PCR buffer, 1 mM β-mercaptoethanol, and 5 mM MgCl$_2$. An Absolute qPCR SYBR Green Rox Mix was used (Thermo Scientific, Hamburg, Germany) for the master mix; primer mix and RNAse-free water were added. Quantitative PCR was carried out in 96-well plates using the following conditions: 15 min at 95 °C for enzyme activation, 15 s at 95 °C for denaturation, 30 s for annealing, 30 s at 72 °C for elongation, followed by a melting curve analysis. Products were checked by agarose gel electrophoresis in selected experiments. Quantification of the PCR fragment was carried out using the Eppendorf realplex2 Mastercycler epgradient S (Eppendorf, Hamburg, Germany). Standard curves were prepared for the amplification specific efficiency correction, and the efficiencies (E) were calculated according to the equation $E = (10^{-1}/m^{-1}) \times 100$, where m is the slope of the linear regression model fitted over log-transformed data of the input cDNA concentrations versus CT values [12,13]. E for actin-beta was 1.9164, and for luciferase = 1.9399. The relative efficiency-corrected mRNA expression of the target gene was calculated based on efficiencies and the CT (Threshold cycle) deviation of an unknown sample versus a positive control (ΔCT) and was expressed in comparison to a reference gene [12,13]. Data were calculated (rel. expression = (E Luc = 1.9164)$^{\Delta CT\ Luc}$/(E actin = 1.9399)$^{\Delta CT\ actin}$) and expressed as percent (the calculated rel. expression 1.0 refers to 100%, the value 0.02 refers to 2%). The luciferase primer was constructed using the firefly luciferase gene from *Photinus pyralis* (GenBank No. AB644228.1, forward: TGAAGAGATACGCCCTGGTT, reverse: CTACGGTAGGCTGCGAAATG; product size 288 bp) and the reference primer for *murine actin-beta* (NM_007393, forward: F: CCACCATGTACCCAGGCATT, reverse: AGGGTGTAAAACGCAGCTCA, product size 253 bp) (Invitrogen, Karlsruhe, Germany). In addition, PCR products were separated by agarose electrophoresis and observed under UV illumination [10].

2.8. Statistical Analysis

The data were expressed as mean ± standard deviation (SD) and were analyzed using an unpaired student's Test or a Mann–Whitney test. For multiple comparisons, analysis of variance (ANOVA) with Bonferroni's multiple comparison test was used for statistical analysis. p values < 0.05 were considered significant.

3. Results

3.1. Atm-Deficient Mice Exhibited Signs of Lung Disease

Comparison of the lung parenchyma showed slight tendency for alveolar septal thickening and patchy areas of neutrophilic inflammation in *Atm*-deficient mice (Figure 1B,D) compared to wild-type mice (Figure 1A,C) accompanied by significantly increased lung resistance (Rrs) (Figure 1E) and respiratory system elastance (Ers) (Figure 1F) as well as decreased tissue compliance (Figure 1F) in comparison to control mice.

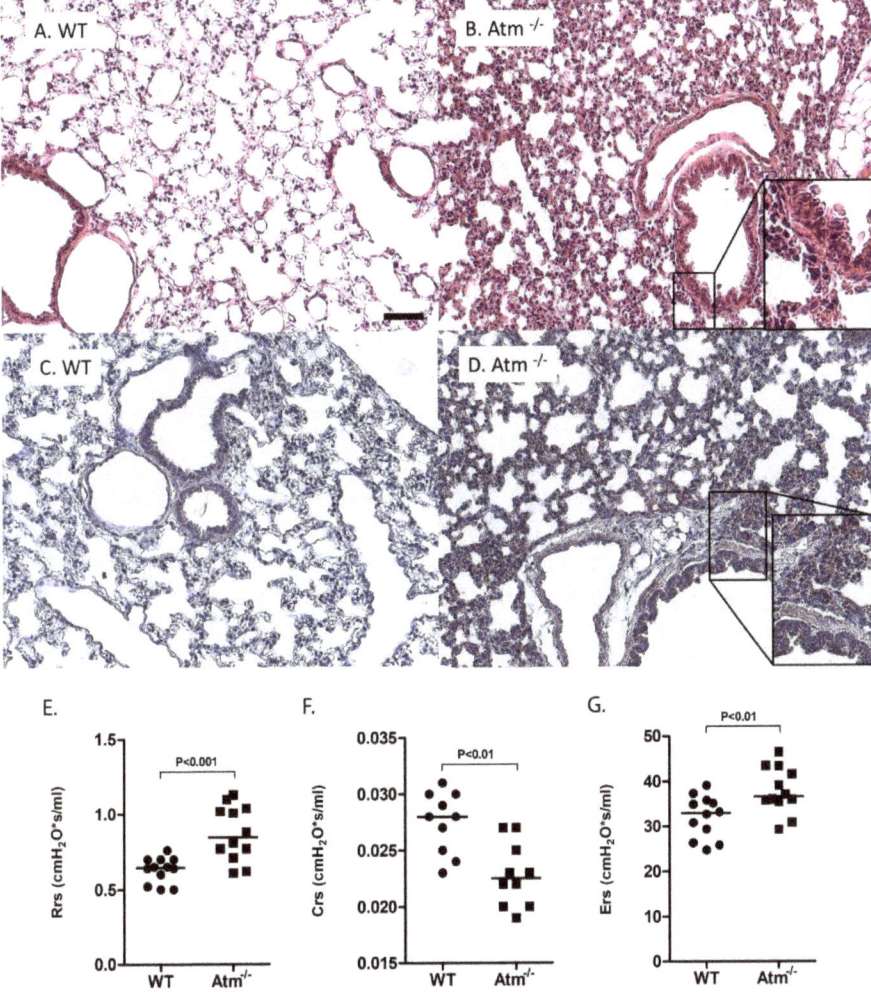

Figure 1. Lung injury in *Atm*-deficient mice. Representative histological lung sections of (**A**,**C**) wild-type (WT) and (**B**,**D**) *Atm*-deficient (Atm$^{-/-}$) mice stained with hematoxylin and eosin (**A**,**B**) or with chloracetate esterase staining (**C**,**D**), respectively. Lung function testing using a FlexiVent mouse ventilator, respiratory system resistance (**E**), compliance (**F**), and elastance (**G**) in *Atm*$^{-/-}$ mice compared to a WT control group (n = 10–12). Bar = 100 µm.

3.2. Luc⁺ mASCs Stayed Longer in Lung Tissue of Atm-Deficient Mice Compared to Wildtype Mice

Examination of in vivo luciferase expression showed a positive bioluminescent signal in all transplanted mice on day one after transplantation with no differences between *Atm*-deficient and wildtype mice (Figure 2A). After three days, the bioluminescent signal in wildtype mice rapidly dropped down and disappeared completely on day six. In contrast, the transplanted *Atm*-deficient mice showed a strong bioluminescent signal even after nine days. At day 14, the bioluminescence signal decreased to undetectable levels in all mice including the four *Atm*-deficient mice (data not shown).

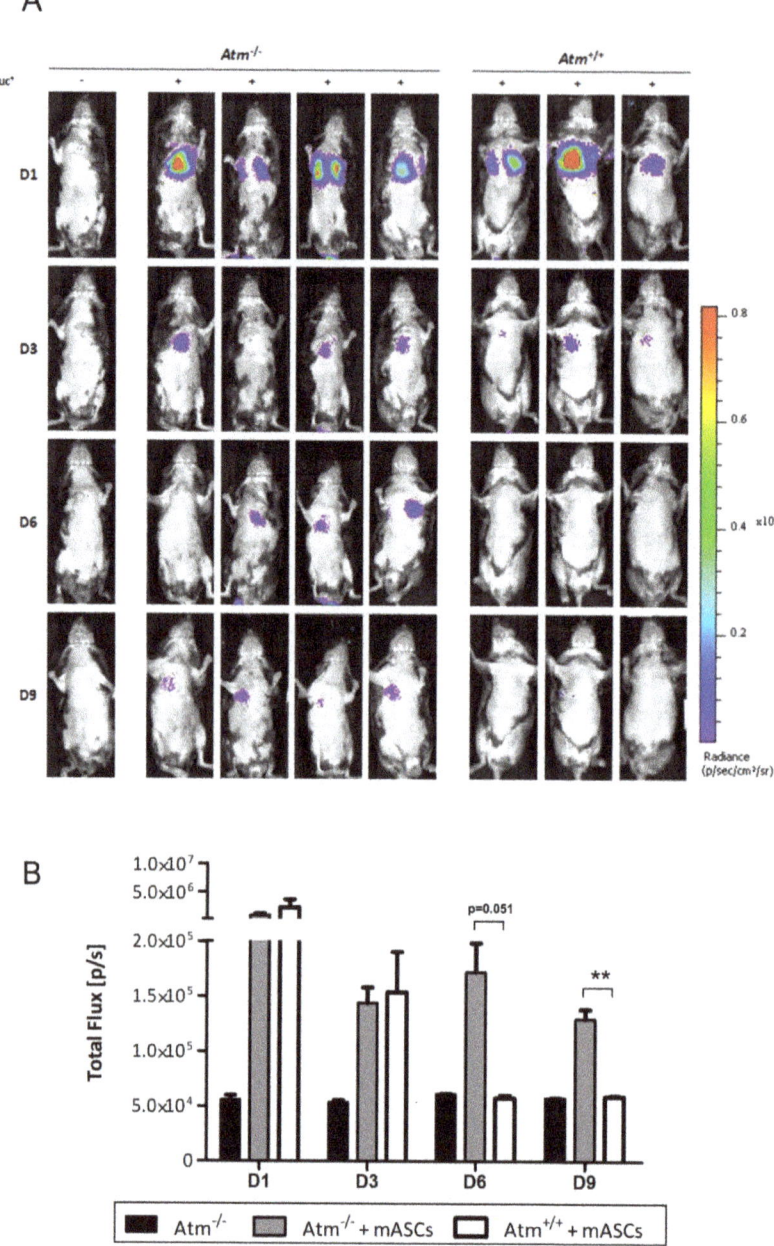

Figure 2. Retention of adipose-derived mesenchymal stromal/stem cells (ASCs) isolated from luciferase transgenic mice (mASCs) into the lung tissue of *Atm*-deficient mice. (**A**) Bioluminescence imaging of mASCs transgenic for the firefly luciferase gene (Luc$^+$) in the lung tissue of *Atm*-deficient mice ($Atm^{-/-}$, $n = 4$) and wild type mice ($Atm^{+/+}$, $n = 3$). MSCs were analyzed at days 1, 3, 6, and 9 after transplantation. (**B**) Quantitative analysis of the light emission data of the analyzed bioluminescence signals from untransplanted $Atm^{-/-}$ mice (black bars, $n = 3$), Luc$^+$ mASCs transplanted $Atm^{-/-}$ mice (grey bars, $n = 4$), and $Atm^{+/+}$ mice (white bars, n=3). ** $p < 0.01$.

Quantification of the light emission of the analyzed bioluminescence signals confirmed the above findings (Figure 2B). A strong signal was seen on day one for both genotypes after transplantation, whereas the mock-transplanted animals, which were signal negative in the overlay recordings, showed a constant-low total flux background value on all days. Up to day three, the total flux of the bioluminescent signal revealed no differences between MSC-transplanted *Atm*-deficient and wildtype mice. After that, the signal in transplanted wildtype mice dropped down to the level of the untransplanted mice. In contrast, the total flux signal maintained in the MSC-transplanted *Atm*-deficient mice.

3.3. Transplanted mASCs Exhibited a Long Retention Time in the Lung Parenchyma of Atm-Deficient Mice

Quantitative real-time PCR was used on days 15 and 50 to follow the retention time of Luc$^+$ mASCs after the bioluminescence signal disappeared (Figure 3). After transplantation of Luc$^+$ mASCs, *Atm*-deficient mice showed a 50-fold higher luciferase gene expression in lung parenchyma compared to wildtype mice ($Atm^{-/-}$: 2.0% ± 0.59; $Atm^{+/+}$: 0.04% ± 0.004, $p < 0.05$), whereas no differences could be detected in the kidney and the thymus (Figure 3).

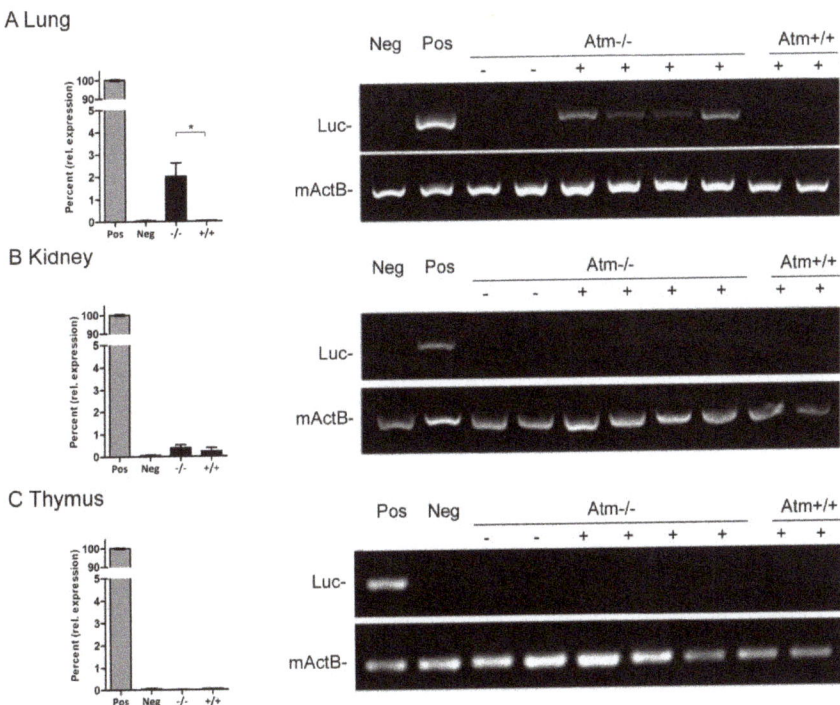

Figure 3. Detection of Luc$^+$ mASCs on day 15 after transplantation of *Atm*-deficient ($Atm^{-/-}$, $n = 4$) and wild type mice ($Atm^{+/+}$, $n = 3$) knock-out using PCR. Quantitative analysis of the relative expression (expressed as percent; MW ± SEM) (left side) and results of the gel electrophoresis of lungs, kidney, and thymus (right side). Controls: RNA from Luc negative tissue (Neg), RNA from Luc positive tissue (Pos = 100%). Luc=luciferase, mActB= murine actine-beta. * $p < 0.05$.

An exemplary examination of long-term stay revealed still a positive Luc-signal in the lung parenchyma of the *Atm*-deficient mouse at day 50 ($n = 1$). Although the Luc signal in the lungs decreased on day 50 compared to day 15, it was still detectable (Figure 4). While a very slight increase of the signal was observed in the kidney at day 50, no signal was detected in the thymus on day 15 or day 50.

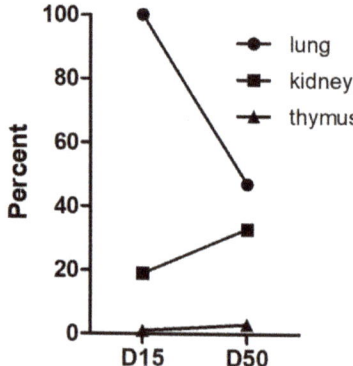

Figure 4. Detection of Luc$^+$ mASCs on day 15 (D15, $n = 4$) and on day 50 (D50, $n = 1$) after transplantation in $Atm^{-/-}$ mice. Graph shows fold Luc$^+$ expression in lung, kidney, and thymus at days 15 and 50 in relation to Luc+ expression in the lung at day 15 (quantitative analysis of the relative Luc-mRNA amounts (percent of signal, lung D15 = 100%)).

4. Discussion

Respiratory disease accounts for significant morbidity and mortality in patients with A-T [14]. Major phenotypes include recurrent respiratory tract infections and bronchiectasis, aspiration, respiratory muscle abnormalities, interstitial lung disease, and pulmonary fibrosis [15]. Aside from the immunodeficiency, it has been proposed that ongoing low grade inflammation and oxidative stress might be responsible for the clinical pathogenesis causing lung failure [1,16]. Recent studies further demonstrated restricted lung function, high sensitivity to inflammatory agents, and a significant amount of oxidative DNA damage in the lung parenchyma of Atm-deficient mice, especially after triggering inflammation [3,11].

Cell therapy using MSCs might be a promising approach for tissue regeneration in A-T. MSCs have been shown to integrate into the damaged sites in a variety of tissues, including lung tissue, showing positive effects on tissue regeneration [7]. There are recent studies using administration of MSCs or their derivates (e.g., extracellular vesicles) in in vivo studies [17] or human clinical trials to treat pulmonary fibrosis [18]. Averyanov and co-workers evaluated the safety and the tolerability of repeated infusions of high doses of MSCs up to the total cumulative dose of two billion cells in subjects with rapidly progressing idiopathic pulmonary fibrosis. They showed that the treatment was safe and well tolerated. Transplanted patients had an increased lung function compared to the placebo group, where a sustained decrease in lung function was observed. Currently, it could be shown that MSCs improved the outcome of patients with COVID-19 pneumonia [19]. Transplantation of MSCs was shown to cure or significantly improve the functional outcomes of seven COVID-19 patients without observed adverse effects. The pulmonary function and symptoms of seven patients were significantly improved in two days after MSC transplantation [19]. Nevertheless, it should be noted in this context that others reported that reduced migration of transplanted MSCs correlated with decreased fibrosis in the lungs [20].

However, lung disease in A-T is a creeping process that slowly develops over time, and experience with MSCs in A-T is scarce. Even in the Atm-mouse model, lung damage is difficult to determine without induction of experimental inflammation, as the mice died from thymic lymphomas within 3–6 months before lung failure could occur. This prompted us to investigate whether mASCs remained in the lung parenchyma of Atm-deficient mice in an increased manner compared to healthy controls.

It is important to note that the mice were housed in individually ventilated cages to protect them from any harmful microorganism.

Although tissue damage and inflammation are hard to detect in *Atm*-deficient mice without exogenous trigger, our present data showed signs of lung disease and damage in *Atm*-deficient mice [3,4]. These findings are underlined by our in vivo imaging and qPCR results, which demonstrated increased retention of MSCs into the lung parenchyma of *Atm*-deficient mice compared to wild-type. Because MSCs preferentially migrate into injured or inflamed tissues, such as during wound healing or in association with tumors, these findings together with the pathological changes in lung function parameters indicate that the *Atm*-deficient mouse has some kind of ongoing pulmonary damage [21]. It should be mentioned that signals in the lung do not necessarily reflect transgenic donor cells. They may derive from inflammatory host cells (e.g. macrophages or others) in the lung, which have phagocytosed donor cells. Nevertheless, our results shown here are in line with earlier findings showing an engraftment of $CD31^+CD45^-$ endothelial cells and EpCAM+ epithelial cells into the lung tissue of *Atm*-deficient mice after bone marrow transplantation [4]. In addition, impaired lung resistance and respiratory system elastance in *Atm*-deficient mice has also been described in other studies without the presence of inflammation [3,11]. In this regard, an earlier study from our group also showed increased spontaneous oxidative stress and damage in the lung tissue of *Atm*-deficient mice and alveolar basal epithelial cells in the presence of the ATM-kinase inhibitor KU55933 [3,16]. Thus, in the absence of inflammatory signals, oxidative stress could attract MSCs in our experimental setting. Due to their ability to counteract reactive oxygen species, further experiments investigating the effect of MSCs on oxidative stress should be performed. Luc-based real-time PCR together with BLI is an important tool for cell tracking after transplantation in models of inflammatory lung diseases such as A-T [10].

In conclusion, tracking of transplanted Luc^+ mASCs, by a combination of luciferase-based PCR together with BLI showed an increased migration into lung parenchyma accompanied by a significantly longer retention time in *Atm*-deficient mice, pointing to ongoing pulmonary damage in the lung tissue in these animals. To what extent these cells improve the regeneration of damaged lung tissue in $Atm^{-/-}$ mice will now be investigated in further studies. Therefore, further experiments are necessary to confirm the regenerative impact of MSCs on lung disease in A-T.

Author Contributions: Investigation, P.C.B., J.S., E.U., R.S.; conceptualization, P.C.B., H.G., S.Z., R.S.; formal analysis, P.C.B., J.S., R.P.D., R.S.; writing, review, and editing, P.C.B., R.P.D., P.B., S.Z., H.G., R.S. All authors have read and agreed to the published version of the manuscript.

Funding: This research received no external funding.

Acknowledgments: The authors thank Jochen Früh and Katja Stein for their assistance in bioluminescence measurements.

Conflicts of Interest: The authors declare no conflict of interest.

Abbreviations

A-T	Ataxia-telangiectasia
Atm	Ataxia-telangiectasia mutated
BLI	Bioluminescence imaging
Luc	Luciferase
mASC	Murine adipose-derived stromal/stem cells
MSC	Mesenchymal stromal/stem cells
PCR	Polymerase chain reaction
qRT-PCR	Quantitative real-time polymerase chain reaction

References

1. McGrath-Morrow, S.A.; Collaco, J.M.; Detrick, B.; Lederman, H.M. Serum Interleukin-6 Levels and Pulmonary Function in Ataxia-Telangiectasia. *J. Pediatr.* **2016**, *171*, 256–261.e1. [CrossRef] [PubMed]
2. Overstreet, J.M.; Samarakoon, R.; Cardona-Grau, D.; Goldschmeding, R.; Higgins, P.J. Tumor suppressor ataxia telangiectasia mutated functions downstream of TGF-β1 in orchestrating profibrotic responses. *FASEB J.* **2015**, *29*, 1258–1268. [CrossRef] [PubMed]
3. Duecker, R.; Baer, P.; Eickmeier, O.; Strecker, M.; Kurz, J.; Schaible, A.; Henrich, D.; Zielen, S.; Schubert, R. Oxidative stress-driven pulmonary inflammation and fibrosis in a mouse model of human ataxia-telangiectasia. *Redox Biol.* **2018**, *14*, 645–655. [CrossRef] [PubMed]
4. Pietzner, J.; Baer, P.C.; Duecker, R.P.; Merscher, M.B.; Satzger-Prodinger, C.; Bechmann, I.; Wietelmann, A.; Del Turco, D.; Doering, C.; Kuci, S.; et al. Bone marrow transplantation improves the outcome of Atm-deficient mice through the migration of ATM-competent cells. *Hum. Mol. Genet.* **2013**, *22*, 493–507. [CrossRef] [PubMed]
5. Baer, P.C.; Geiger, H. Adipose-derived mesenchymal stromal/stem cells: Tissue localization, characterization, and heterogeneity. *Stem Cells Int.* **2012**, *2012*, 812693. [CrossRef] [PubMed]
6. Da Silva Meirelles, L.; Chagastelles, P.C.; Nardi, N.B. Mesenchymal stem cells reside in virtually all post-natal organs and tissues. *J. Cell Sci.* **2006**, *119*, 2204–2213. [CrossRef] [PubMed]
7. Huleihel, L.; Levine, M.; Rojas, M. The potential of cell-based therapy in lung diseases. *Expert Opin. Biol. Ther.* **2013**, *13*, 1429–1440. [CrossRef] [PubMed]
8. Sinclair, K.; Yerkovich, S.T.; Chambers, D.C. Mesenchymal stem cells and the lung. *Respirology* **2013**, *18*, 397–411. [CrossRef]
9. Hsiao, S.T.-F.; Asgari, A.; Lokmic, Z.; Sinclair, R.; Dusting, G.J.; Lim, S.Y.; Dilley, R.J. Comparative analysis of paracrine factor expression in human adult mesenchymal stem cells derived from bone marrow, adipose, and dermal tissue. *Stem Cells Dev.* **2012**, *21*, 2189–2203. [CrossRef] [PubMed]
10. Schubert, R.; Sann, J.; Frueh, J.T.; Ullrich, E.; Geiger, H.; Baer, P.C. Tracking of Adipose-Derived Mesenchymal Stromal/Stem Cells in a Model of Cisplatin-Induced Acute Kidney Injury: Comparison of Bioluminescence Imaging versus qRT-PCR. *Int. J. Mol. Sci.* **2018**, *19*, 2564. [CrossRef] [PubMed]
11. Eickmeier, O.; Kim, S.Y.; Herrmann, E.; Döring, C.; Duecker, R.; Voss, S.; Wehner, S.; Hölscher, C.; Pietzner, J.; Zielen, S.; et al. Altered mucosal immune response after acute lung injury in a murine model of Ataxia Telangiectasia. *BMC Pulm. Med.* **2014**, *14*, 93. [CrossRef] [PubMed]
12. Pfaffl, M.W. A new mathematical model for relative quantification in real-time RT–PCR. *Nucleic Acids Res.* **2001**, *29*, e45. [CrossRef] [PubMed]
13. Fleige, S.; Walf, V.; Huch, S.; Prgomet, C.; Sehm, J.; Pfaffl, M.W. Comparison of relative mRNA quantification models and the impact of RNA integrity in quantitative real-time RT-PCR. *Biotechnol. Lett.* **2006**, *28*, 1601–1613. [CrossRef] [PubMed]
14. McGrath-Morrow, S.A.; Gower, W.A.; Rothblum-Oviatt, C.; Brody, A.S.; Langston, C.; Fan, L.L.; Lefton-Greif, M.A.; Crawford, T.O.; Troche, M.; Sandlund, J.T.; et al. Evaluation and management of pulmonary disease in ataxia-telangiectasia. *Pediatr. Pulmonol.* **2010**, *45*, 847–859. [CrossRef] [PubMed]
15. Schroeder, S.A.; Zielen, S. Infections of the respiratory system in patients with ataxia-telangiectasia. *Pediatr. Pulmonol.* **2014**, *49*, 389–399. [CrossRef] [PubMed]
16. Pietzner, J.; Merscher, B.M.; Baer, P.C.; Duecker, R.P.; Eickmeier, O.; Fußbroich, D.; Bader, P.; Del Turco, D.; Henschler, R.; Zielen, S.; et al. Low-dose irradiation prior to bone marrow transplantation results in ATM activation and increased lethality in Atm-deficient mice. *Bone Marrow Transplant.* **2016**, *51*, 560–567. [CrossRef]
17. Mansouri, N.; Willis, G.R.; Fernandez-Gonzalez, A.; Reis, M.; Nassiri, S.; Mitsialis, S.A.; Kourembanas, S. Mesenchymal stromal cell exosomes prevent and revert experimental pulmonary fibrosis through modulation of monocyte phenotypes. *JCI Insight* **2019**, *4*, e128060. [CrossRef]
18. Averyanov, A.; Koroleva, I.; Konoplyannikov, M.; Revkova, V.; Lesnyak, V.; Kalsin, V.; Danilevskaya, O.; Nikitin, A.; Sotnikova, A.; Kotova, S.; et al. First-in-human high-cumulative-dose stem cell therapy in idiopathic pulmonary fibrosis with rapid lung function decline. *Stem Cells Transl. Med.* **2020**, *9*, 6–16. [CrossRef]

19. Leng, Z.; Zhu, R.; Hou, W.; Feng, Y.; Yang, Y.; Han, Q.; Shan, G.; Meng, F.; Du, D.; Wang, S.; et al. Transplantation of ACE2- Mesenchymal Stem Cells Improves the Outcome of Patients with COVID-19 Pneumonia. *Aging Dis.* **2020**, *11*, 216–228. [CrossRef]
20. Epperly, M.W.; Franicola, D.; Zhang, X.; Nie, S.; Wang, H.; Bahnson, A.B.; Shields, D.S.; Goff, J.P.; Shen, H.; Greenberger, J.S. Reduced irradiation pulmonary fibrosis and stromal cell migration in Smad3$^{-/-}$ marrow chimeric mice. *In Vivo* **2006**, *20*, 573–582. [PubMed]
21. Herzog, E.L.; van Arnam, J.; Hu, B.; Krause, D.S. Threshold of lung injury required for the appearance of marrow-derived lung epithelia. *Stem Cells* **2006**, *24*, 1986–1992. [CrossRef] [PubMed]

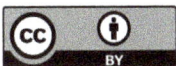

© 2020 by the authors. Licensee MDPI, Basel, Switzerland. This article is an open access article distributed under the terms and conditions of the Creative Commons Attribution (CC BY) license (http://creativecommons.org/licenses/by/4.0/).

MDPI
St. Alban-Anlage 66
4052 Basel
Switzerland
Tel. +41 61 683 77 34
Fax +41 61 302 89 18
www.mdpi.com

Cells Editorial Office
E-mail: cells@mdpi.com
www.mdpi.com/journal/cells

www.ingramcontent.com/pod-product-compliance
Lightning Source LLC
LaVergne TN
LVHW070141100526
838202LV00015B/1872